MODERN ARTHROSCOPY

Edited by **Jason L. Dragoo**

Modern Arthroscopy
Edited by Jason L. Dragoo

Published by InTech
Janeza Trdine 9, 51000 Rijeka, Croatia

Publishing Process Manager Ivona Lovrić

Technical Editor Teodora Smiljanic

Cover Designer InTech Design Team

Additional hard copies can be obtained from orders@intechopen.com

Modern Arthroscopy, Edited by Jason L. Dragoo
p. cm.
ISBN 978-953-307-771-0

For EU product safety concerns:
IN TECH d.o.o., Prolaz Marije Krucifikse Kozulić 3, 51000 Rijeka, Croatia,
info@intechopen.com or visit our website at intechopen.com.

Meet the editor

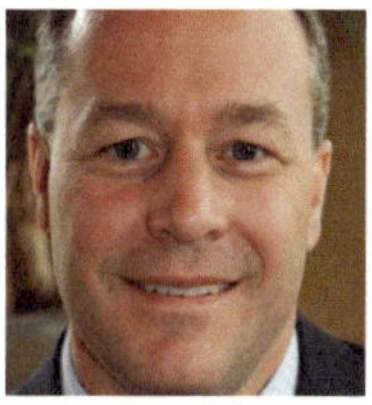

Dr. Jason L. Dragoo, MD is a board certified Orthopaedic Surgeon, specializing in Sports Medicine at Stanford University. He serves as a team physician for numerous elite athletic associations including the US Ski Team, US Olympic Committee and Stanford University Athletics. For many years, he has educated a variety of specialists including orthopaedic surgeons, physical therapists, athletic trainers, and coaches on sports medicine concepts and techniques. Dr. Dragoo's basic science and clinical research has led to new methods of cartilage regeneration using adult stem cells, as well as pioneering new methods of prevention and treatment of anterior cruciate ligament (ACL) injuries and stiff and painful joints.

Contents

Preface

Staying current in the rapidly changing field of arthroscopic surgery presents a challenge for practitioners and students. Books and review articles are often outdated on the day of release. Recently, rapidly published on-line books have filled an educational void, assisting millions of practitioners to stay updated on the latest techniques.

The chapters in this book entitled *Modern Arthroscopy* were written by a panel of international experts in the various disciplines of arthroscopy. The goals of this text are to present the classical techniques and teachings in the fields of Orthopaedics and Dentistry, but also to include new, cutting-edge applications of arthroscopy, such as temporomandibular arthroscopy and extra-articular arthroscopy of the knee, just to name a few. The InTech online publishing format allows rapid publishing of these new techniques to keep the content accurate and up to date.

The chapters are organized anatomically, with the first chapters introducing basic arthroscopic techniques, while later chapters describe newer, more advanced techniques. The surgical technique sections of the chapters are clearly labeled for easy reference.

It is my hope that this book will either assist readers in learning the current techniques of arthroscopic surgery, or serve as a springboard to stimulate the creation of new techniques, which have yet to be described. On behalf of the authors and InTech Publishing we thank you for your interest in this book, and hope *Modern Arthroscopy* becomes a core reference for your arthroscopic surgery practice.

Jason L. Dragoo, MD
Assistant Professor
Department of Orthopaedic Surgery and Sports Medicine
Stanford University,
USA

Part 1

Arthroscopy of the Temporomandibular Joint

1

Temporomandibular Joint Arthroscopy

Edvitar Leibur[1,2], Oksana Jagur[1] and Ülle Voog-Oras[1]
[1]*Department of Stomatology,*
[2]*Department of Internal Medicine,*
Tartu University, University Hospital
Estonia

1. Introduction

Arthroscopy is a technique for direct visual inspection of internal joint structures, including biopsy and other surgical procedures performed under visual control. In 1918 Takagı first described arthroscopy of the knee joint examinations using cystoscope (Tag, 1939). Onishi in 1970 was the first to report arthroscopy of the human temporomandibular joint (TMJ) and the first results were published by him (Onishi, 1975, 1980). The progress in research and applications of TMJ arthroscopy in joint disease have led to the acceptance of small operative procedures as a safe, minimally invasive means of effectively treating a number of intra-articular and degenerative TMJ problems (McCain, 1992; Holmlund &Axelsson, 1996; Holmlund et al., 2001). Arthroscopic surgery has been an effective treatment for TMJ disorders refractory to nonsurgical treatments (Ohnuki et al., 2003; Gonzalez-Garcia et al., 2008, Leibur et al., 2010). TMJ arthroscopy has been variously reported as successful in up to 80% of cases where outcome of arthroscopic surgery to the TMJ correlates with the stage of internal derangement (K. Murakami et al., 2000; Sanroman, 2004). Studies have been variable in their scientific method and some long-term outcomes studies have been completed where both quality of life and functional outcome have been assessed (Voog et al., 2003a; Undt et al., 2006; Jagur et al., 2011). For enabling direct comparison of the clinical results following arthroscopic surgery and open surgery a retrospective study comparing two centers´ results using the Jaw Pain and Function Questionnaire (Clark et al., 1989) has been performed and these treatment results of open surgery were comparable with arthroscopic treatment results (Undt et al., 2006).

2. Anatomy of the temporomandibular joint

The temporomandibular joint is the articulation between the mandible and the cranium. The mandibular head (condyle), glenoid (mandibular) fossa, and articular eminence form the TMJ. These joints serve as one anatomic control for both mandibular movement and the occlusion, surrounded by a capsule which consists of fibrous material, and a synovial lining. The capsule is quite thin anteromedially and medially ~ 0,7 mm and thick laterally and posteriorly ~ 1,8 mm. The inner layer of the capsule or synovial membrane is highly vascularized layer of endothelial origin cells, producing synovial fluid. The capsule stretches from the edge of the mandibular fossa to the neck of the mandible, proximal to the pterygoid fovea, and envelops the articular eminence. TMJ is reinforced by the temporomandibular and sphenomandibular ligaments. The articular surface of the

mandible is the upper and anterior surface of the condyle, lined by dense, avascular fibrous connective tissue. A layer of hyaline cartilage covers the articulating cortical bone. The adult human condyle is about 15 to 20 mm from side to side and 8 to 10 mm from front to back. The articular surface is convex when viewed from the side and less when viewed from the front. Glenoid fossa is the concavity within the temporal bone. The anterior wall is formed by the articular eminence of the temporal bone and its posterior wall by the tympanic plate, which also forms the anterior wall of the external auditory meatus. An articular disc is interposed between the temporal bone and the mandible, dividing the articular space into upper and lower compartments. The interposed fibrocartilaginous disc has a bow-tie-shaped biconcave morphology. The anterior and posterior ridges of the disc are termed anterior and posterior bands and are longer in the mediolateral than in the anteroposterior dimension. The smaller anterior band attaches to the articular eminence, condylar head, and joint capsule. The posterior band blends with highly vascularized, loose connective tissue, the bilaminar zone, and the capsule, the bilaminar zone residing in the retrodiscal space in the mandibular fossa and attaching to the condyle and temporal bone. Medially and laterally, the disc is firmly attached to the capsule and the condylar neck. Anteromedially, it is attached to the superior part of the pterygoid muscle. In a physiologic joint, the disc is positioned between the mandibular head inferiorly and the articular eminence anteriorly and superiorly when the jaw is closed. The posterior band of the disc lies within 10° of the 12 o'clock position. The medial and lateral corners of the disc align with the condylar borders and do not bulge laterally or medially. When the jaw is opened, the disc slides into a position between the mandibular head and articular eminence. The loose tissue of the bilaminar zone allows the remarkable range of motion of the disc. The attachments of the disc prevent luxation during opening. A triangular lateral ligament acts as a strong lateral stabilizer and inhibits the posterior translation of the mandibular head (Fig. 1).
The muscles of mastication are responsible for the complex movement of the jaw. The temporal, medial pterygoid, and masseter muscles facilitate jaw closure. Mouth opening is effected by coordinated action of the lateral digastric, mylohyoid, and suprahyoid muscles. The lateral pterygoid muscle and part of the fibers of the masseter and medial pterygoid muscles effect the anterior translation of the mandible. The superior belly of the lateral pterygoid muscle originates from the greater sphenoid wing and inserts on the disc. Subsequently, the superior belly plays a key role in upholding the physiologic position of the disc as it pulls the disc forward when the jaw is opened, in a combined translation and rotation. The inferior head of the lateral pterygoid muscle stretches from the lateral lamina of the pterygoid process to the pterygoid fovea. The medial pterygoid muslcle originates from the pterygoid fossa and inserts near the medial aspect of the mandibular angle (Sommer et al., 2003). The blood supply to the TMJ, outer and inner ear is provided mainly by branches from the internal maxillary artery as follows: temporal superficial artery, superior auricular artery, anterior tympanic artery and pterygoid artery. Innervation is provided by the auriculotemporal nerve (sensory branch of the mandibular nerve), deep temporal nerve, masseteric nerve. Sensory cervical sympathetic ramifications are going to the disc and capsule. The auriculotemporal nerve runs medial to the joint, then runs laterally, crossing the condylar neck, where it divides into branches to innervate the capsule, disc attachments, the tympanic membrane, the anterior surface of the cochlea, the upper part of the auricle, the tragus of the ear, the skin lining the external auditory meatus, the temporal region,. Nerve receptors as Ruffin receptors, Golgi tendon organs, Vater-Pacini corpuscules free nerve endings are in the capsule and substance P nerve fibres are also available in both the auriculotemporal and masseteric nerves, and have been demonstrated in the capsule, disc attachments but they are not present in the disc (Fig. 2).

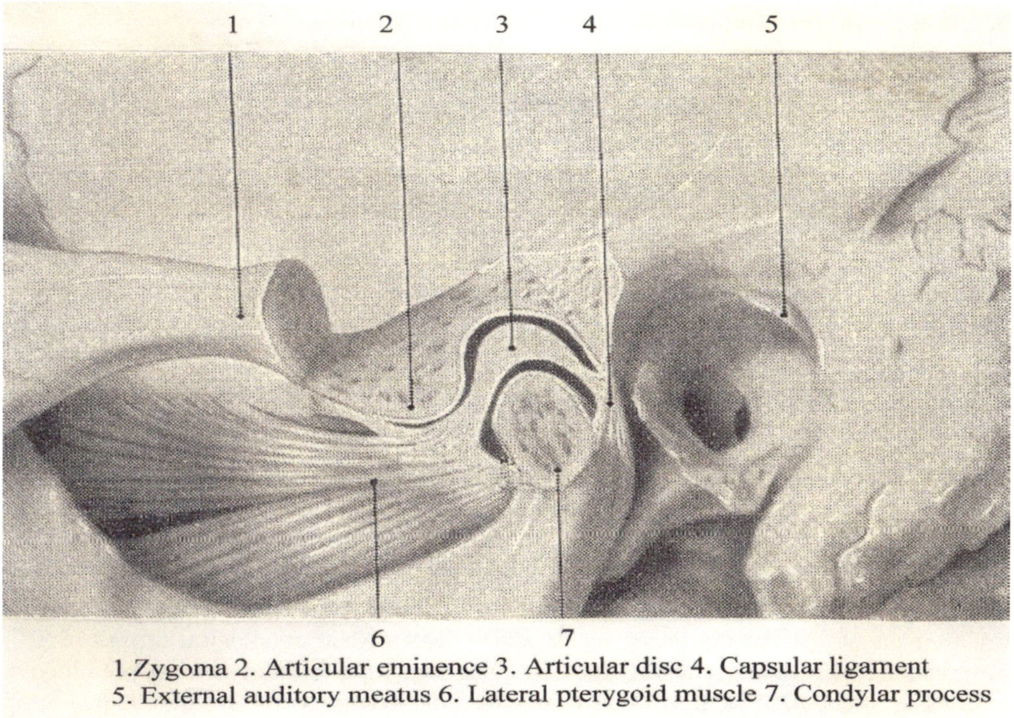

Fig. 1. A sagittal section through the left temporomandibular joint .

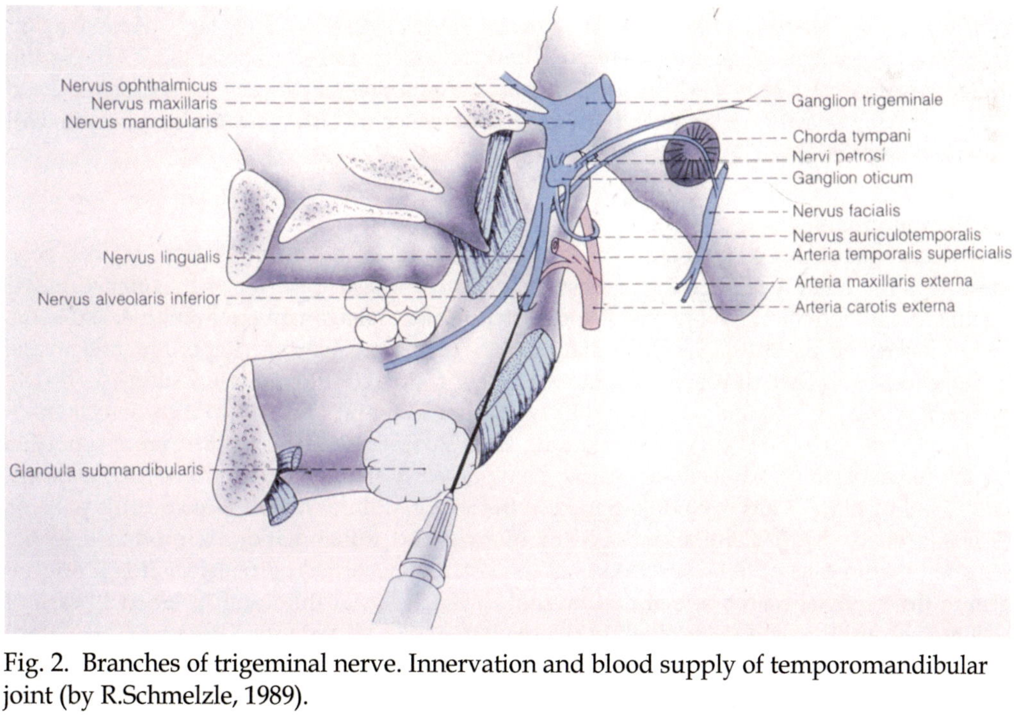

Fig. 2. Branches of trigeminal nerve. Innervation and blood supply of temporomandibular joint (by R.Schmelzle, 1989).

3. Classification of temporomandibular joint disorders:

- Arthritis- acute, chronic, infectious (specific, nonspecific)
- Osteoarthritis/arthrosis - most often disorder
- Injuries - luxations, concussion, fracture
- Ankylosis (fibrous, fibro-osseous, osseous)
- Tumours (benign and malignant)
- Congenital disturbances: I & II branchial arch malformations, condylar hypo-, hyperplasia
- Idiopathic condylar resorption
- Systemic conditions affecting the TMJ (rheumatoid arthritis, psoriasis, pseudogout etc.)

4. Aetiology and pathogenesis of temporomandibular disorders

4.1 Aetiology

Most scientists regard osteoarthritis as an inflammatory process, being most frequent TMJ disorder, characterised with proliferative changes in the synovia and primary degeneration of the cartilage and surrounding tissues with destruction of the bone structures. (Holmlund & Axelsson, 1996; Emshoff , 2005). It is found that 28% of the adult population have signs of temporomandibular joint disorder. In systemic diseases (rheumatoid arthritis, psoriasis etc.) involvement of TMJ occurs (Voog et al., 2003b; 2004). Main aetiological factors of TMJ disorders are as follows: systemic diseases (rheumatoid arthritis, psoriasis, pseudogout, ankylosing spondylitis etc.), secondary inflammatory component from the neighbouring regions (otitis, maxillary sinusitis, tonsillitis), trauma (chronical), prevalence of dental arch defects e.g. missing of molar teeth, (Tallents et al. 2002), malocclusion, endocrinological disturbances, odontogenic infections (third molars). Presence of specific bacterial species as *Staphylococcus aureus, Streptococcus mitis, Mycoplasma fermentas, Actinobacillus actinomycetemcomitans (Aa)* in the synovial fluid have been found (Kim et al., 2003). Serum antibodies against *Chlamydia spp.* in patients with monoarthritis of the TMJ have been occurred. An association may exist between the presence of *Chlamydia trachomatis* and TMJ disease (Paegle et al., 2004).

4.2 Pathogenesis

Knowledge about the pathogenesis on a molecular level of disorders of the TMJ has been improved in recent years giving a possibility to use these data for the evidence based treatment. Inflammation mainly affects the posterior disc attachement (Holmlund & Axelsson, 1996; Leibur et al., 2010). Several inflammatory mediators play an important role in the pathogenesis of TMJ diseases as tumor necrosis factor α (TNFα), interleukin-1β (IL-1β), prostaglandin E_2 (PGE_2), leukotrien B_4 (LkB_4), matrix metalloproteinases (MMP_s), serotonin- 5-hydroxytryptamine (5-HT), (Alstergren et al., 1999; Voog et al., 2003b). MMP_s are responsible for the metabolism of extracellular matrix, being an early marker to determine TMJ arthritis. High level of MMP-3 has been determined in the synovial fluid in TMJ osteoarthritis patients (Kamada et al., 2000). Serotonin, mediator of pain and inflammation, is produced in the enterocromaffin cells of the gastrointestinal mucosa and absorbed by platelets. It is produced also in the synovial membrane and is present in the synovial fluid and in blood in case of rheumatoid arthritis and is involved in the mediation of TMJ pain in systemic inflammatory joint diseases (Alstergren & Kopp, 1997; Voog et al., 2000). It plays a role also in bone metabolism (Warden & Haney, 2008). Tissue response in case of inflammation is as follows:

vasodilatation, extravasation, releasing of mediators, activation of nociceptors, release of neuropeptides as substance P (SP), neuropeptide Y (NPY), which stimulate releasing of histamin and serotonin from afferent nerve endings and hyperalgesia in TMJ occurs.

5. Diagnostics of the temporomandibular disorders

5.1 Clinical data

The most frequent complaint is pain and a decrease in the maximal interincisal opening (MIO), which normal values are between 35 - 50 mm (Fig. 3).
The following symptoms as pain (at rest, during maximum mouth opening and upon chewing), tenderness to digital palpation of the joint, sounds (clicking, crepitation), restricted mandibular mobility e.g. difficulty in opening the mouth, intermittent lock, closed lock, stiffness in the morning are observed. The stages of disease are usually classified according to Wilkes (1989; Table 1) by reviewing the case histories, clinical data, radiological records (computerized tomography images, magnetic resonance images, ortopantomography and/or plain radiographs by Schüller, Parma).

I. Early stage	
a.	Clinical: No significant mechanical symptoms other than opening reciprocal clicking; no pain or limitation of motion
b.	Radiologic: Slight forward displacement , good anatomic contour of the disc, negative tomograms, no bone structure changes
c.	Pathoanatomy: Excellent anatomic form; slight anterior displacement, passive in-coordination demonstrable
II. Early intermediate stage	
a.	Clinical: One or more episodes of pain: beginning major mechanical problems consisting of mid-to-late opening loud clicking; transient catching and locking
b.	Radiologic: Slight forward displacement; beginning disc deformity, slight thickening of posterior edge; negative tomograms, no bone structure changes
c.	Pathoanatomy: Anterior disc displacement; early disc deformity; good central articulating area
III. Intermediate stage	
a.	Clinical: Multiple episodes of pain; major mechanical symptoms consisting of locking (intermittent or fully closed): restriction of motion, function difficulties
b.	Radiologic: Anterior disc displacement with significant deformity or prolapse of disc (increased thickening of posterior edge), negative tomograms, no bone structure changes
c.	Pathoanatomy: Marked anatomic disc deformity with anterior displacement; no hard tissue changes
IV. Late intermediate stage	
a.	Clinical: Slight increase in severity over intermediate stage
b.	Radiologic: Increase in severity over intermediate stage; positive tomograms showing early-to-moderate degenerative changes - flattening of eminence, deformation of condylar head, erosions, sclerosis
c.	Pathoanatomy: Increase in severity over intermediate stage; hard tissue degenerative remodelling of both bearing surfaces (osteophyts), multiple adhesions in anterior and posterior recesses; no perforation of disk or attachments

V. Late stage	
a.	Clinical: Characterized by crepitus; variable and episodic pain; chronic restriction of motion and difficulty with function
b.	Radiologic: Disc or attachment perforation, filling defects, gross anatomic deformity of disc and hard tissues, positive tomograms with essentially degenerative arthritic changes
c.	Pathoanatomy: Degenerative changes of disc and hard tissues; perforation of posterior attachement; multiple adhesions, osteophyts, flattening of condyle and eminence, subcortical cyst formation

Table 1. Classification for internal derangement of the TMJ by Wilkes (1989).

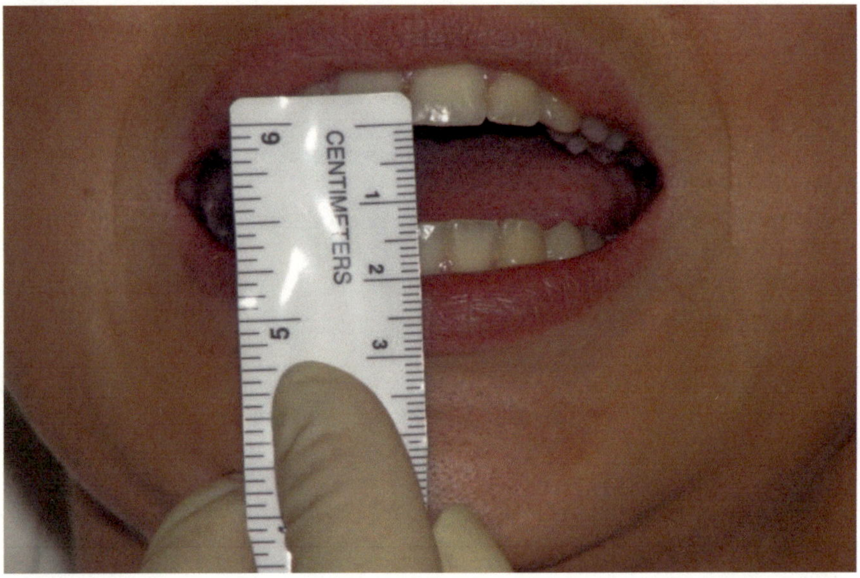

Fig. 3. Maximal interincisal opening (MIO) is 13 mm.

Symptom related factors obtained by questionnaire, the scores pre- and posttreatment maximal interincisal opening (MIO) and visual analogue scale (VAS) for pain are to be documentated and compared. Joint pain is assessed with 100 mm visual analogue scale with end points marked „no pain" and „worst pain ever experienced". The absence of pain is scored as 0. If pain is present the patient is asked to select marked field from 1mm to 100 mm.

It is known that inflammation often is accompanied by pain. Evaluation and estimation of the impact of pain is a complicated matter, since pain has many different ways to interfere with everyday life. The impact of pain on the health status and quality of life in patients with chronic inflammatory joint diseases has been recognized, but there is a lack of knowledge about the specific impact of TMJ pain on daily activities in patients with clinical involvement of the TMJ. A scale for measuring the activity of daily living (ADL), (List & Helkimo, 1995) is a useful tool for assessment of the restriction of activities of patients with TMJ disorders in their everyday life (Voog et al., 2003a; Kaselo et al., 2007; Jagur et al., 2011).

5.2 Radiographic investigations

Radiological changes of the TMJ are evaluated by orthopantomography (OPTG), computed tomography (CT), magnet resonance imaging (MRI) (Ohnuki et al. 2003; Voog et al., 2003b, 2004; Whyte et al., 2006) as well as ultrasonography (C.A. Landes et al., 2007).

OPTG is mainly used to demonstrate the structural bone changes in the TMJ and it has the advantage of being easily available but gaves limited information about the above mentioned joint being an alternative method to other radiological methods. To obtain a more detailed anatomic picture, CT or MRI are recommended. By evaluating the OPTGs the following radiographic signs of bone structural changes can be achieved such as presence of erosions, flattening and osteophytes of the condyle as well as temporal bone (Rohlin et al., 1986). Erosion in condyles in the radiographs is scored according to Helenius et al. (2004) as follows: score 1 - very slight erosion; score 2 - erosion on top of the condyle; score 3 - half of condyle is eroded; score 4 - condyle totally eroded. The first report of TMJ CT was published by Suarez et al. (1980) and this method is superior to plain transcranial or transmaxillary imaging for detecting bone changes. CT allows detailed three-dimensional examination of the TMJ and it is capable to detect even small bone changes not demonstrable by conventional tomographic procedures (Raustia et al., 1985; Larheim & Kolbensvedt, 1990). The CT sections are evaluated for presence of radiographic signs of bone changes within three regions (lateral, central and medial) of the mandibular and temporal part (eminence) of the TMJ. The recording of the signs is made in the axial, coronal and sagittal views (Emshoff et al., 2003; Voog et al., 2003). The changes are defined as follows: erosion - a local area with decreased density of the cortical joint surface including or not including adjacent subcortical bone (Fig.4), sclerosis - a local area with increased density of the cortical bony joint surface that may extend into the subcortical bone (Fig. 5), subchondral pseudocyst - a well defined, local area of bone rarefication underneath an intact cortical outlining of the joint surface, flattening - a flat bony contour deviating from the convex form (Fig. 6), osteophyte - a marginal bony outgrowth (Fig. 6). The grade of the total changes of the TMJ can be evaluated according to the scoring system developed by Rohlin & Petersson (1989) as well.

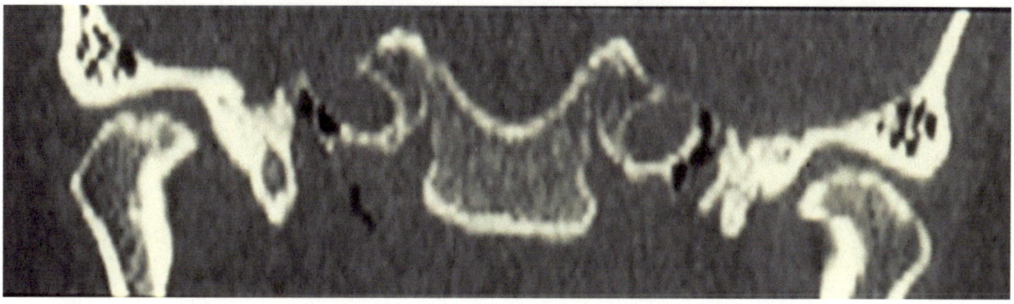

Fig. 4. Osteoarthritis of the TMJ. Signs of erosions on the surfaces of the condyles in a coronal view of the CT. An irregular outline is revealed on the condyles. The bone structure of the both glenoid fossa is normal.

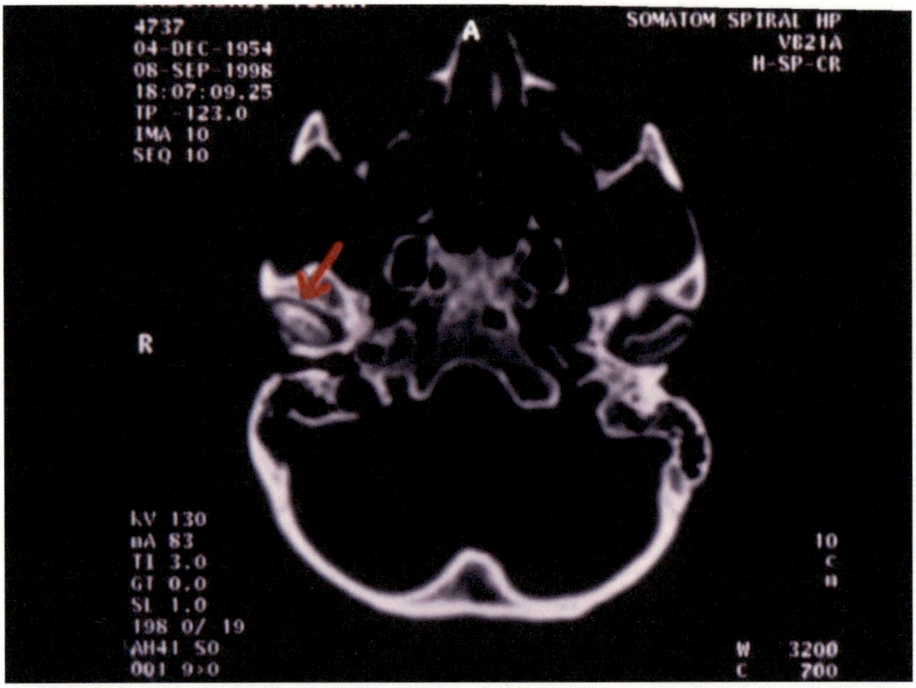

Fig. 5. Axial view of the CT. Sign of sclerosis in the medial and central parts of the right condyle of the mandible (arrow) . Reduced space is seen.

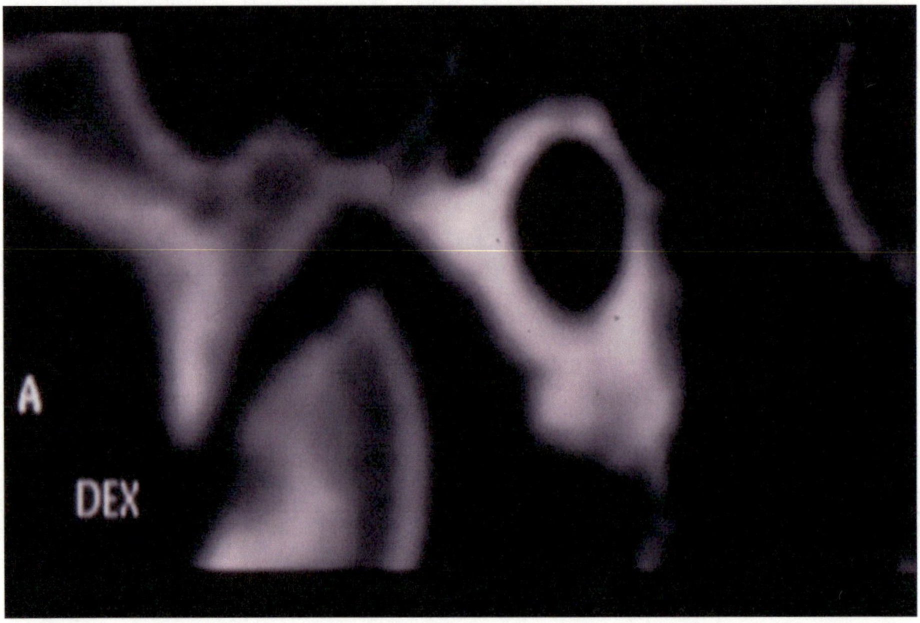

Fig. 6. Sagittal view of the CT from the left temporomandibular joint. Sign of flattening of the condyle.

MRI has a diagnostic value for internal derangements of the TMJ and rapidly surpassing CT as the imaging method of choice. MRI can detect not only TMJ soft tissue abnormalities like disc displacements, pathology of synovial membrane or capsule, pathology in the posterior attachement but also hard tissue morphologic changes can be demonstrated with MRI (Lieberman et al., 1996; Larheim et al., 1999). Sections in the oblique sagittal plane (i.e. perpendicular to the horizontal long axis of the mandibular condyle) and oblique coronal plane (i.e. parallel with the long axis of the condyle), and bilateral temporomandibular base surface coils are used (Larheim et al., 2001) for obtaining the images (Fig. 8).
The biting device (MEDRAD; Pittsburg) which enables dynamic imaging can be used as bite blocks during the open jaw phase of the imaging procedure (Gaggl et al.,1999). Dynamic magnetic resonance imaging is a recent method that investigate directly in vivo articular function and shows much promise as a noninvasive method of the disc function, however this limitation should diminish with continuing technological advances in the imaging field. Ultrasonography has been a helpful diagnostic approach for patients with TMJ disorders, having a possibility to diagnose with considerable reliability when compared with MRI and being a sensitive tool for assessing joint function (C. Landes et al., 2000; C.A. Landes et al., 2006).

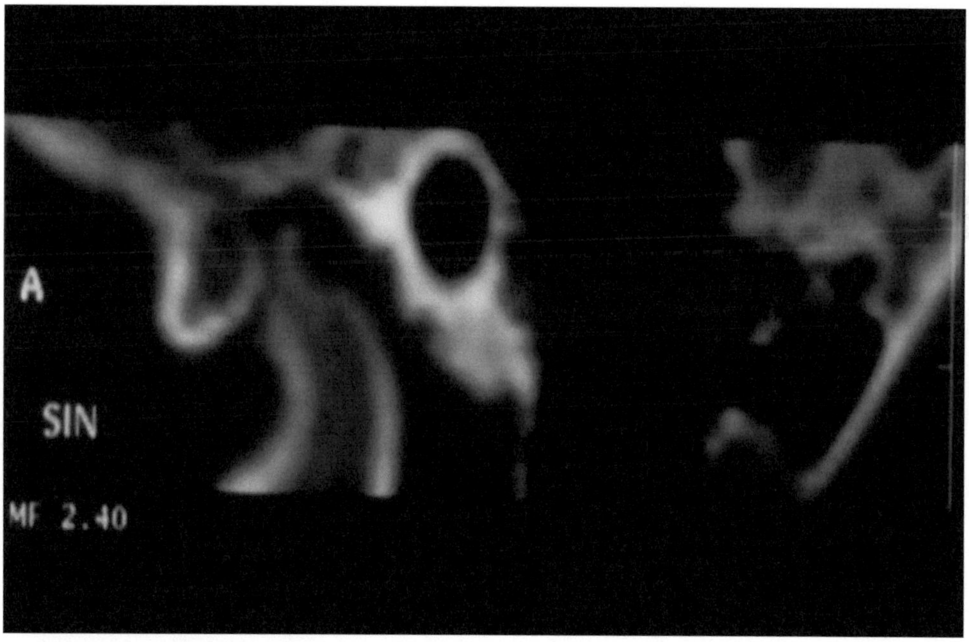

Fig. 7. An osteophyte in the medial part of the right mandibular condyle in a sagittal view of the CT., cortical destruction of the glenoid fossa surface.

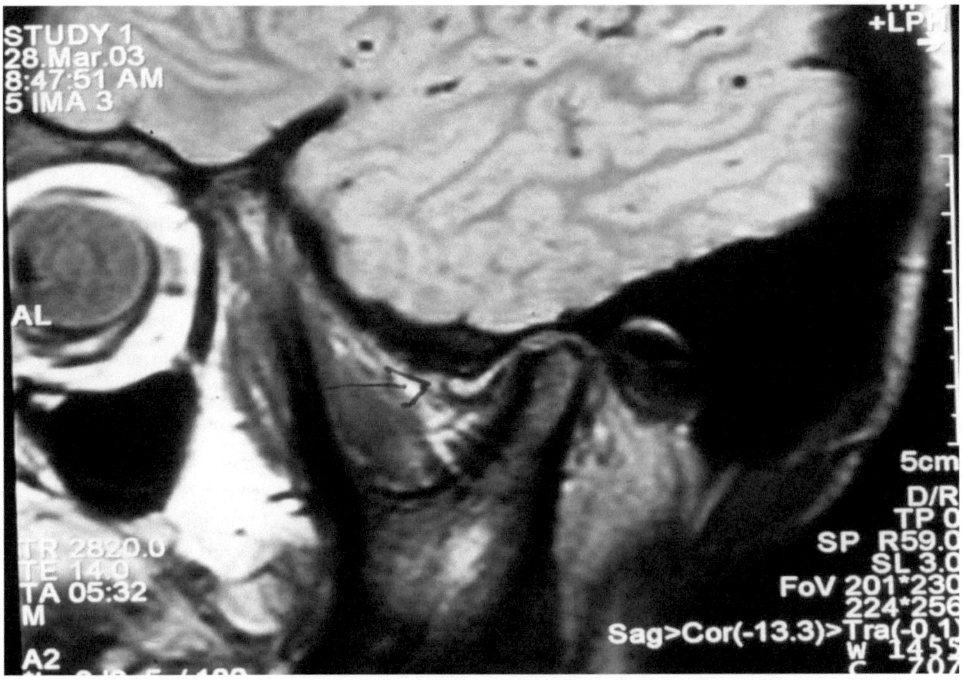

Fig. 8. Sagittal view of the MRI in a patient with internal derangement of the left TMJ. Anterior disc displacement (arrow), destruction of the disc. Changes of bone structures, effusion in the anterior recess.

6. Temporomandibular joint arthroscopy

6.1 Indications for arthroscopy

Indications for arthroscopy are radiological bone changes in TMJ characteristic to osteoarthritis with disc displacement or deformity and non effectiveness of conservative treatment with NSAIDs, intraoral splints or arthrocentesis. In practice, the decision to operate and the choice of the method seems to be a matter of the individual surgeon´s training, experience, and attitude toward the surgical management of TMJ disorders. Involvement of the TMJ in patients with rheumatoid arthritis or other connective tissue diseases is rather common and arthroscopy with simultaneous biopsy is indicated in these situations. Posttraumatic complaints may also be an indication for arthroscopy. Arthroscopy is contraindicated in case of acute arthritis. In these situations as large medial osteophyts on the condyle, large central cartilaginous perforations, fibrous, fibro-osseous, osseous ankylosis are better to handle *via* open reduction. Arthocentesis is considered as an intervening treatment modality between nonsurgical treatment and arthroscopic surgery. All cases for arthroscopy are usually classified as advanced Wilkes (1989) stages IV and V, in rare cases stage III (Table 1).

6.2 Technique for arthroscopy

Arthroscopy is performed under nasotracheal general anaesthesia which makes possible to manipulate the mandible during the operation. First the zygomatic arch and the condyle are palpated. The condyle is then forced in anterior position by the assistant and the preauricular concavity is formed in the skin, marking a point for the injection. Usually arthroscope KARL STORZ GmbH & Co.KG is used. Although various arthroscopic approaches to the TMJ have been described, the one most commonly used is the posterolateral approach to the upper joint space. After the condylar head of the TMJ has been determined , a marking line and puncture points are made on the skin surface (Fig. 9)

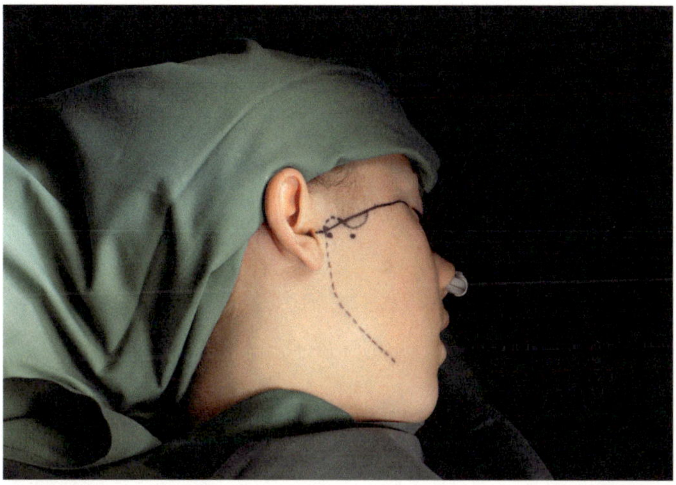

Fig. 9. A marking line and the puncture points on the skin surface for TMJ arthroscopy

The puncture site is located by manipulating the mandible anterio-inferiorly. For distension of the superior compartement and in order to avoid iatrogenic damage to the cartilaginous surfaces during introduction of the trocar, 1% lidocain solution 2,0 mL is inserted. The needle is aimed in a medial and slightly anteriosuperior direction until the contact with the glenoid fossa is achieved. The posterior recess of the superior joint space is reached when there is a backflow into the syringe of the solution injected into the joint space (Fig.10).

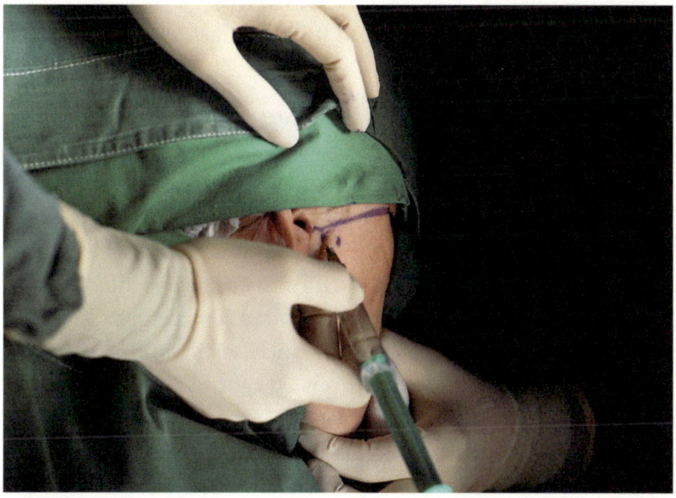

Fig. 10. Distension of the superior compartment of the right temporomandibular joint with 2% lidocaine solution.

Through the small skin incision 0,75 - 1,0 cm from the center of the *tragus* at the injection site the lateral capsule is punctured with a sharp trocar in an arthroscopic sheath inserted in the same direction as the previous injection needle. The sharp trocar is exchanged for a blunt one and the arhroscopic sheath is advanced further into the upper joint space. Puncture with arthroscope sheath (trocar) with a blunt obturator inserted into upper posterior recess is performed angling it medially upward ~ 2,5 cm. Another skin incision is made ~ 0,75 cm from the first skin incision in anterolateral direction for outflow cannula to be inserted into the upper joint anterior recess.
Following insertion of the trocar (diameter 1,8 mm, length 4 cm) into the joint space, blunt obturator is removed and forward-oblique telescope 30° (HOPKINS®), diameter 1,9 mm, length 6,5 cm, fiber optic light transmission incorporated is inserted (Fig. 11).

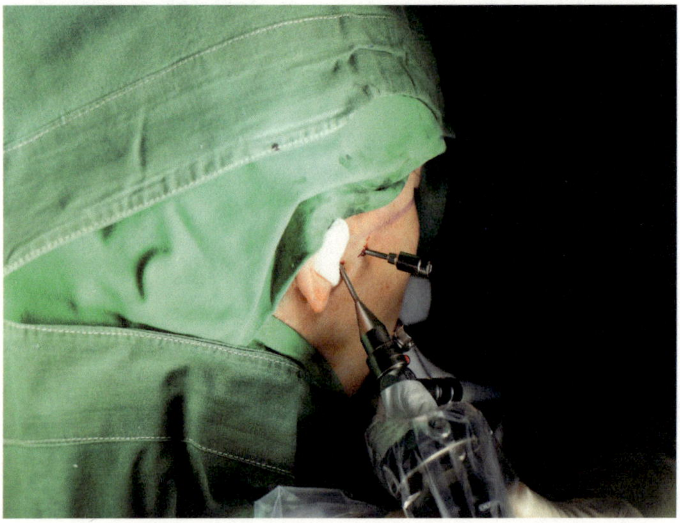

Fig. 11. Forward - oblique telescope 30° (HOPKINS®) fiber optic light transmission incorporated and outflow cannula are inserted into the right upper temporomandibular joint space.

Initial recognition of anatomical structures as the superior surface of the disc, articular fossa, and internal aspects of the posterior and medial capsule is performed. The fluid level in the arthroscope sheath should move with the jaw, confirming that the sheath is correctly positioned in the joint upper space.The upper joint compartment is examined from the posterior pouch *via* the intermediate zone to the anterior pouch. Disc may give the impression of being obstructed against the arthrotic surface of the temporal cartilage. The anterior part of the disc surface looks usually smooth and collagen fibres could clearly seen. The condylar cartilage is normally smooth, but in case of pathology e.g. in osteoarthritis where irregularities of the surface as erosions, osteophyts can be seen. Sever arthrotic changes of both fossa cartilage and disc may also observed. Adhesions between the disc and glenoid fossa are quite common. In rare cases the arthrotic or inflammatory changes are found in the anterior recess. Upper compartment is swept clear under constant irrigation with isotonic saline solution. This manipulation allow translation of the disc along the eminence, allowing the condyle to complete its natural path. After the diagnostic arthroscopy has been completed, either forceps, palpation hook or blunt probe are used to cut fibres, mainly fibers of the pterygoid muscle anterior to the disc, in order to reduce pull in the anterior direction and facilitate repositioning of the disc. Cutting of adhesions facilitate repositioning of the disc. During arthroscopy a sweeping procedure between the disc and fossa release the adhesions and fibrillations increasing the mobility in the joint. Release of the adhesions and fibrillations of the superior suface of the disc and shaving the surface of articular fossa in the upper joint compartment are performed with the aid of a blunt obturator or hook and with grasping forceps, scissors or double-edged knife. Removal of the superficial layer of cortical bone induces capillar bleeding stimulating formation of fibrocartilage on bone. Quite often a displaced disc may be found during arthroscopy. Surgical procedure is completed by irrigating the joint space to remove small tissue fragments. The outflowing fluid is collected and may be retained for diagnostic purposes. Arthroscopic lysis and lavage includs also a lateral release of the upper joint compartment performed with the aid of the blunt obturator or hook.Thus the locked disc could be mobilized sufficiently. Clinical, radiographic and arthroscopic findings in patients who underwent arthroscopy are given in Table 2 (Leibur et al. 2010).

Signs and symptoms	Sum	% abn	Radiographic findings	Sum	% abn	Arthro-scopic findings	Sum	% abn
Pain	25	86	Flattening	10	34	Adhesions	29	100
Hypomo-bility	23	79	Bone cyst / Subchondral pseudocycts	9	31	Chondro-matosis	5	17
Closed lock	5	17	Erosions	20	69	Fibrillations	22	76
Intermittent lock	5	17	Reduced space	10	34	Synovitis	9	31
Deviation	4	14	Sclerosis	8	27	Eburneation of fossa	15	52
			Hypomobilityof condyle Osteophyts	4 5	14 17	Displaced disc	23	23

Sum = total number of patients with findings; % abn = percentage of individuals with abnormal findings.

Table 2. Clinical, radiographic and arthroscopic findings in patients who underwent arthroscopy (N=29).

Arthroscopic findings are as follows: irregularities of joint surfaces, foldings and synovitis - hyperaemia of the inner wall, localising also in the posterior part of the disc, intra-articular fibrous adhesions, intracapsular adhesions, fibrillations of superior surface of the disc and arthrotic lesions of temporal cartilage, pseudowalls, foreign bodies - chondromatosis (Fig. 12, 13, 14, 15).

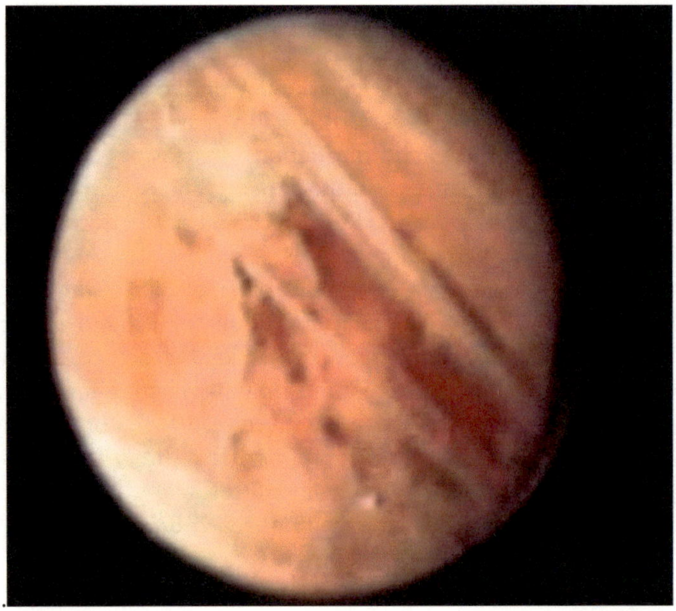

Fig. 12. Posterior recess of the superior compartment of the right TMJ. Fibrillations and pronounced adhesions with appearance irregularities of condylar surface, hyperaemia in the posterior capsular wall.

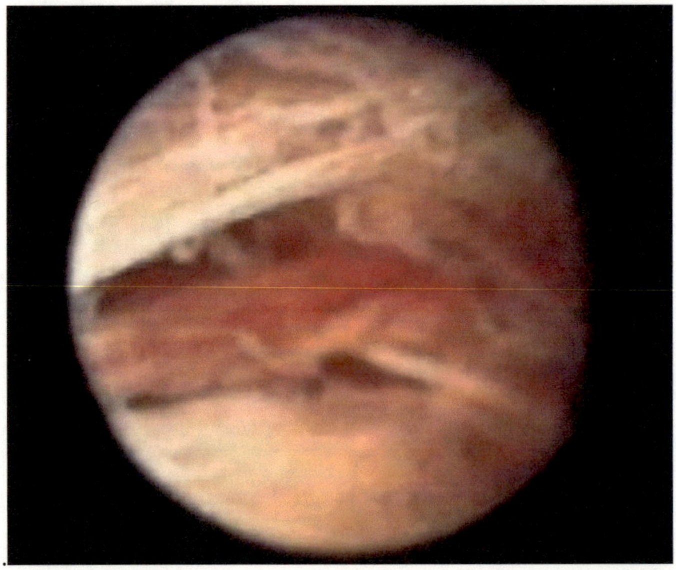

Fig. 13. Posterior recess of the superior compartment of the left TMJ. Eburneation of glenoid fossa, adhesions and fibrillations with „crab meat" appearance, mild granulations, irregularities of condylar surface, hyperaemia of the posterior attachment can be determined.

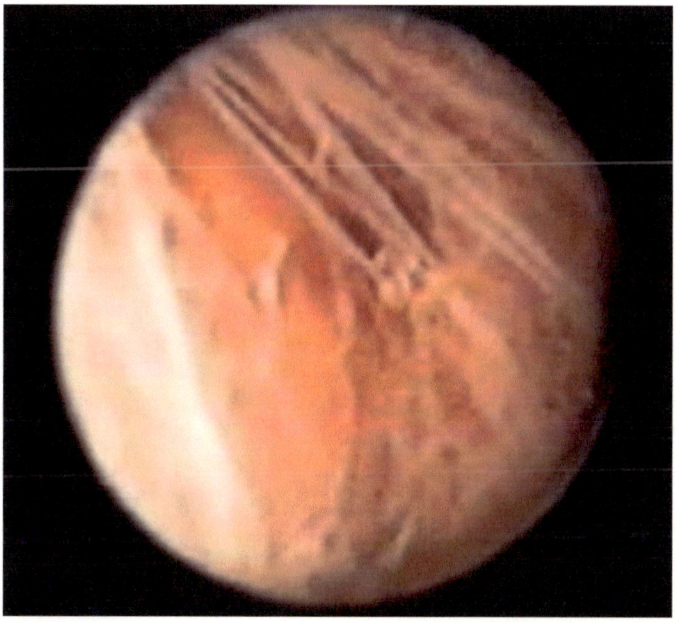

Fig. 14. Posterior recess of the superior compartment of the right TMJ. Fibrous adhesions, fibrillations and smooth fibres seen clearly. Synovial inflammation is obvious, localizing in the posterior part of the disc.

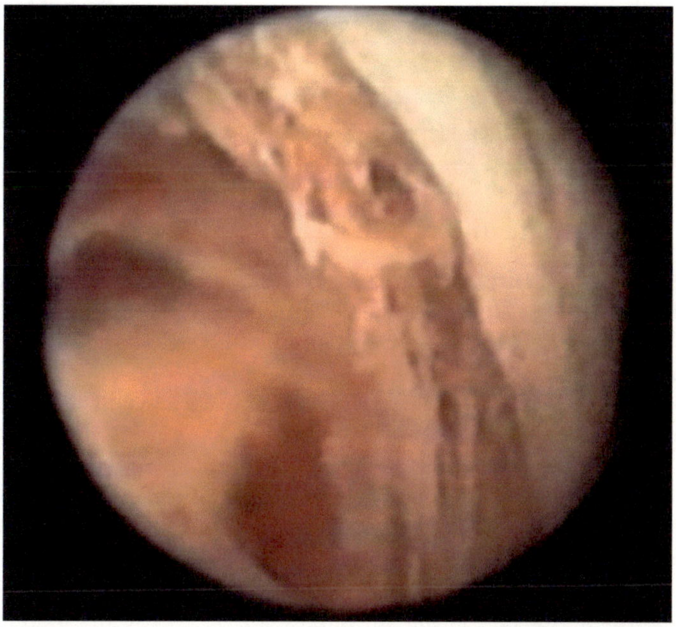

Fig. 15. Posterior recess of the superior compartment of the left TMJ. Debris on the posterior glenoid fossa wall can be seen. Fibrillations, adhesions and increased vascularization in the posterior capsular wall.

The patients are to be followed up after 6 months and approximayely 5 years after the operation. Intravenous antibiotics at the beginning of the procedure is recommended. Concepts of irrigation are to maintain the capsule distended through the procedure. Continuous irrigation constantly cleanses a joint debris and blood, increases mobility, reliefing symptoms. It is also important to use of adjunctive therapy postoperatively to obtain maximum success with arthroscopic surgery e.g. physical therapy especially in case of haemorrage, as it may prolong healing time. A pressure dressing during the first couple of hours after the operation is recommended.

6.3 Summary of arthroscopic findings

A number of arthroscopic findings as fibrous adherences mainly between the disc and fossa, fibrillations with „crab meat" appearance, mild granulations, irregularities of condylar surface, foreign bodies, increased vascularisation are to be found. Synovitis in the upper joint space of the TMJ has been observed during arthroscopy and this inflamed synovium may cause pain. The alterations in the constituents of the synovial fluid affect lubrication of the joint causing stickness and decreased mobility. Synovial chondromatosis has been found in the joint space (Mercuri, 2008; Leibur *et a*l. 2010; González-Pérez et al., 2011). Synovial chondromatosis of the TMJ in both the superior and inferior joint compartments have found due to osteoarthritis during long period ~ 10 years (Sato et al., 2002).

6.4 Possible complications

Intra- and postoperative complications for arthroscopy are rare. Bleeding may be from branches of the temporal vein during puncture. Extravasation of irrigation fluid into surrounding tissues may be occur sometimes due to leakage of the irrigating fluid into the surrounding tissues caused by accidental perforation of the TMJ capsule. This situation is easily controled if the surgeon always check the out-flow from out-flow cannula. From postoperative complications a few cases with otologic complications and nerve damage have been reported (Appelbaum et al.,1988; McCain et al., 1992). Injurie of superficial branches of facial nerve resulting to paraesthesia in the preauricular region was observed in two cases. These symptoms disappeared during one month (Leibur et al. 2010).

7. Analysis of clinical data and results

It has been shown that during arthroscopy several inflammatory and pain mediators causing destructive changes, foreign bodies as grains of chondromatosis are washed out elicitating joint noises (Shibuya et al., 2002; González-Pérez et al., 2011). For the patients with episodic signs and symptoms a noninvasive conservative approach is indicated (Wilkies stages I-III). Procedures currently used for the TMJ derangements as osteoarthritis/arthrosis (Wilkies stages IV and V) are: arthrocentesis, arthroscopy, arthrotomy or TMJ replacement. From arthroscopic findings fibrillation seemed to be the most common ~76% (Dimitroulis, 2002). Arthroscopic lysis and lavage has been an effective treatment for TMJ disorders refractory to nonsurgical treatments (Ohnuki et al., 2003; Sanroman, 2004; Politi et al., 2007). An evaluation following temporomandibular joint arthroscopic surgery with lysis and lavage after 2 to 10,8 years treatment showed that arthroscopic surgery of the temporomandibular joint is successful in the long term for patients in case of osteoarthritis and painful motion (Sorel & Piecuch, 2000). Assessment of symptoms reported by the patient as well as of objective signs noted on clinical examination confirms resolution of pain on movement and increased vertical opening. A significant and maintained improvement in maximal interincisal opening (MIO) and visual analogue scale (VAS) is also observed over the 5 years period of time (Fig. 16, 17), (Leibur et al. 2010).

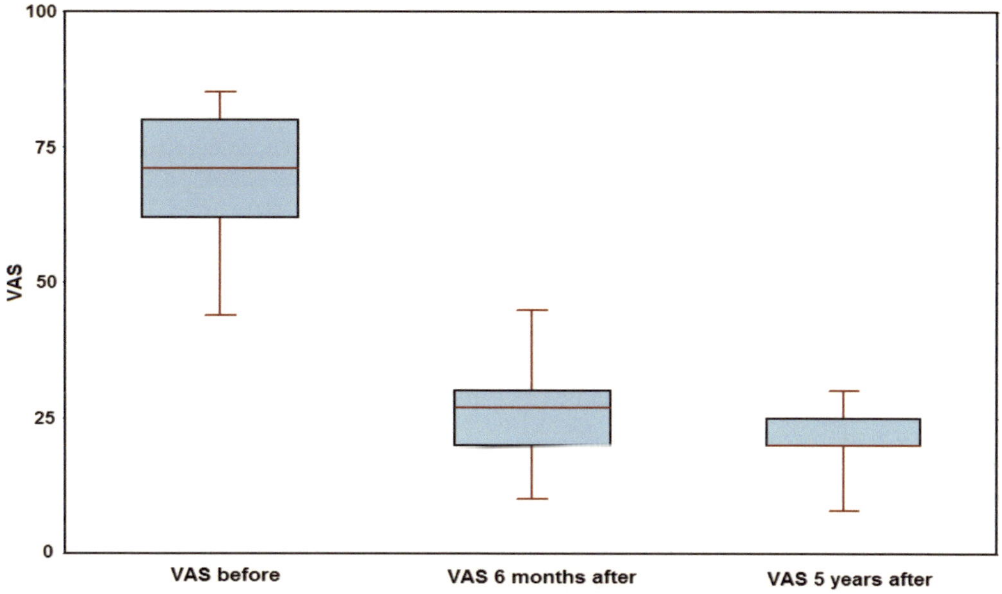

Fig. 16. Graphical representation of VAS values (median) before treatment and after 6 months and 5 years treatment in patients (n = 29).

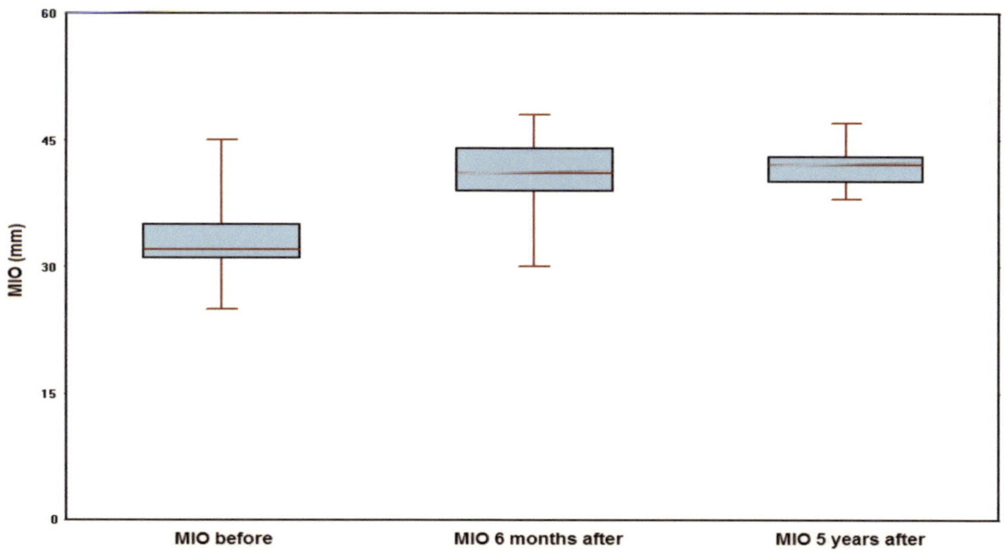

Fig. 17. Graphical representation of MIO values (median) before treatment and after 6 months and 5 years after treatment in patients (n = 29).

TMJ arthroscopy is especially useful when the disc has not yet been deformed. Superior joint compartment adhesions and disc immobility can be treated during arthroscopic

procedure, leading to resolution of symptoms and return of joint function (Leibur et al. 2010). The adhesions may cause retention of the disc in its anteriorly displaced position, which may explain the failure to respond to conservative treatment.
An adherence of the disc to the fossa may be caused by an alteration of the normal lubrication of the joint as a result of intermittent joint overloading, with secondary activation of oxidative species and degradation of hyaluronic acid. Anchored Disc Phenomen could be one of the first clinical symptoms observed in the chain events that would end in a more severe internal derangement (Sorel & Piecuch, 2000; Krug et al. 2004). Long-term results of TMJ arthroscopy have been analysed demonstrating a high accuracy for adhesions, fibrillations and degenerative changes of the bone structures. The adhesions may cause retention of the disc in its anteriorly displaced position, which may explain the failing response to conservative treatment. It has been shown that during this procedure several inflammatory and pain mediators causing destructive changes and chondromatosis are washed out elicitating joint noises (Emshoff et al., 2003; Voog et al., 2003b; Leibur et al., 2010). It is important to select the procedure with the highest probability of success and least morbidity. For the patients with episodic signs and symptoms a noninvasive , conservative approach is indicated (Wilkies stages I-III). Procedures currently used for the TMJ derangements as osteoarthritis/arthrosis (Wilkies stages IV and V) are: arthrocentesis (Sanroman, 2004), arthroscopy, arthrotomy or TMJ replacement (McCain et al.,1992; Smolka & Iizuka, 2005). Pain and hypomobility seems to be a part of a wide spectrum of symptoms appearing in the context of chronic dysfunction of the TMJ. Some authors have reported that the major symptom has been closed lock phenomenon (Dimitroulis, 2002; Sanroman, 2004). From arthroscopic findings (Dimitroulis 2002) fibrillation seemed to be the most common - 76%. In other study (Leibur et al. 2010) closed lock was found in 17,2 % and fibrillations in 75,8 % of cases. Several authors (K.Murakami et al., 2000; Sorel & Piecuch, 2000) performed long-term evaluation following temporomandibular joint arthroscopic surgery with lysis and lavage covering 10 years. On the bases of assessment of symptoms reported by the patients as well as objective signs noted on clinical examination confirmed resolution of pain on movement and increased maximal interincisial opening.. In a later study also lysis and lavage improved translation of the joint, decreased or eliminated pain. The chief presenting complaint for most patients (86,2%) was pain preoperatively. A significant maintained decrease in VAS score was achieved after 6 months and also after 5 years follow-up. A significant and maintained improvement in MIO was also observed over the same period of time (Leibur et al., 2010).The results are comparable to those reported in the other papers (Sorel and Piecuch, 2000; Smolka and Iizuka, 2005). It is important to take into account that the sympathetic and sensory nerve fibres within the temporomandibular joint are located in the anterior recess and the retrodiscal tissue of the upper compartment. Anterior disc release may reduce the number of these nerve fibres in arthroscopic procedures, thus influencing pain dynamics. The advantages of arthroscopy compared with open joint surgery using the Jaw Pain and Function Questionnaire are that arthroscopic surgery is less invasive and associated with lower morbidity (Undt et al., 2006). No statistical differences were also observed between arthroscopic lysis and lavage and operative arthroscopy in relation to postoperative pain or MIO at any stage of the follow-up period (Gonzalez - Garcia et al., 2008). The limitation in condylar movement probably originates from changes in the upper compartement that restricts the sliding motion of the disc. Arthroscopy improved the condylar movement. Arthroscopic lysis and lavage has been found effective in 84% of patients in case of osteoarthritis of TMJ (Dimitroulis, 2005). Multiple adhesions also develop skeletal changes, with a shortened ramus. If the condition develops rapidly enough, open

bite and rethrognathia may occur (Emshoff et al., 2003; Emshoff, 2005; Hamada et al., 2005). During arthroscopic surgery nodules of TMJ synovial chondromatosis are able to pass through the cannula by lavage with saline solution (Shibuy*a* et al., 2002). Based on the present findings, it follows that a displaced disc, by itself, is of only limited significance. This is not surprising because the majority of individuals with derangement of the TMJ are asymptomatic (Holmlund et al., 2001; Hamada et al., 2005). The intriguing question that remains is why lavage and lysis of adhesions or high-pressure irrigation of the upper joint space should be therapeutic. The answer is, that during this procedure several inflammatory mediators available in the synovial fluid as prostaglandins (K.I. Murakam*i* et al., 1998), cytokines (Kardel et al., 2003; Voog et al., 2003b), serotonin as pain mediator (Voog et al., 2000) etc. are washed out. In episodes of closed lock , the limitation in condylar movement probably originates from changes in the upper compartment that restrict the sliding motion of the disc. This course of events may explain the efficacy of lysis and lavage of only this joint space, as this manipulation allows translation of the disc along the eminence, allowing the condyle to complete its natural path. The data in the literature have stated that the most frequent disc displacements were anterior and anteromedial (Sorel & Piecuch, 2000). In episodes of closed lock , the limitation in condylar movement probably originates from changes in the upper compartment that restrict the sliding motion of the disc. The data in the literature have stated that the most frequent disc displacements were anterior and anteromedial. Using MRI pre- and postoperatively revealed that disc position remained anteriorly without reduction, disc mobility increased and deformity of the discs progressed after arthroscopic surgery (Ohnuki et al. 2003). Improvement in joint symptoms and function is not attributed so much as to the restoration of disc position as to possible release of the lateral capsular fibrosis during arthroscopy (Moses & Lo,1992; Sorel & Piecuch, 2000).

8. Arthroscopy vs. arthrotomy

There is still a group of patients whom an arthrotomy and disc surgery are necessary e.g. to treat painful clicking in patients with anteriorly displaced, nonreducing discs and limited mouth opening, irreparable disc perforation or if it is misshaped , shortened, rigid (Laskin, 2006). Large medial osteophyts on the condyle are very difficult to shave arthroscopically, and in these situations they are better to handle *via* arthrotomy. Large central cartilaginous perforations may need an arthrotomy and possibly discectomy, although there are data about healing of disc perforations as the bilaminar zone undergoes metaplastic changes forming pseudodisc (Moses & Lo, 1992). The importance of disc position and shape is emphasized by many authors (Ohnuki et al., 2003; Politi et al., 2007). As a result, open joint procedures are developed to reposition the displaced disc (Holmlund et al., 2001; González - Garcia et al., 2008). Direct comparison of the clinical results are achieved in patients following arthroscopic surgery with a group of patients who underwent open surgery. The postoperative follow-up period ranged 5 to 6 years and 9 months. These results following open and arthroscopic surgery measured with the Jaw Pain and Function Questionnaire a self rating scale, originally published by Clark et al., 1989; and differentiated by Wilkes´(1989) stages. No significant difference was noted when comparing the groups 5 years postoperatively (Undt et al., 2006).

9. Summary

Clinical success of arthroscopy is based on several factors. Lysis and lavage remove intraarticular inflammatory and pain mediators. The release of fibrillations and adhearences as well as improvement in discal mobility allows to distrbute the functional stresses on the articular tissues and adverse loading on the joints is decreased. The long-term outcome of TMJ arthroscopic surgery with lysis and lavage is considered to be acceptable and effective. Fibrillations and fibrous adhesions are the most usual pathological signs of arthroscopic findings in patients with internal derangement of the TMJ. Arthroscopic releasing of these restrictive bands improves the joint mobility and contributes to reducing pain level. The results of arthroscopy offer favourable long-term stable results with regard to increasing MIO and reducing pain and dysfunction. The improvement in joint mobility and disc mobility will lead to adaptive changes in the hard tissues .This may implay that the arthroscopic procedure with mechanics may stop the process of further TMJ degeneration. The advantages of arthroscopy compared with open joint surgery are that arthroscopic surgery is less invasive, procedure needs less time and associated with lower morbidity.

10. References

Alstergren, P. & Kopp. S. (1997). Pain and synovial fluid concentration in arthritic temporomandibular joints. *Pain* , Vol.72, No. 1-2 (August 1997), pp. 137-143, ISSN 0304-3959

Alstergren, P.; Kopp, S. & Theordosson, E. (1999). Synovial fluid sampling from the temporomandibular joint: sample quality criteria and levels of interleukin- 1 beta and serotonin. *Acta Odontologica Scandinavica*,Vol.57, No.1 (January 2003), pp. 278-282, ISSN 0001- 6357

Appelbaum, E.L.; Berg, L.F.; Kumar, A. & Mafee, M.F. (1988). Otologic complications Following temporomandibular joint arthroscopy. *Annals of Otology, Rhinology, Laryngology*, Vol.97, No. 6 (November-December 1988), pp. 675-679, ISSN 0003-4894

Clark, GT.; Seligman, D.; Solberg, W.K. & Pullinger, A.G. (1989). Guidlines for the examination and diagnosis of temporomandibular disorders. *Journal of Craniomandibular Disorders*, Vol.3, No.1 (Winter 1989), pp. 7-14, ISSN 0890-2739

Dimitroulis, G. (2002). A review of 56 cases of chronic closed lock treated with temporomandibular joint arthroscopy. *Journal of Oral and Maxillofacial Surgery*, Vol.60, No.5 (May 2002), pp. 519-524, ISSN 0278-2391

Dimitroulis, G.(2005). The prevalence of osteoarthrosis in cases of advanced internal derangement of the Tempoomandibular Joint: a clinical, surgical and histological study. *International Journal of Oral & Maxillofacial Surgery*, Vol.34, No. 2 (February 2005), pp. 345-349, ISSN 0901–5027

Emshoff, R.; Brandlmaier, I.; Bertram, S.& Rudish, A.(2003). Relative odds of temporomandibular joint pain as a function of magnetic resonance imaging findings of internal derangement, osteoarthrosis, effusion, and bone marrow edema. *Oral Surgery Oral Medicine Oral Pathology Oral Radiology Endodontics*, Vol. 95, No.4 (April 2004), pp. 437-445, ISSN 0904-2512

Emshoff, R.(2005). Clinical factors affecting the outcome of arthrocentesis and hydraulic distension of the temporomandibular joint. *Oral Surgery Oral Medicine Oral Pathology Oral Radiology Endodontics*, Vol.100, No.4 (October 2005), pp.409-414, ISSN 0904-2512

Gaggl, A.; Schults, G.; Santler, G.; Kärcher, H. & Simbrunner, J. (1999). Clinical and magnetic resonance findings in the temporomandibular joints of patients before and after orthognathic surgery. *The British Journal of Oral & Maxillofacial Surgery, Vol. 37, No.1 (February 1999), pp. 41-45, ISSN 0266-4356*

González-Garcia, R.; Rodriguez-Campo, FJ.; Monje, F.; Sastre-Perez, J.& Gil-Diez Usandizaga JL. (2008). Operative versus simple arthroscopic surgery for chronic closed lock of the temporomandibular joint: a clinical study of 344 arthroscopic procedures. *International Journal of Oral &Maxillofacial Surgery,* Vol.17, No.9 (September 2008), pp. 790-796, ISSN 0901-5027

González-Pérez, L.M., Concregado-Córdoba, J.& Salinas-Martin, M.V. (2011). Temporomandibular joint synovial chondromatosis with a traumatic etiology. *International Journal of Oral & Maxillofacial Surgery,* Vol.40, No.3 (March 2011), pp. 330-334, ISSN 0901-5027

Hamada, Y.; Kondoh, T.; Holmlund, A.B.; Iino, M.; Kobayashi, K.& Seto, K. (2005). Influence of arthroscopically observed fibrous adhesions before and after joint irrigation on clinical outcome in patients with chronic closed lock of the temporomandibular joint. *International Journal of Oral & Maxillofacial Surgery,* Vol.34, No.7 (October 2005), pp. 727-732., ISSN 0901-5027

Helenius, L.; Hallikainen, D.; Meurman, J.; Koskimies, S.; Tervahartiala, P.; Kivisaari, L.; Hietanen, J.; Suuronen, R.; Lindqvist, C. & Leirisalo-Repo, M. (2004). HLA-DRB1* alleles and temporomandibular joint erosion in patientes with rheumatic disease. *Scandinavian Journal of Rheumatology* ,Vol 33, No.1 (January 2004), pp. 24-29, ISSN:0300-9742

Holmlund, A.B.& Axelsson S. (1996). Temporomandibular arthropathy: correlation between clinical signs and symptoms and arthroscopic findings. *International Journal of Oral & Maxillofacial Surgery,* Vol.25, No.3, (June 1996), pp. 266-271, ISSN 0901 - 5027

Holmlund, A.B.; Axelsson, S.& Gynther, G.W. (2001).A comparison of discectomy and arthroscopic lysis and lavage for the treatment of chronic closed lock of the temporomandibular joint: a randomized outcome study. *Journal of Oral and Maxillofacial Surgery,* Vol.59, No.9 (September 2001), pp. 972-977, ISSN 0278-2391

Jagur, O.; Kull, M.; Leibur, E.; Kallikorm, R.; Loorits, D.; Lember, M.& Voog-Oras, Ü. (in print 2011). The impact of pain in TMJ on activities of daily living and bone status. *Stomatologija. Baltic Dental and Maxillofacial Journal,* (in print, 2011), ISSN 1392-8589

Kamada, A.; Kakudo, K.; Arika, T.; Okazaki, J.; Kano, M.& Sakaki, T.(2000). Assay of synovial MMP-3 in temporomandibular joint diseases. *Journal of Cranio-Maxillo-Facial Surgery,* Vol.28, No.3 (June 2000), pp.247-248, ISSN 1010-5182

Kardel, R.; Ulfgren, A.K.; Reinholt, F.P.& Holmlund, A.B. (2003). Inflammatory cell and cytokine patterns in patients with painful clicking and osteoarthritis in the temporomandibular joint. *International Journal of Oral & Maxillofacial Surgery,* Vol. 32, No.5 (May 2003), pp. 390-396, ISSN 0901-5027

Kaselo, E.; Jagomägi, T.& Voog, U. (2007). Malocclusion and the need for orthodontic treatment in patients with temporomandibular dysfunction. *Stomatologija. Baltic Dental and Maxillofacial Journal,* Vol.9, No.3, (Autum 2007), pp.79-85, ISSN 1392-8589

Kim, S.J.; Park, Y.H.; Hong, S.P.; Cho, B.O.; Park, J.W.& Kim, S.G. (2003). The presence of Bacteria in the synovial fluid of the temporomandibular joint and clinical significance: preliminary study. *Journal of Oral and Maxillofacial Surgery,* Vol.61, No.10 (October 2003), pp. 1156-1161, ISSN 0278-2391

Krug, J.; Jirousek, Z.; Suchmova, H.& Germakova, E. (2004). Influence of discoplasty and discectomy of the temporomandibular joint on elimination of pain and restricted mouth opening. *Acta Medica (Hradec Kralove),* Vol.47, No.1 (January 2004), pp. 47-53, ISSN 1211-4286

Landes, C.; Walendzik, H. & Klein, C. (2000). Sonography of the temporomandibular joint from 60 examinations and comparison with MRI and axiography. *Journal of Cranio-Maxillo-Facial Surgery,* Vol.28, No.6 (December 2000), pp.352-361, ISSN 1010-5182

Landes, C.A.; Goral, W.A.; Sader, R.& Mack, M.G. (2007). 3-D sonography for diagnosis of disc dislocation of the temporomandibular joint compared with MRI. *Ultrasound Medical Biology,* Vol.32, No.5 (May 2007), pp. 633-639, ISSN 0301-5629

Larheim, T.A. & Kolbenstvedt, A. (1990). Osseous temporomandibular joint abnormalities in rheumatic disease. Computed tomography versus hypocycloidal tomography. *Acta Radiologica,* Vol 31, No.4 (July 1990), pp.383-387, ISSN 0284-1851.

Larheim, T.A.; Westesson, P.- L.; Hicks, D.G.; Eriksson, L. & Brown, D.A. (1999). Osteonecrosis of the temporomandibular joint: correlation of magnetic resonance imaging and histology. *Journal of Oral and Maxillofacial Surgery,* Vol.57, No.8 (August 1999), pp. 888-898, ISSN 0901-5027.

Larheim, T.A.; Westesson, P. & Sano, T. (2001). Temporomandibular Joint Disk Displacement: Comparison in Asymptomatic Volunteers and Patients. *Radiology,* Vol.218, No.2 (February 2001), pp. 428-32, ISSN 0033-8419.

Laskin, D.M. (2006).Surgical Management of Internal Derangements, In: *Temporomandibular Disorders. An Evidence-Based Approach to Diagnosis and Treatment,* D.M. Laskin; C.S. Green; W.L. Hylander (Ed.), 469-481, Quintessence Publishing Co. Inc, ISBN 0-86715-447-0

Leibur, E.; Jagur, O.; Müürsepp, P.; Veede, L. & Voog-Oras, Ü. (2010). Long-term evaluation of arthroscopic surgery with lysis and lavage of temporomandibular disorders. *Journal of Cranio-Maxillo-Facial Surgery,* Vol.38, No.8 (December 2010), pp.615-620, ISSN 1010-5182

Lieberman, J.M.; Gardner, C.L.; Motta, A.O. & Schwartz, R.D. (1996). Prevalence of bone marrow signal abnormalities observed in the temporomandibular joint using magnetic resonance imaging. *Journal of Oral and Maxillofacial Surgery* , Vol.54, No. 4 (April 1996), pp. 434-439, ISSN 0901-5027..

List, T. & Helkimo, M. (1995). A scale for measuring the activities of daily living (ADL) of patients with craniomandibular disorders. *Swedish Dental Journal,* Vol.19, No.1 (January 1995), pp. 33-40, ISSN 0001-6357.

McCain, J.P.; Sanders, B.; Koslin, M.G.; Quinn, J.H.; Peters, P.B. & Indresano, A.T. (1992). Temporomandibular joint arthroscopy : a 6-year multicenter retrospective study of 4,831 joints. *Journal of Oral and Maxillofacial Surgery,* Vol.50, No.9 (September 2002), pp.926-930, ISSN 0278-2391

Mercuri, L.G. (2008). Synovial chondromatosis of the temporomandibular joint with medial cranial fossa extension. *International Journal of Oral & Maxillofacial Surgery,* Vol.37, No.7 (July 2008), pp. 684-685, ISSN 0901 - 5027

Moses, J.J. & Lo, H. (1992). The treatment of internal derangement of the temporomandibular joint - an arthroscopic approach. *Oral Surgery Oral Diagnosis,* Vol.3 (1992), pp. 5-11, ISSN 0788-6020

Murakami, K.I.; Shibata, T.; Kubota, E.& Maeda, H. (1998). Intra-articular levels of prostaglandin E_2 , hyaluronic acid, and chondroitin - 4 and - 6 sulfates in the temporomandibular joint synovial fluid of patients with internal derangement. *Journal of Oral and Maxillofacial Surgery,* Vol.56, No.2 (February 1998), pp. 199-203, ISSN 0278-2391

Murakami, K.; Segami, N.; Okamoto, I.; Takahashi, K. & Tsuboi, Y. (2000). Outcome of arthroscopic surgery for internal derangement of the temporomandibular joint: long - term results covering 10 years. *Journal of Cranio-Maxillo-Facial Surgery*, Vol.28, No.3 (March 2000), pp. 264 - 271, ISSN 1010-5182

Onishi, M. (1975). Arthroscopy of the temporomandibular joint (author´s transl.). *Journal of Japanese Stomatological Association*, No.42, (June 1975), pp. 207-213, ISSN 0300-9149

Onishi, M. (1980).Clinical application arthroscopy in the temporomandibular joint diseases. *Bulletin Tokyo Medical Dental University*. No. 27(1980), pp. 141-148.

Ohnuki, T.; Fukuda, M.; Iino, M. & Takahahshi, T. (2003). Magnetic resonance evaluation of the disk before and after arthroscopic surgery for temporomandibular disorders. *Oral Surgery Oral Medicine Oral Pathology Oral Radiology Endodontics*, Vol.96, No.2 (February 2003), pp.141-148. ISSN 0904-2512

Paegle, D.I.; Holmlund, A.B.; öStlund, M.R. & Grillner, L. (2004). The occurence of antibodies against Chlamydia species in patients with monoarthritis and chronic closed lock of the temporomandibular joint. *Journal of Oral and Maxillofacial Surgery*, Vol.62, No.4 (April 2004), pp. 435-439, ISSN 0278-2391

Politi, M.; Sembronio, S.; Robiony M.; Costa, F.; Toro, C. & Undt, G. (2007). High condylectomy and disc repositioning compared to arthroscopic lysis, lavage and capsular strech for the treatment of chronic closed lock of the temporomandibular joint. *Oral Surgery Oral Medicine Oral Pathology Oral Radiology Endodontics*, Vol. 103, No.1 (January 2007), pp.27 - 33. ISSN 0904-2512

Raustia, A.M.; Pyhtinen, J.& Virtanen, K.K. (1985). Examination of the temporomandibular joint by direct sagittal computed tomography. *Clinical Radiology*, Vol. 36, No. 3 (May 1985), pp. 291-296, ISSN 0009-9260.

Rohlin, M.; Åkerman, S.; & Kopp, S. (1986). Tomography as an aid to detect macroscopic changes of the temporomandibular joint. *Acta Odontologica Scandinavica*, Vol. 44, No.3 (June 1986), pp.131-140,ISSN 0001-6357

Rohlin, M. & Petersson, A. (1989). Rheumatoid arthritis of the temporomandibular joint: radiologic evaluation based on standard reference films. *Oral Surgery, Oral Medicine, and Oral Pathology*, Vol. 67, No. 5 (May 1989), pp. 594-599, ISSN0030-4220.

Sanroman, J.F. (2004). Closed lock (MRI fixed disc): a comparison of arthrocentesis and arthroscopy. *International Journal of Oral & Maxillofacial Surgery*, Vol.33, No.4 (April 2004), pp. 344-348, ISSN 0901 - 5027

Sato, J.; Segami, N.; Suzuki, T.; Yoshitake, Y.& Nishikawa, K. (2002).The expression of fibroblast growth factor receptor 1 in chondrocytes in synovial chondromatosis of thetemporomandibular joint. Report of two cases. *International Journal of Oral & Maxillofacial Surgery*, Vol.31, No.7 (July 2002), pp. 532-536, ISSN 0901 - 5027

Schmelzle, R. (1989). Lokalanästhesie. In: *Zahnärztliche Chirurgie*. 2. Auflage Urban & Schwarzenberg. München-Wien Baltimore, p.19, ISBN 3-541-15290-7

Shibuya, T.; Kino, K.; Yoshida, S. & Amagasa, T. (2002). Arthroscopic removal of nodules of synovial chondromatosis of the temporomandibular joint. *Cranio*, Vol.20, No.4 (October 2002), pp. 304-306, ISSN 0886-9634

Smolka, W. & Iizuka, T. (2005). Arthroscopic lysis and lavage in different stages of internal derangement of the temporomandibular joint: correlation of preoperative staging to arthroscopic findings and treatment outcome. Journal of Oral and Maxillofacial Surgery, Vol.63, No.4 (April 2005), pp. 471-478, ISSN 0278-2391

Sommer, O.J.; Aigner, F.; Rudisch, A.; Gruber, H.; Fritsch, H.; Millesi, W. & Stiskal, M. (2003). Cross-sectional and functional imaging of the temporomandibular joint: radiology, pathology, and basic biomechanics of the jaw. *Radiographics.*,Vol. 23, No.6 (November-December 2003), pp. e14, ISSN 0271-5333

Sorel. B. & Piecuch, J.F. (2000). Long-term evaluation following temporomandibular joint arthroscopy with lysis and lavage. *International Journal of Oral & Maxillofacial Surgery*, Vol.29, No.4 (August 2000), pp. 532-536, ISSN 0901 - 5027

Suarez, F.R.; Bhussry, B.R.; Neff, P.A.; Huang, H.K. & Vaughn, D. (1980). A preliminary study of computerized tomographs of the temporomandibular joint. *The Compendium on continuing education in general dentistry*, Vol. 1, No. 3 (May-June 1980), pp.217-222, ISSN 0196-1756.

Tag, H. (1939). Arthroscope. *Journal of Japanese Orthopedic Association*, No.14, pp.359 - 362.

Tallents, R.H.; Macher, D.J.; Kyrkanides, S.; Katzberg, R.W. & Moss, M.E. (2002). Prevalence of missing posterior teeth and intraarticular temporomandibular disorders. *Journal of Prosthetic Dentistry*, Vol. 87, No.1 (January 2002), pp. 45-50, ISSN 0022-3913

Undt, G.; Murakami, K.I.; Rasse, M & Ewers, R. (2006). Open versus arthroscopic surgery for internal derangement of the temporomandibular joint: A retrospective study comparing two centers results using Jaw Pain and Function Questionnaire. *Journal of Cranio-Maxillo-Facial Surgery*, Vol.34, No.4 (June 2006), pp.234-241, ISSN 1010-5182

Voog, Ü.; Alstergren, P., Leibur, E.; Kallikorm, R. & Kopp, S. (2000). Immediate effect of the serotonin antagonist granisetron on temporomandibular joint pain in patients with systemic inflammatory disorders. *Life Sciences*, Vol.68, No.5, (December 2000), pp. 591-602, ISSN 0024-3205

Voog, Ü.; Alstergren, P.; Leibur, E.; Kallikorm, R. & Kopp, S. (2003a). Impact of temporomandibular joint pain on activities of daily living in patients with rheumatoid arthritis. *Acta Odontologica Scandinavica*,Vol.61, No.5 (October 2003), pp. 278-282, ISSN 0001- 6357

Voog, Ü.; Alstergren, P.; Eliasson, S.; Leibur, E.; Kallikorm, R. & Kopp, S. (2003b). Inflammatory mediators and radiographic changes in temporomandibular joints in patients with rheumatoid arthritis. *Acta Odontologica Scandinavica*, Vol.61, No.1 (January 2003), pp. 57-64, ISSN 0001- 6357

Voog, Ü.; Alstergren, P.; Eliasson, S.; Leibur, E.; Kallikorm, R. & Kopp, S. (2004). Progression of radiographic changes in the temporomandibular joints of patients with rheumatoid arthritis in relation to inflammatory markers and mediators in the blood. *Acta Odontologica Scandinavica*, Vol.62, No.1 (January 2004), pp. 7-13, ISSN 0001- 6357

Warden, S.J. & Haney, E.M. (2008). Skeletal effects of serotonin (5-hydroxytryptamine) transporter inhibition: evidence from in vitro and animal-based studies. *Journal of Musculoskeletal Neuronal Interaction*,Vol.8, No.2 (February 2008), pp. 121-132, ISSN 1108-7161

Whyte, A.M.; McNamara, D.; Rosenberg, I. & Whyte, A.W. (2006). Magnetic resonance imaging in the evaluation of temporomandibular joint disc displacement. *International Journal of Oral & Maxillofacial Surgery*, Vol.35, No.8 (August2006), pp.696-703, ISSN 0901 - 5027

Wilkes, C.H. (1989).Internal derangements of the temporomandibular joint. Pathological variations. *Archives of Otolaryngology, Head Neck Surgery*, Vol.115, No.4 (April 1989), pp. 469-477, ISSN 0886-4470

Part 2

Arthroscopy of the Upper Extremity

2

Arthroscopic Treatment of Recurrent Anterior Glenohumeral Instability

Michael Hantes and Alexandros Tsarouhas
Orthopaedic Department, University Hospital of Larissa
Greece

1. Introduction

The glenohumeral joint achieves the greatest mobility compared with all other joints in the human body. Due to its complex anatomy, its stability is conferred by a combination of bone, soft tissue and muscular structures. It is therefore the most commonly dislocated joint, with an overall incidence of approximately 17/100.000 per year (Kroner et al, 1989). The classification of shoulder instability is complex, depending on the cause (traumatic vs. atraumatic), degree (dislocation, subluxation, or microinstability), direction (anterior, posterior, inferior or multidirectional), and chronology (acute, chronic, or acute on chronic). Traumatic glenohumeral instability is defined as occurring after an inciting event that results in subjective or objective subluxation or dislocation that is reduced either spontaneously or by a health professional (Cadet, 2010). Atraumatic instability occurs as the sequel of generalized ligamentous laxity or repetitive motion, as in overhead throwing athletes. Inferior and multidirectional instabilities are less common than anterior and posterior ones and have been described to combine the presence of a sulcus sign or inferior subluxation of the humeral head with symptoms of pain or instability (Neer & Foster, 1980).
Anterior shoulder instability accounts for 95% of acute traumatic dislocations. Although many patients who suffer an initial shoulder dislocation never experience a second episode of instability, a significant percentage present with recurrent instability that results in morbidity and decreased functionality in respect to the demands placed on the joint during everyday, occupational and athletic activities.

2. Anatomy and biomechanics of the glenohumeral joint

Both static structures and dynamic stabilizers of the glenohumeral joint interact to produce stability. Static stabilizers include the bony anatomy, labrum, capsule, glenohumeral ligaments and rotator interval. Dynamic stabilizers include the rotator cuff, long head of the biceps, deltoid and scapular muscles. Negative pressure within the joint also contributes to stability by producing the "suction cup effect", which helps center the humeral head independently of muscular forces and is primarily important in the midrange, where the capsule and ligaments are not under tension.
The bony anatomy of the glenohumeral joint also plays a significant role in stability. The glenoid is more concave in the superoinferior than the anteroposterior direction. In addition, the articular cartilage is thicker towards the periphery of the glenoid, thus increasing the

depth of the concavity. Because the size of the glenoid is limited compared with the humeral head, even a relatively small bone loss may reduce considerably the surface area for articulation and consequently compromise stability. A bone loss that exceeds 20% of the glenoid surface is considered critical for the recurrence of instability (Burkhart & De Beer, 2000; Tauber et al, 2004).

The labrum is a fibrocartilaginous structure attached to the glenoid rim. It functions to increase the anteroposterior and superoinferior depth of the glenoid and the surface contact area for the humeral head. Specifically, it increases the concavity of the glenoid up to 9mm in the superior-inferior direction and the anteroposterior depth to 5mm (Howell et al, 1988). Labral resection reduces resistance to translation by 20% (Lippitt & Matsen, 1993). The labrum also provides an attachment site for the glenohumeral ligaments. Two types of labral attachments to the glenoid have been described. The first, around the periphery through a fibrocartilaginous transition zone, which creates mobility along the central border similar to the knee meniscus. The second is securely attached both peripherally and centrally. The anteroinferior attachment of the labrum to the glenoid is normally tight. On the contrary, the superior attachment inserts directly into the biceps tendon distal to the insertion on the supraglenoid tubercle, it is loose and anatomically variant. Isolated lesions of the superior labrum do not result in instability. However, if the biceps insertion is also destabilized, significant translation occurs (Pagnani et al, 1995).

The glenohumeral capsuloligamentous system provides a restraint to excessive translation in varying positions of the joint. In particular, the anterior band of the inferior glenohumeral ligament (AIGHL) attaches to the anteroinferior labrum and primarily resists anteroinferior translation in the abducted externally rotated shoulder position.

The rotator cuff compresses the humeral head into the glenoid throughout the range of motion. An association between undersurface rotator cuff tears and instability has been described (Jobe & Bradley, 1989). The rotator interval (RI), between the leading edge of the supraspinatus and the superior edge of the subscapularis, has also been implicated in glenohumeral instability. Closure of a large defect in the RI has been shown to decrease inferior instability. There may be an inverse relationship between the size of the RI and the superior glenohumeral ligament (SGHL) contributing to the instability (Nobuhara & Ikeda, 1987).

3. Natural history of anterior instability

The natural history of anterior shoulder instability has been studied extensively and recurrence has been correlated with a younger age at the time of first dislocation. In a large cohort of 255 patients with primary traumatic anterior dislocation, who were treated with a sling for 4 weeks, there was a 55% incidence of an additional episode of instability within 2 years of the initial traumatic dislocation. Furthermore, 66% of the patients had an episode of instability within 5 years (Robinson et al, 2006). In another study, 324 shoulders were followed for at least 10 years after primary anterior dislocation. Ninety-four percent of the patients younger than 20 years had a recurrence compared with 14% of those older than 40 years. The patients without shoulder immobilization had a 70% recurrence rate that decreased to 26% to 46% when immobilized for 1 to 3 weeks (Rowe, 1956). These findings suggest that younger patients with primary anterior dislocations have a significantly higher rate of recurrence.

The effectiveness of rehabilitation is still in debate. In a study evaluating the effect of rehabilitation, 115 patients with traumatic and atraumatic recurrent shoulder subluxation, underwent a muscle-strengthening exercise regimen (Burkhead & Rockwood, 1992). Sixteen percent of the shoulders with traumatic etiology had excellent or good results in contrast to 80% of those with atraumatic etiology. The authors highlighted the importance of identifying the etiology of instability to ascertain a successful result out of conservative treatment. In a prospective randomized clinical trial, active patients aged less than 30 years who were treated with supervised physical therapy showed recurrence rates of 17 to 96% whereas arthroscopic instability repair had failure rates between 4% and 22% (Bottoni et al, 2002). These findings indicate that young, highly active patients would benefit from early, arthroscopic repair after first-time traumatic anterior shoulder dislocation compared with conventional nonoperative treatment.

4. Type of associated pathology

A **Bankart lesion** is the commonest sequel of an anterior dislocation and the main cause of instability. It is defined as a labral complex avulsion from the scapular periosteum. It usually includes some degree of capsular stretch and injury. When the lesion involves a fracture of the antero-inferior glenoid rim in addition to the soft tissue avulsion it is referred to as **bony Bankart** (Fig 1).

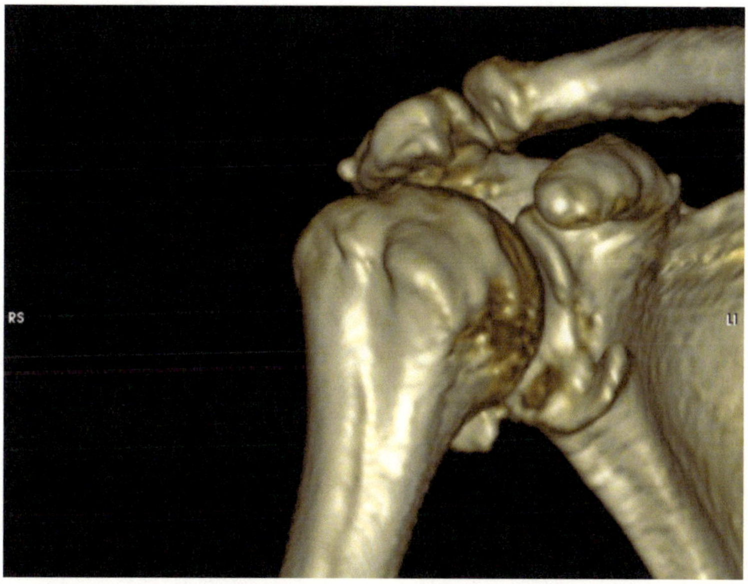

Fig. 1. A three-dimensional reconstruction CT-image demonstrating a bony-Bankart lesion.

Humeral avulsion of glenohumeral ligaments (HAGL) occurs when the capsuloligamentous structures are avulsed and torn off the humeral head and not the glenoid. An external rotation force in addition to hyperabduction commonly results in this lesion in contrast to a hyperabduction and impaction force that may produce a Bankart lesion (Matsen et al, 2006). The incidence of HAGL lesions after a traumatic dislocation has been reported at 39% (Bokor et al, 1999). A bony HAGL lesion occurs when the glenohumeral ligament is avulsed along with a bone fragment of the humeral head (Oberlander et al, 1996).

Anterior labral periosteal sleeve avulsion (ALPSA) is a soft-tissue or bony Bankart lesion that has healed in a medially displaced position on the glenoid rim and therefore, does not restrain adequately the anterior translation of the humeral head (Fig 2). In this case, the avulsed periosteum has not raptured, causing medial and inferior displacement of the labroligamentous structures (Neviaser, 1993).

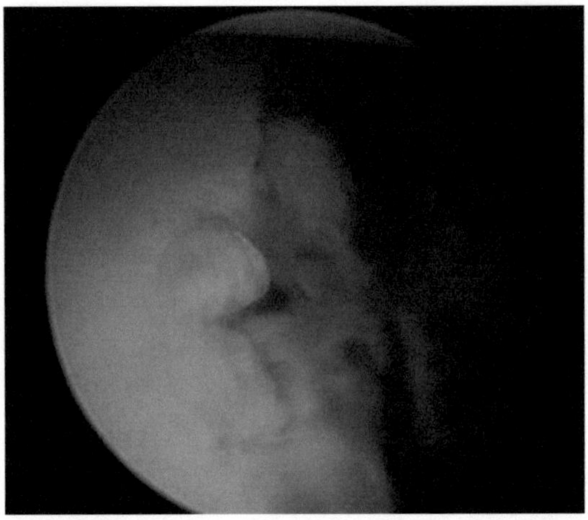

Fig. 2. An ALPSA lesion as seen from the anterosuperior arthroscopic portal. The labrum and periosteum have been avulsed and displaced medially.

A **Perthes lesion** is an incomplete avulsion without displacement of the antero-inferior labrum with a medially striped but intact periosteum.

Glenoid labral articular disruption (GLAD) lesion occurs when there is a defect in the articular cartilage of the anteroinferior glenoid in addition to the labral tear. The torn labrum I usually not fully detached from the glenoid and therefore, the predominant symptom is this case is not instability but pain.

A **Hill-Sachs lesion** is an impression fracture at the posterosuperior aspect of the humeral head that results from its impact on the glenoid rim when the humeral head dislocates anteriorly (Fig 3). They occur at 47 to 80% of anterior dislocations and in almost all cases of recurrent instability. If the posterolateral humeral head engages the anterior glenoid when abducted and externally rotated the Hill-Sachs lesion is defined as engaging (Burkhart & De Beer, 2000). The size and location of the defect mainly determine the likelihood of engagement. Although usually insignificant, in patients with glenoid bone loss a Hill-Sachs lesion can become more significant and engage the glenoid with much less force and anterior translation than those without glenoid bone loss.

A **superior labrum anterior posterior (SLAP)** lesion includes a spectrum of pathologic conditions of the superior labrum that may extend to the biceps root (Fig 4). Classification of these lesions was extended by Maffet et al to include 7 subtypes (Table 1). Type II tears are the commonest in most large series. On average, 40% of patients with Bankart lesions have an additional type II SLAP lesion (Hantes et al, 2009). SLAP lesions have been associated with glenohumeral stability. Forty-three percent of patients with SLAP lesions were found to have increased humeral head translation on examination under anesthesia (Maffet et al, 1995).

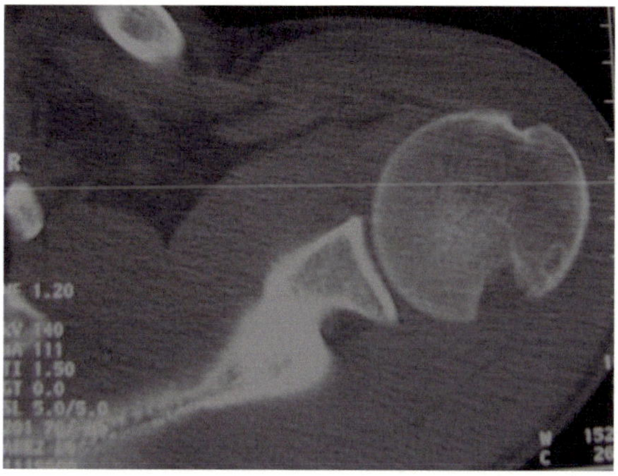

Fig. 3. A transverse plane CT image demonstrating a large Hill-Sachs lesion of the humeral head.

Type 1	Fraying of the anterosuperior labrum
Type 2	Superior labrum-biceps complex detachment from glenoid rim
Type 3	Bucket-handle tear of the labrum with an intact biceps anchor
Type 4	Bucket-handle tear of the labrum with detachment of the biceps complex
Type 5	Bankart lesion continues superiorly and includes separation of the biceps complex
Type 6	Unstable flap tear of the labrum with an unstable biceps complex insertion
Type 7	Labrum-biceps complex separation extending beneath the middle glenohumeral ligament

Table 1. Maffet classification of SLAP lesions (modified Snyder).

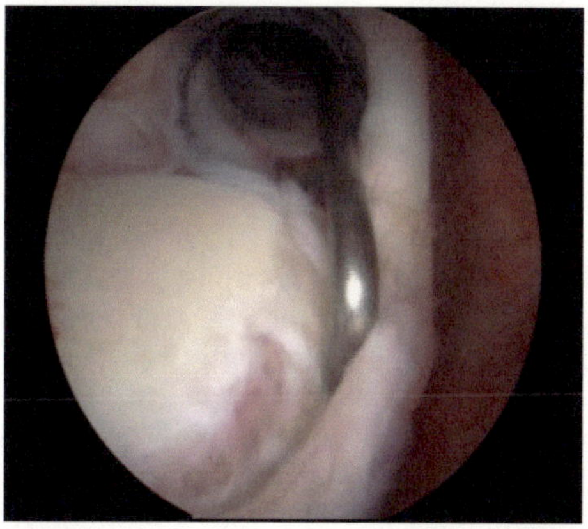

Fig. 4. A type II SLAP lesion as seen during arthroscopy.

5. Evaluation and decision-making

5.1 Patient history

The examiner should obtain a thorough history, which should offer information regarding symptoms, type and direction of instability, age and time elapsed from the initial dislocation, number of instability episodes, need for medical assistance for reduction versus self-reduction, activity level and prior treatment.

The provocative position for dislocation is indicative of the direction of instability. Patients with anterior traumatic instability generally describe the event occurring with the arm in the abducted, extended and externally rotated position. Patients who do not recall a specific dislocation event may have pathologic instability due to generalized ligamentous laxity. Pain may also be associated with instability. For example, overhead-throwing athletes with anterior instability may complain of pain due to repetitive stress on the anteroinferior capsulolabral complex.

Patients who present with a long history of recurrent instability episodes, high-energy trauma leading to dislocation, a progressive ease of symptoms or demonstrate instability in the midrange of motion should be meticulously evaluated for glenohumeral bone deficiencies. The ability to voluntarily dislocate the shoulder should be thoroughly examined because it may be attributed to psychological factors and, secondly, is generally associated with increased rates of recurrence after surgery. Similarly, patients with multiple dislocation events or whose shoulders slip out with limited force (during sleep or when reaching overhead) may have a significant glenohumeral bone defect or other pathology, such as multidirectional laxity or glenoid hypoplasia. Therefore, they would necessitate a different surgical plan. Finally, the degree of disability and loss of functionality should be thoroughly evaluated as part of decision making.

5.2 Physical examination

Both shoulders are exposed for visual inspection and comparative examination. Testing for range of motion and overall muscle strength, and neurovascular examination are performed. The opposite shoulder and other joints are examined to assess the degree of ligamentous laxity normally present in any individual. Clinical tests for glenohumeral laxity and provocative or instability tests are the hallmarks in the physical examination of an unstable shoulder.

Examination for glenohumeral laxity includes the anterior and posterior drawer, and the anterior and posterior load and shift tests, which quantitate the amount of anterior and posterior humeral head translation respectively. The Gagey hyperabduction test is used to measure the laxity of the inferior glenohumeral ligament complex. The sulcus sign also evaluates glenohumeral laxity at the inferior direction when an inferior stress is applied with the arm in adduction and both neutral and 30° external rotation. It is important for the surgeon to discern between pathologic shoulder instability and normal laxity. Instability is generally described as symptomatic laxity, which requires the patients subjectively experiencing the shoulder subluxating or recalling a frank dislocation event. On the contrary, laxity is the normal translation between the components of the glenohumeral joint to achieve full normal range of motion (Bigliani et al, 1996).

Testing for instability includes the apprehension-relocation, and the anterior release and surprise tests. The apprehension test is positive when the patient experiences pain and has a subjective feeling of the arm dislocating when the shoulder is progressively moved to abduction and external rotation. It is especially important to determine the ease with which the shoulder begins to dislocate and engage on the glenoid. If this occurs even with limited external rotation it is highly likely that there exists an engaging hill-Sachs lesion or osseous glenoid defect. Similarly, patients with engaging Hill-Sachs lesions report episodes of instability in the midrange of shoulder abduction and external rotation.

5.3 Imaging

Routine radiographic imaging of the shoulder should include a true anteroposterior, axillary and scapular-Y views. Hill-Sachs lesions can be best appreciated on the anteroposterior view in internal rotation and the notch view (Hall et al, 1959). Avulsion fractures and glenoid bone deficiencies can be visualized with the Velpeau or West point axillary views (Rokous et al, 1972).

Advanced imaging has offered an improved ability to evaluate soft tissue lesions as well as glenohumeral deficiencies following shoulder dislocation. MRI has become the gold standard in evaluating glenohumeral instability demonstrating a high accuracy for detecting labral tears using noncontrast, enhanced imaging techniques (Ng et al, 2009). MR arthrography, however, has been found to present the highest sensitivity in detecting labral pathology compared with plain MRI and CT arthrography (Chandnani et al, 1993). It also achieved the best visualization of the inferior glenohumeral ligament and labrum. Both MRI and MR arthrography can also be helpful in evaluating bone loss. However, recently volume-rendering three-dimensional CT scans have offered a highly accurate method of measuring glenoid deficiencies and Hill-Sachs lesions. The humeral head can be digitally subtracted to allow for preoperative measurement of the inferior glenoid surface and the percentage of bone missing (Fig 5). Glenoid bone defects occur along a line parallel to its long axis. The inferior two thirds of the glenoid have been described as a well-conserved circle and the amount of bone missing is assessed in respect to surface area loss of the circle. Glenoid bone loss of between 6 to 8 mm of the anteroposterior diameter corresponds to 20-25% of the surface of the inferior glenoid. In a similar fashion, the extent and morphology of a Hill-Sachs lesion can be evaluated to assess the degree of engagement.

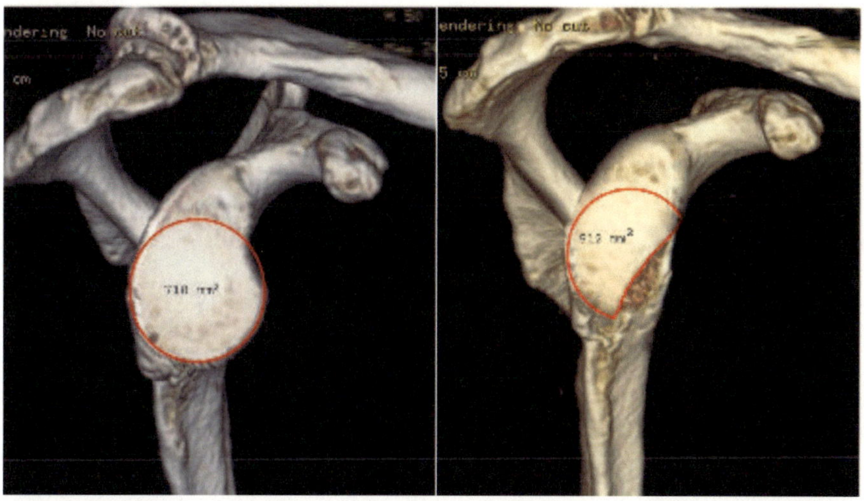

Fig. 5. Volume-rendering 3D reconstructed image of a cadaveric shoulder before (left image) and after (right image) artificially creating a glenoid bone defect. The surface area of the inferior glenoid is being measured.

6. History of the procedure

Bankart lesions, which are most commonly seen after recurrent shoulder dislocations, were first described in 1923 as "shearing of the fibrous capsule of the joint from its attachment to the fibro-cartilaginous glenoid ligament". For decades, open repair of Bankart lesions was considered the gold standard, with success rates reaching up to 97% (Rowe et al, 1978).

Arthroscopic techniques for the repair of these lesions were not introduced until 1982, when Johnson first described the arthroscopic use of staples as a modification of the open procedure (Johnson, 1980). However, this technique produced unacceptably high rates of recurrence along with hardware loosening or migration, which subsequently limited its use. Transosseous sutures for arthroscopic Bankart repair were introduced in 1987 (Morgan & Bodenstab, 1987). The sutures were passed through the scapular neck, exited posteriorly and were tied over the posterior fascia. Although excellent results were reported originally, they were not confirmed by follow-up studies. Disadvantages of this technique included the need for knot tying over the posterior fascia and the risk of iatrogenic injury to the suprascapular nerve. Removable arthroscopic rivets and absorbable cannulated bio-tacks have also been used with promising results but without gaining wide popularity.

Suture anchors present the latest technological advance in arthroscopic shoulder instability repair. They were first introduced in 1993 (Wolf, 1993). The advantages of their use include multiple points of fixation, no posterior glenoid penetration and increased pullout strength, which in the case of later-generation suture anchors is comparable to transosseous suture fixation. Suture anchors traditionally used for labral repairs are either push-in or screw-in anchors.

Each anchor commercially available is unique with regard to its pull-out strength, type of suture, retrievability, bioabsorbability, insertion technique and cost. The ideal characteristics include strength and sturdiness at the time of insertion, fixation strength and safe biologic replacement of the glenoid as the anchor resorbs. Various types of suture anchors are currently available, including metal, bioabsorbable, and bioinert. Metallic anchors have raised concerns of migration or potentially complicating revision surgery. Absorbable anchors were developed later, but concerns remain regarding bone giant cell reaction during the dissolving process. An additional concern is raised by the friction of the sliding knots, which may increase the temperature adjacent to the eyelet of most anchors currently available, and consequently compromise fixation.

7. Arthroscopic or open treatment?

Recent advances in suture technology and instrumentation and increasing surgeon experience have broadened the application of all-arthroscopic shoulder stabilization techniques. Open surgical procedures were thought to restrict external rotation and lead to secondary osteoarthritis. Additional disadvantages included wide surgical dissection and scarring. On the contrary, arthroscopic procedures were associated with reduced post-operative pain, earlier rehabilitation and less restriction of movement (Green & Christensen, 1993). Shoulder arthroscopy also provides improved articular visualization intra-operatively and allows for the preservation of the subscapularis.

Although initial results from comparison studies between arthroscopic and open procedures indicated significantly higher rates of recurrence (13%-70% compared with

0%-30% respectively), improvements in patient selection and operative technique have steadily decreased recurrence rates to match that of open procedures (Geiger et al, 1997; Roberts et al, 1999; Fabbriciani et al, 2004). In a systematic meta-analysis, which included 62 studies and 3044 arthroscopic operations, no difference was found in failure rates between open and arthroscopic treatment of anterior shoulder instability with suture anchors or bio-absorbable tacks. On the contrary, there was a higher rate of failure compared with open techniques when staples or transglenoid sutures were used arthroscopically (Hobby et al, 2007).

However, data from prospective randomized trials are still limited. Fabbriciani et al found no difference between open and arthroscopic repair of isolated Bankart lesions in a group of 60 patients at 2-year follow-up (Fabbriciani et al, 2004). Similarly, Bottoni et al found no differences in functional scores and recurrence rates between open and arthroscopic techniques for isolated anterior instability repair. However, a trend was established towards improved external rotation and forward flexion as well as significantly reduced operative time in the group of arthroscopic repair. The authors concluded that the latter was equivalent to the open surgical technique for anterior shoulder instability repair (Bottoni et al, 2006).

8. Suture anchor surgical technique for anterior shoulder instability repair

8.1 Examination under anaesthesia

A meticulous examination under anaesthesia should be performed in all cases before arthroscopy. A sensitivity of 100% and specificity of 93% have been found for this examination as confirmed by the actual arthroscopic findings (Cofield et al, 1993). The examination should be performed either in the supine or beach chair positions. Passive range of motion is recorded first with the arm at the side and 90° of abduction. With the arm abducted at 90°, posterior and anterior forces are applied to provoke translation of the humeral head in relation to the glenoid. A sulcus sign is tested in adduction and external rotation, and also at 45° abduction that tightens the inferior capsule. Persistent sulcus sign in both positions is abnormal and indicative of rotator interval pathology.

8.2 Patient positioning

The patient can be positioned in either the lateral decubitus or beach chair positions, which is mainly based on surgeon preference. The beach chair position affords several advantages including the ease to address concomitant rotator cuff pathology and the ability to convert to open surgery if necessary. However, it is often easier to address the pathology at the anteroinferior capsulolabral complex with the patient in the lateral decubitus position, because it provides a wider distension of the glenohumeral joint (Fig 6). The arm is usually placed at 45° abduction and traction is applied both in the axial and lateral directions. One of the disadvantages of this patient setup is the difficulty to achieve rotational control during the repair. For example, subscapularis repair and rotator interval closure are best performed in 30° to 45° of external rotation, which cannot be easily done at the lateral position.

8.3 Instrumentation

Basic equipment for shoulder arthroscopy includes a tower containing a video monitor, control box, light source, shaver power and electrocautery source, and irrigation pump. A

30-degree arthroscope is usually adequate for most arthroscopic procedures in the shoulder. Fluid pressure within the joint should be kept around 30mmHg and may increase up to 70mmHg for viewing the subacromial space. Maintaining a systolic arterial pressure below 100mmHg improves visualization. Increased fluid pressure or flow may cause extravasation of fluid into the surrounding soft tissue, distort the anatomy intra-operatively and increase morbidity postoperatively.

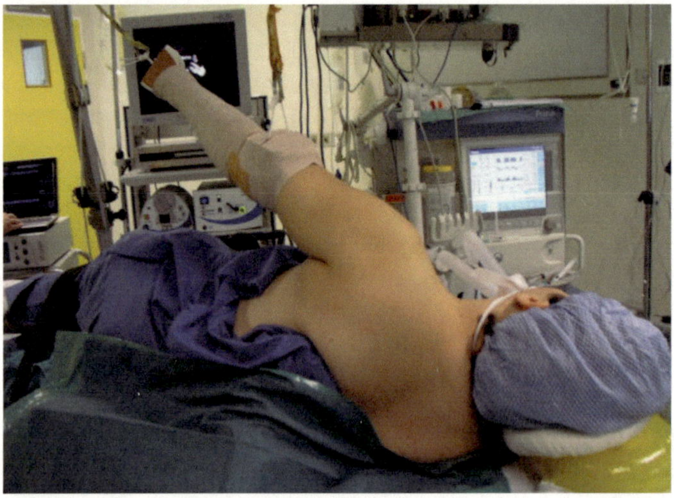

Fig. 6. Lateral decubitus setup for arthroscopic instability repair. Axial and lateral traction is applied with the arm at approximately 45° abduction.

8.4 Arthroscopic portals

Initially, a standard posterior portal is used for diagnostic arthroscopy. It can be created in line with the lateral edge of the acromion and 1cm inferior to its posterior tip to have an improved trajectory in relation to the glenoid. This portal is used for diagnostic glenohumeral arthroscopy and to localize the pathology to be addressed. An anterior-superior portal is then created with an inside-out or outside-in technique between the biceps tendon and superior edge of the subscapularis. This portal is used for mobilization of the capsulolabral complex and for subsequent suture management. It is always advisable to assess the intra-articular pathology through the anterior-superior portal as well, to better evaluate the extent of labral tear posteriorly or glenoid bone loss and avoid missing a possible ALPSA lesion. A second anterior-inferior portal is placed just above the superior edge of the subscapularis to allow for inferior placement of suture anchors on the lower aspect of the glenoid neck. Both anterior portals are created within the rotator interval and there should ideally be enough skin bridge between them (2-3cm) to allow for easier handling of arthroscopic instruments (Fig 7). Alternative portals have been described, such as a transubscapularis portal described by Davidson and Tibone or a 7-o-clock posteroinferior portal for accessing the most inferior aspect of the glenoid.

Working cannulas are inserted into the two working portals to facilitate instrumentation handling. A wider (8mm) cannula is preferable for the anterior-inferior portal to allow for curved suture hooks, while a 5.5mm cannula is adequate for the superior portal for grasping instruments to be inserted.

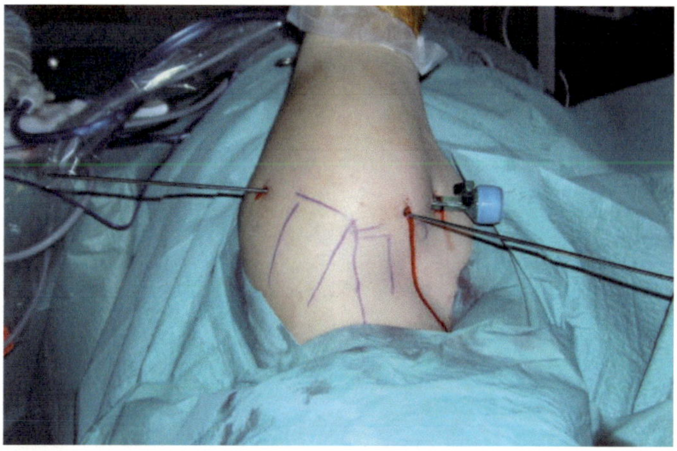

Fig. 7. Typical posterior, anterior-superior and anterior-inferior portals for arthroscopic anterior instability repair. A working cannula is inserted in the anterior-inferior and Wissinger rods in the remaining two portals.

8.5 Glenoid and labrum preparation

Assessment of the mobility of the capsuloligamentous complex is crucial to determine if the soft tissues have been displaced or are scarred in a medial position on the neck of the glenoid. A combination of probes, rasps, motorized shavers and periosteal elevators are used to mobilize the medially displaced soft tissues from the glenoid neck. Care must be taken not to debride normal tissue needed for the repair. During this step, the subscapularis muscle must be visualized underneath the mobilized labral tissue. It is recommended to release tissue inferiorly to the 6 o'clock position on the glenoid face for optimal mobilization. Attention is then turned towards the glenoid. An abrader or rasp is used to decorticate the glenoid edge while preserving the bone stock. It is important to ensure that the soft tissue remnants have been removed and there is a bleeding bed of bone at the repair site to enhance healing.

8.6 Suture anchor placement

A hole is created along the anterior and anteroinferior articular margin and the anchors are inserted below the articular surface. Accurate positioning of the anchors is critical to restore the depth of the glenoid. Ideally, the anchors are placed at 45° angle relative to the glenoid surface, perpendicular to the superior-inferior axis, and 2 to 3 mm inside the anterior glenoid rim (Fig 8). Eight to 10 mm intervals between the anchor holes are considered to limit the stress risers for more secure fixation (Abrams, 2007).

Glenoid anchors are commonly smaller than those used in rotator cuff repair because bone quality is usually better. Our current preference in our department is 2.8mm, absorbable, screw-in anchors loaded with permanent, reinforced braided sutures.

The number and positioning of suture anchors used across the glenoid rim is still controversial. A standard arthroscopic Bankart repair typically requires three anchors. Others however have suggested the routine use of four anchors, because a three-anchor configuration was associated with increased failure rates (Boileau et al, 2006). Typically, the anchors are placed below the 3 o'clock position beginning inferiorly and then progressing superiorly. In general, it is acceptable to insert as many anchors as needed to achieve an adequate restoration of the capsulolabral restraint to anterior humeral head translation.

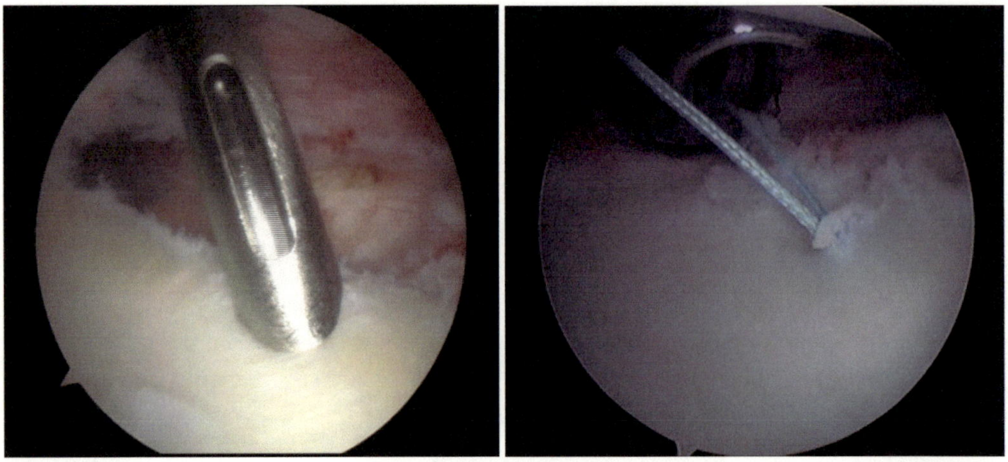

Fig. 8. Correct positioning of the suture anchor drill guide relative to the glenoid (left). The suture anchor has been inserted below the articular cartilage (right) with one arm facing the detached labrum.

Suture management is a challenge for arthroscopists performing reconstructive surgery. The anchors should be properly oriented to prevent unnecessary twists in the suture arms. Single- or double-loaded anchors may be used and should be inserted so that a single arm of the suture is facing the anticipated repair. A soft-tissue penetration device (suture passer or suture hook) is used to facilitate suture passage. We prefer to use a curved Spectrum suture hook (ConMed Linvatec, Largo, FL) and perform two separate passes though the capsule and then under the detached labrum towards the glenoid margin. A suture shuttle or a no1 monofilament suture is advanced through the hook and retrieved through the other working portal. The arm of the braided suture is passed through the eyelet of the shuttle or tied at the end of the monofilament suture and then pulled backwards to incorporate the piece of labrum and capsule (Fig 9). Sliding knots are then preformed and tied using a knot pusher and a knot cutter. The capsulolabral tissue is seen re-approximating the glenoid rim (Fig 10).

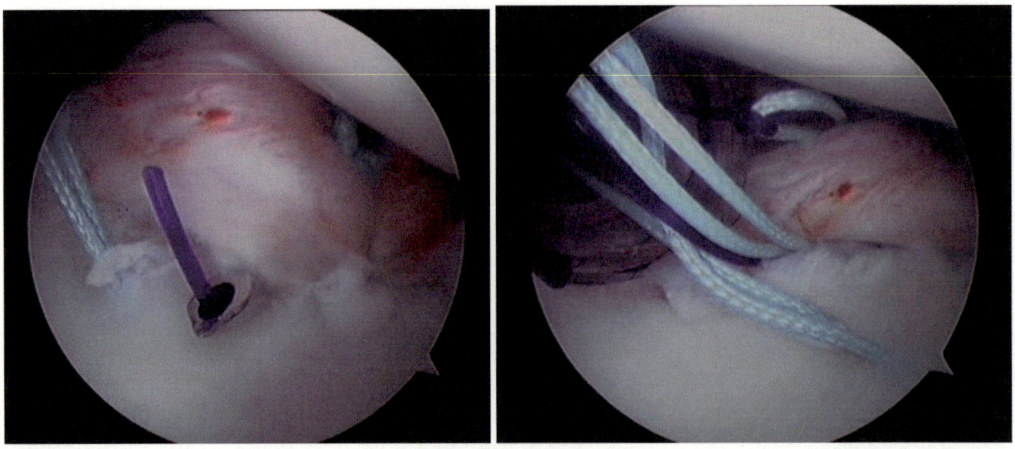

Fig. 9. Using a Spectrum suture hook, a PDS suture is passed (left) and tied (right) to the arm of the braided suture.

Capsular plication is an important aspect of correcting plastic deformation of the capsule. Sutures can be passed using suture hooks and shuttles along the posterior inferior labrum, anterior inferior pouch, and mid anterior capsule to reinforce the capsular thickness in vulnerable areas. These sutures can close defects, reinforce capsule thickness, and obliterate a pouch that developed as a result of capsular stretching. The capsule can be plicated either directly to the labrum or to itself.

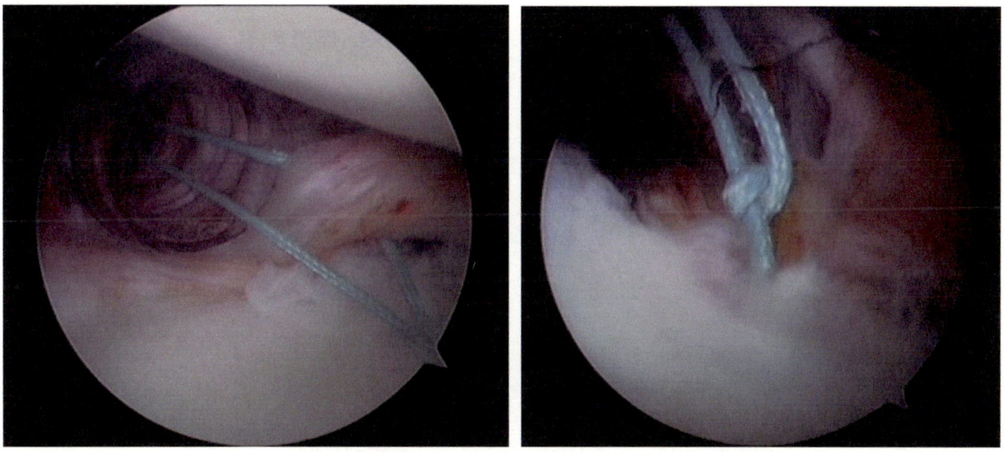

Fig. 10. The arm of the braided suture has been passed through the labrum (left) and a sliding knot is being performed.

Rotator interval closure is advisable when residual inferior translation is evident during the examination under anaesthesia or after Bankart repair. Typical Bankart repair does not require RI closure but may benefit from it. One or two sutures are passed from the middle glenohumeral ligament to the capsule anterior to the biceps tendon and tied. Consequently, the sides of this triangular interval are approximated.

Associated SLAP tears are addressed simultaneously. Typical treatment of these lesions (type II and above) involves the placement of one or two suture anchors to reattach the superior labrum and biceps root to the glenoid rim. An accessory anterior portal is commonly created lateral to the biceps tendon within the rotator interval to provide the optimal approach angle for anchor insertion (Hantes et al. 2009). Alternatively, a trans-rotator cuff portal can be used. When the lesion extends to the posterior labrum a posterolateral acromial (Wilmington) portal is created 1cm anterior and 1cm lateral to the posterolateral edge of the acromion. After debridement of the superior glenoid and labrum, suture anchors are properly placed at the superior margin of the articular cartilage and sutures are tied as described above to restore all avulsed structures.

After all suture anchors are placed, the repair is evaluated from both the posterior and anterior portals (Fig 11). It is a good practice to remove the arm and evaluate the humeral head position and rotation, to best understand the tensioning effect of the repair. The head should appear well centered on the glenoid and any Hill-Sachs lesion should rotate posteriorly. Ideally, this lesion will not come in contact with the articular surface in any position of the shoulder.

8.7 Postoperative management and rehabilitation

Following surgery, the arm is placed in a sling in slight abduction and reduced internal rotation. Passive external rotation is restricted to 0 degrees. Active flexion and extension of the elbow is encouraged. After 3 weeks, the sling is discontinued, forward flexion is increased and external rotation is allowed to 30 degrees. Isotonic rotator cuff and scapular muscles strengthening is initiated after the 6th week. The return to unrestricted activity and full contact sports is determined on an individual basis and usually is not anticipated until 4 to 6 months.

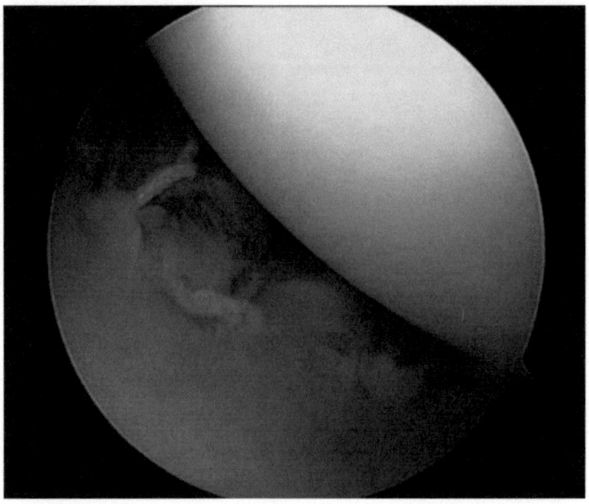

Fig. 11. Final view of the re-approximated capsulolabral complex.

8.8 Complications

The most common complication is the recurrence of instability, which may be attributed to diagnostic and technical errors, or to additional trauma. Misdiagnosis may occur when a significant glenohumeral bone loss is not properly evaluated or a multidirectional component escapes diagnosis. Inadequate capsular tensioning and restoration of the glenoid concavity are the commonest technical errors met. It is therefore crucial to reassess range of motion and humeral head alignment after the repair. In athletes, the risk of recurrence increases with return to sports, since the demands placed on the shoulder are analogous to those that caused the initial injury.

Hardware failure commonly involves misplacement of the suture anchors. Absorbable implants have reduced the occurrence of late anchor displacement and complications during revision surgery. However proper anchor placement is mandatory and a careful evaluation should be performed whenever symptoms appear. Osteopenia along the glenoid rim has been correlated with absorbable anchors along with disuse during the postoperative period.

Nerve injury is not common. Structures at risk, however, include the axillary nerve that lies 1-1.5 cm below the inferior glenohumeral capsule and the musculocutaneous nerve situated 5-8 cm below the coracoid. Manipulation at the extremes of the range of motion should be avoided.

A recent concern after arthroscopic instability repair has been chondrolysis (Levine et al, 2005). Although rare, it is devastating because it often requires additional surgery and potentially causes permanent deficits. Intra-articular use of thermal devices, articular pain pumps, and local anesthetics within the articular space, as well as increased articular pressure during surgery have been implicated in the pathogenesis of chondrolysis.

9. Contraindications to arthroscopic instability repair

Numerous pathologic conditions have been suggested as contraindications to arthroscopic shoulder instability repair, including capsular attenuation, humeral avulsion of the glenohumeral ligament (HAGL) lesions, failure of previous stabilization, and instability in a collision athlete. However, sizeable glenohumeral bone defects represent the most important contraindication to arthroscopic shoulder stabilization.

9.1 Glenohumeral bone defects

Studies have shown that compression fractures of the posterior superior humeral head (Hill-Sachs lesion) can occur in 32% to 51% of initial anterior dislocations, while anteroinferior glenoid deficiency in 22% of primary dislocations (Rowe et al, 1978; Rowe et al, 1984). The incidence of both glenoid and humeral head bone defects approaches 100% in cases of chronic anterior shoulder instability (Burkhart and De Beer 2000).

A critical decision on shoulder stabilization today focuses on the degree of bone loss and whether soft tissue reconstruction can be successful. Diagnostic pearls for clinical and imaging evaluation of glenohumeral bone defects have been discussed above. Bone defects between 20% and 30% of the inferior glenoid have shown a high recurrence rate after arthroscopic Bankart repair. However, the size and orientation of glenoid and humeral head defects can be extremely variable, making preoperative assessment and decision making difficult. It is currently suggested that patient with glenoid bone deficiency exceeding 20 to 25% of the articular surface should better be treated with a bone-substituting procedure (Provencher et al, 2010).

Bone grafting procedures, such as iliac bone-block or distal tibia transfer, glenoid allograft augmentation and the Bristow procedure have been advocated to restore osseous glenoid defects and shoulder stability. The Latarjet procedure was introduced in 1954. It delineates an osteotomy of the coracoid just proximal to its angle, which comprises the horizontal part of the coracoid and provides a 2 to 3cm bone segment. This is then transferred along with the attached conjoined tendon and the released coracoacromial ligament through a horizontal division of the subscapularis tendon and fixed at the antero-inferior glenoid, preferably with two screws (Fig 12).

The Latarjet procedure has shown excellent and reliable results both in biomechanical testing and the clinical setting. Quantitative Computed Tomography (qCT) has shown this technique to adequately restore a mean defect of up to 28% the intact inferior glenoid (Hantes et al, 2010). Compared with a structural bone graft, it resulted in significantly less anterior and anteroinferior translation at 60° of abduction. Satisfactory clinical results have also been reported with shoulder function ranging from good to excellent with recurrence rates between 0% and 7%. Complications include bony nonunion, graft displacement, progressive impingement and hardware loosening or migration. Improper graft placement, due to lack of experience or surgical exposure, may predispose to recurrent dislocation (when placed too medially or high) or osteoarthritis (too laterally).

Routinely, the Latarjet procedure is performed through a standard deltopectoral approach. However, an all-arthroscopic alternative has been advocated recently as a consequence of the success of the open procedure and the advancements in arthroscopic instrumentation and techniques. This procedure offers the potential advantages of more accurate graft placement, management of associated joint pathology, such as bidirectional shoulder instability, ease of technique conversion, and faster rehabilitation with decreased joint stiffness and better cosmetic result (Lafosse et al, 2010). Although there is inevitably a steep learning curve, excellent results with good graft positioning and minimal complications have also been reported with arthroscopic Latarjet repair.

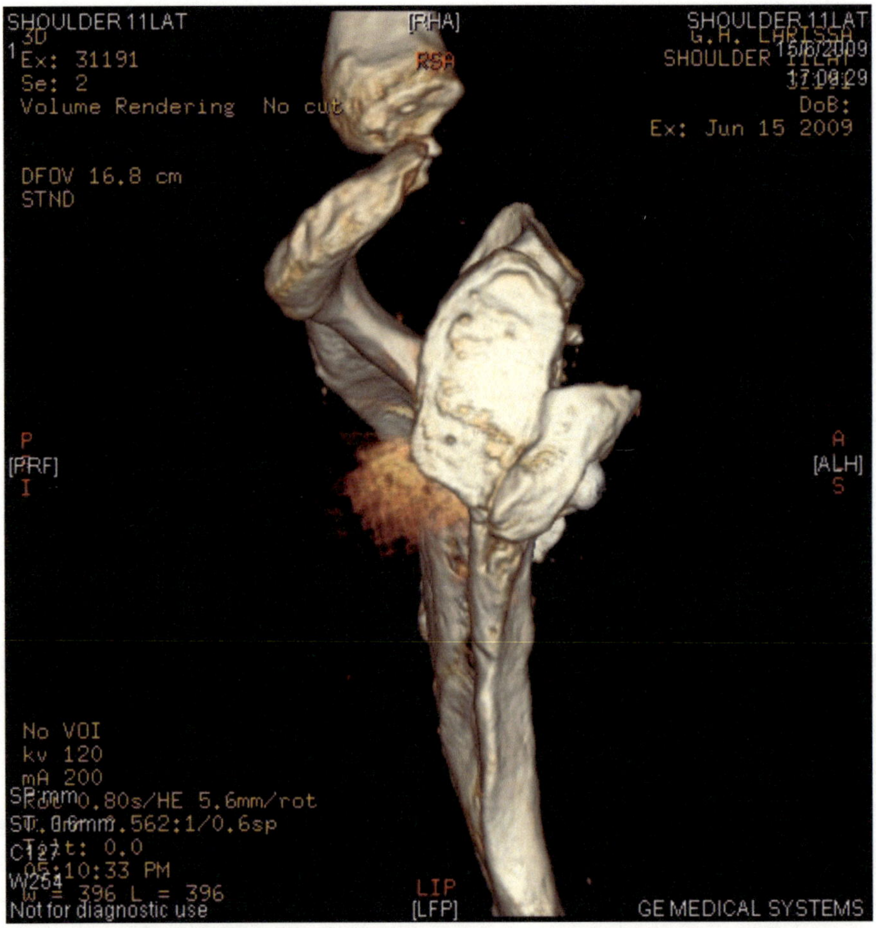

Fig. 12. The Latarjet procedure. Notice how the coracoid process graft supplements the articular surface of the original "inverted pear" glenoid to increase its anteroposterior diameter.

Significant humeral Hill-Sachs lesions also raise concerns on the success of soft-tissue instability repairs. There is a debate on what size humeral head defects require treatment with bony reconstruction. Some authors suggest that defects involving over 12.5% of the humeral head diameter should raise concerns as potentially significant lesions (Kropf et al, 2007). Open allograft humeral head or autograft transfer reconstructions are indicated for the treatment of engaging Hill-Sachs lesions through deltopectoral or mini-open approaches. The Latarjet procedure has also been used successfully in such cases. Recently, an arthroscopic "remplissage" technique was introduced consisting of an arthroscopic capsulotenodesis of the posterior capsule and infraspinatus tendon to fill the Hill-Sachs lesion (Purchase et al, 2008). In light of such progress, glenohumeral bone loss should no longer be considered an absolute contraindication for arthroscopic instability repair.

10. Conclusions

Arthroscopic treatment of shoulder instability has evolved considerably over the past decades. A detailed patient history and thorough physical examination are still considered the milestones for successful treatment planning. Advanced MRI imaging has offered a more accurate diagnosis and improved understanding of the pathology to be addressed. Presently, suture anchor stabilization is the operation that best duplicates the time-tested open procedure. Patient selection criteria, improved surgical techniques and implants available have contributed to the enhancement of clinical and functional outcomes to the point that arthroscopic treatment is considered nowadays the standard of care. However, arthroscopic techniques are demanding and there is a steep learning curve. Bone loss issues, including Hill-Sachs and glenoid rim lesions, remain a concern and a challenge for arthroscopists to manage.

11. References

Abrams, J. S. (2007). Role of arthroscopy in treating anterior instability of the athlete's shoulder. *Sports Med Arthrosc* 15(4): 230-238.

Bigliani, L. U., R. Kelkar, et al. (1996). Glenohumeral stability. Biomechanical properties of passive and active stabilizers. *Clin Orthop Relat Res*(330): 13-30.

Boileau, P., M. Villalba, et al. (2006). Risk factors for recurrence of shoulder instability after arthroscopic Bankart repair. *J Bone Joint Surg Am* 88(8): 1755-1763.

Bokor, D. J., V. B. Conboy, et al. (1999). Anterior instability of the glenohumeral joint with humeral avulsion of the glenohumeral ligament. A review of 41 cases. *J Bone Joint Surg Br* 81(1): 93-96.

Bottoni, C. R., E. L. Smith, et al. (2006). Arthroscopic versus open shoulder stabilization for recurrent anterior instability: a prospective randomized clinical trial. *Am J Sports Med* 34(11): 1730-1737.

Bottoni, C. R., J. H. Wilckens, et al. (2002). A prospective, randomized evaluation of arthroscopic stabilization versus nonoperative treatment in patients with acute, traumatic, first-time shoulder dislocations. *Am J Sports Med* 30(4): 576-580.

Burkhart, S. S. and J. F. De Beer (2000). Traumatic glenohumeral bone defects and their relationship to failure of arthroscopic Bankart repairs: significance of the inverted-pear glenoid and the humeral engaging Hill-Sachs lesion. *Arthroscopy* 16(7): 677-694.

Burkhead, W. Z., Jr. and C. A. Rockwood, Jr. (1992). Treatment of instability of the shoulder with an exercise program. *J Bone Joint Surg Am* 74(6): 890-896.

Cadet, E. R. (2010). Evaluation of glenohumeral instability. *Orthop Clin North Am* 41(3): 287-295.

Chandnani, V. P., T. D. Yeager, et al. (1993). Glenoid labral tears: prospective evaluation with MRI imaging, MR arthrography, and CT arthrography. *AJR Am J Roentgenol* 161(6): 1229-1235.

Cofield, R. H., J. P. Nessler, et al. (1993). Diagnosis of shoulder instability by examination under anesthesia. *Clin Orthop Relat Res,* (291): 45-53.

Fabbriciani, C., G. Milano, et al. (2004). Arthroscopic versus open treatment of Bankart lesion of the shoulder: a prospective randomized study. *Arthroscopy* 20(5): 456-462.

Geiger, D. F., J. A. Hurley, et al. (1997). Results of arthroscopic versus open Bankart suture repair." *Clin Orthop Relat Res (*337): 111-117.

Green, M. R. and K. P. Christensen (1993). Arthroscopic versus open Bankart procedures: a comparison of early morbidity and complications. *Arthroscopy* 9(4): 371-374.

Hall, R. H., F. Isaac, et al. (1959). Dislocations of the shoulder with special reference to accompanying small fractures. *J Bone Joint Surg Am* 41-A(3): 489-494.

Hantes, M. E., A. Venouziou, et al. (2010). Repair of an anteroinferior glenoid defect by the latarjet procedure: quantitative assessment of the repair by computed tomography. *Arthroscopy* 26(8): 1021-1026.

Hantes, M. E., A. I. Venouziou, et al. (2009). Arthroscopic repair for chronic anterior shoulder instability: a comparative study between patients with Bankart lesions and patients with combined Bankart and superior labral anterior posterior lesions. *Am J Sports Med* 37(6): 1093-1098.

Hobby, J., D. Griffin, et al. (2007). Is arthroscopic surgery for stabilisation of chronic shoulder instability as effective as open surgery? A systematic review and meta-analysis of 62 studies including 3044 arthroscopic operations. *J Bone Joint Surg Br* 89(9): 1188-1196.

Howell, S. M., B. J. Galinat, et al. (1988). Normal and abnormal mechanics of the glenohumeral joint in the horizontal plane. *J Bone Joint Surg Am* 70(2): 227-232.

Jobe, F. W. and J. P. Bradley (1989). The diagnosis and nonoperative treatment of shoulder injuries in athletes. *Clin Sports Med* 8(3): 419-438.

Johnson, L. L. (1980). Arthroscopy of the shoulder. *Orthop Clin North Am* 11(2): 197-204.

Kroner, K., T. Lind, et al. (1989). The epidemiology of shoulder dislocations. *Arch Orthop Trauma Surg* 108(5): 288-290.

Kropf, E. J., F. P. Tjoumakaris, et al. (2007). Arthroscopic shoulder stabilization: is there ever a need to open? *Arthroscopy* 23(7): 779-784.

Lafosse, L., S. Boyle, et al. (2010). Arthroscopic latarjet procedure. *Orthop Clin North Am* 41(3): 393-405.

Levine, W. N., A. M. Clark, Jr., et al. (2005). Chondrolysis following arthroscopic thermal capsulorrhaphy to treat shoulder instability. A report of two cases. *J Bone Joint Surg Am* 87(3): 616-621.

Lippitt, S. and F. Matsen (1993). Mechanisms of glenohumeral joint stability. *Clin Orthop Relat Res* (291): 20-28.

Maffet, M. W., G. M. Gartsman, et al. (1995). Superior labrum-biceps tendon complex lesions of the shoulder. *Am J Sports Med* 23(1): 93-98.

Matsen, F. A., 3rd, C. Chebli, et al. (2006). Principles for the evaluation and management of shoulder instability. *J Bone Joint Surg Am* 88(3): 648-659.

Morgan, C. D. and A. B. Bodenstab (1987). Arthroscopic Bankart suture repair: technique and early results. *Arthroscopy* 3(2): 111-122.

Neer, C. S., 2nd and C. R. Foster (1980). Inferior capsular shift for involuntary inferior and multidirectional instability of the shoulder. A preliminary report. *J Bone Joint Surg Am* 62(6): 897-908.

Neviaser, T. J. (1993). The anterior labroligamentous periosteal sleeve avulsion lesion: a cause of anterior instability of the shoulder. *Arthroscopy* 9(1): 17-21.

Ng, A. W., C. M. Chu, et al. (2009). Assessment of capsular laxity in patients with recurrent anterior shoulder dislocation using MRI. *AJR Am J Roentgenol* 192(6): 1690-1695.

Nobuhara, K. and H. Ikeda (1987). Rotator interval lesion. *Clin Orthop Relat Res* (223): 44-50.

Oberlander, M. A., B. E. Morgan, et al. (1996). The BHAGL lesion: a new variant of anterior shoulder instability. *Arthroscopy* 12(5): 627-633.

Pagnani, M. J., X. H. Deng, et al. (1995). Effect of lesions of the superior portion of the glenoid labrum on glenohumeral translation. *J Bone Joint Surg Am* 77(7): 1003-1010.

Provencher, M. T., S. Bhatia, et al. (2010). Recurrent shoulder instability: current concepts for evaluation and management of glenoid bone loss. *J Bone Joint Surg Am* 92 Suppl 2: 133-151.

Purchase, R. J., E. M. Wolf, et al. (2008). Hill-sachs "remplissage": an arthroscopic solution for the engaging hill-sachs lesion. *Arthroscopy* 24(6): 723-726.

Roberts, S. N., D. E. Taylor, et al. (1999). Open and arthroscopic techniques for the treatment of traumatic anterior shoulder instability in Australian rules football players. *J Shoulder Elbow Surg* 8(5): 403-409.

Robinson, C. M., J. Howes, et al. (2006). Functional outcome and risk of recurrent instability after primary traumatic anterior shoulder dislocation in young patients. *J Bone Joint Surg Am* 88(11): 2326-2336.

Rokous, J. R., J. A. Feagin, et al. (1972). Modified axillary roentgenogram. A useful adjunct in the diagnosis of recurrent instability of the shoulder. *Clin Orthop Relat Res* 82: 84-86.

Rowe, C. R. (1956). Prognosis in dislocations of the shoulder. *J Bone Joint Surg Am* 38-A(5): 957-977.

Rowe, C. R., D. Patel, et al. (1978). The Bankart procedure: a long-term end-result study. *J Bone Joint Surg Am* 60(1): 1-16.

Rowe, C. R., B. Zarins, et al. (1984). Recurrent anterior dislocation of the shoulder after surgical repair. Apparent causes of failure and treatment. *J Bone Joint Surg Am* 66(2): 159-168.

Tauber, M., H. Resch, et al. (2004). Reasons for failure after surgical repair of anterior shoulder instability. *J Shoulder Elbow Surg* 13(3): 279-285.

Wolf, E. M. (1993). Arthroscopic capsulolabral repair using suture anchors. *Orthop Clin North Am* 24(1): 59-69.

3

Anesthesia for Arthroscopic Shoulder Surgery

Diego Benítez and Luis M. Torres
Department of Anesthesia, University Hospital Puerta del Mar,
Cátedra del Dolor Fundación Grunenthal-Universidad de Cádiz
Spain

1. Introduction

Arthroscopic shoulder surgery is a minimally invasive technique that effectively treats certain diseases and injuries of the shoulder joint. Indeed, new lesions and surgical techniques for their treatment have also been discovered by using this approach.
Controlling post-operative pain in shoulder surgery facilitates early mobilization and fast functional recovery, allowing pain-free muscle contraction. Tissue injury due to the surgical intervention results in the release of many chemical mediators that activate and increase the excitability of nociceptors, producing intra- and post-operative hyperalgesia. Local anesthesia can be used more frequently for less aggressive surgical techniques, particularly in limb surgery, both for intra-operative and post-operative pain.
It is essential to be familiar with the anatomy of the region to be anesthetized in order to minimize the potential risks and recognize them when they occur. The upper limb is innervated by the arms of the cervical spinal nerves (C5-C8) and part of the ventral branch of T1, although anatomical variations may exist. All these sensory, motor and vegetative nerve fibers form an "anastomotic complex of fibers", known as the brachial plexus.
The block of the brachial plexus was first developed in 1884, when Halstead injected cocaine into the exposed roots of the brachial plexus (1). However, it was not until 1911 that Hirschel and Kulenkampff described the percutaneous brachial plexus block first developing the axillary technique and then, the supraclavicular route (2,3). In 1919, Mulley developed a technique aimed at preventing pneumothorax by employing interscalenic approach to the brachial plexus (4). The modern interscalenic approach was perfected by Winnie, using the transverse processes of the 6th cervical vertebra (5) as a reference for needle insertion.
Anesthetic options for shoulder arthroscopic surgery include: general anesthesia, regional anesthesia with or without sedation, and a combination of both general and regional anaesthesia. Regional anesthesia offers many advantages over general anesthesia for arthroscopic shoulder surgery. The most notable advantage is the ability to control perioperative pain by proximally blocking the brachial plexus (supraclavicular approaches). The "Preemptive" analgesia afforded by the blockade and the excellent analgesic conditions can overt the need for intraoperative opioid administration. The patients' perception of pain-free surgery represents a further advantage of this approach. Together, this facilitates earlier hospital discharge with the attendant reduction in the economic cost of the procedure (6,7).

Relaxing the shoulder muscles is essential for successful surgery. We have observed that the muscle relaxation obtained following the interscalene blockage are superior to those observed with general anesthesia, without the need for tracheal intubation and mechanical ventilation due to neuromuscular blockade. Also, there is a decrease in perioperative bleeding associated with regional blockade in shoulder surgery (8). Mechanical ventilation increases intrathoracic pressure and as a consequence, the venous pressure in the upper limbs. This increase in pressure augments venous blood loss, which can be avoided if the patient is breathing spontaneously. In addition, the sympathetic blockade produced by regional blocking, combined with the semi-recumbent position of the patient, decreases venous pressure and bleeding. Hemodynamic stability itself favors regional anesthesia, decreasing mean arterial pressure and bleeding. Moreover, supraclavicular nerve blockage techniques without the need for general anesthesia decrease the possibility of aspiration of stomach contents, making them particularly attractive for emergency surgery.
The total time required does not differ greatly between the different anesthetic techniques, despite the obvious advantages associated with particular approaches. In fact, proximal brachial plexus block, performed by an expert, requires less time than the induction of general anesthesia, especially considering the shorter recovery time associated with regional anesthesia. In addition, the associated latency period can be used to position the patient and prepare the surgical area. The availability of a room for to perform specific preparation before the patient enters the operating theatre also optimizes resources and anesthesia times. Other notable advantages of regional versus general anesthesia include decreased post-operative complications, earlier discharge from the post-operative recovery room, the need for less apparatus, fewer nursing requirements and reduced hospital readmissions (9,10). Together, these advantages make such techniques the better choice for the majority of surgical procedures of the shoulder. The development of modern neurolocalization techniques, such as the use of ultrasound with peripheral nerve blockade, has improved the efficacy and safety of blind techniques, avoiding paresthesia and nerve stimulation, enabling real-time imaging of neural structures.

2. Anatomy of the proximal nerve structures in the upper extremity

As indicated, the brachial plexus is formed by the anterior branches of spinal nerves C5-T1. The union of these fibers is highly variable among individuals and can even be asymmetrical in certain individuals, often also involving fibers C4 and T2. Nevertheless, the organization observed in up to 70% of cadavers involves 3 main trunks: the anterior branch of C5 fusing with that of C6 to form the upper primary trunk; the anterior branch of C7 forms the average primary trunk; and the anterior branch of C8 and T1 join to form the lower primary trunk.
Each of these primary trunks divides into an anterior and posterior branch. The three posterior branches unite to give rise to the posterior cord (the origin of the axillary nerve), circumflex and radial, which is the terminal portion. The anterior branches of the middle and upper primary trunks merge to form the lateral cord, which later gives rise to the musculocutaneous nerve and the lateral portion of the median nerve. The anterior branch of the inferior primary trunk gives rise to the medial cord, which will ultimately separate into the ulnar nerve, medial antebrachial cutaneous nerve and medial cutaneous nerve. The latter two, along with the intercostobrachial nerve, collect sensitivity from the medial arm. The median nerve also receives a portion of the medial cord (Figure 1)

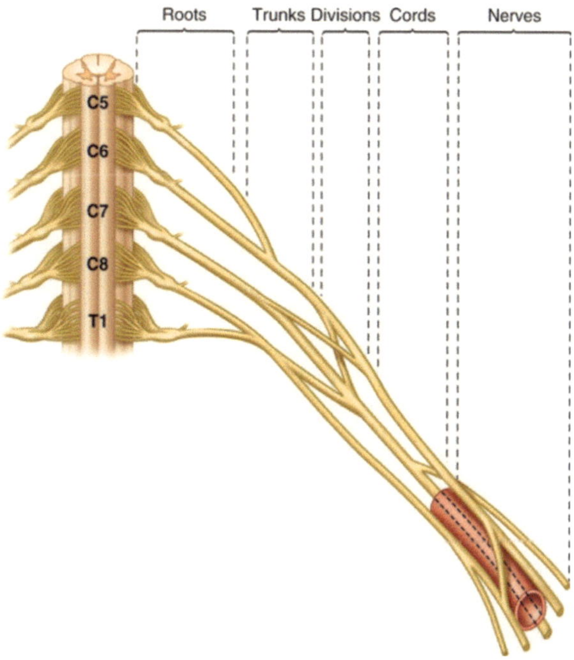

Fig. 1. Schematic representation of the structures of the left brachial plexus.

Situated at the upper surface of the spinous process of the cervical vertebra. From here they run out and down between the anterior and middle scalene muscles to reach the lateral base of the neck, close to the subclavian artery hat is above the pleural dome. They then appear within the costoclavicular axillary canal, closely associated with the vascular bundle.
In the interscalene space, the middle and upper primary trunks are more superficial than the lower trunk. The supraclavicular part of the plexus undergoes its first division in the costoclavicular space, forming a group of clustered secondary trunks lateral and superficial to the subclavian artery, and above the first rib and pleural dome. At the infraclavicular level, the plexus forms a series of bundles or cords (lateral, medial and posterior) around the axillary artery. Distally the terminal branches are individualized, forming the median, ulnar and brachial cutaneous nerves, the medial forearm and the intercostobrachial nerve in the humeral canal. The musculocutaneous nerve and the radial nerve run outside the humeral canal.

3. Preoperative study

Anesthesia visit should be used to carry out both a global study of the surgical-anesthetic risk, and to reduce the patient's anxiety before surgery. Indeed, the treatment of post-operative pain begins in this pre-operative period, with apprehension and anxiety increasing when patients are poorly informed as to the upcoming procedures. In examining the personal background of the patient, it is important to note any previous surgical interventions, particularly those in the cervical and thoracic region.
upper airway should be explored in detail, from the mouth to the base of the neck, noting and missing teeth or dentures that might make ventilation and endotracheal intubation more difficult. Observe whether the patient has a short neck or an increased cervical diameter, which determines the location of skin reference points for locking and positioning if an

ultrasound transducer is employed. It may be difficult to maintain good ventilation in obese patients and to use the neurostimulator to find the brachial plexus in the different supraclavicular approaches. The preanesthesia visit is a good time to perform this exploration. Chronic lung disease may be a relative contraindication to performing a bilateral interscalene block, since phrenic nerve block exacerbates the poor respiratory function in such patients. In such cases additional studies may be necessary, such as chest RX and basic tests of respiratory function (*e.g.*, spirometry).

We explore the contralateral arm to see determine whether the patient has a clear vein network channel for peripheral venous administration, or whether an alternative route of administration will be required. While the patient must fully informed of the technique they are to undergo, if told "a needle will be inserted into your neck" their levels anxiety are likely to rise. However, a correct explanation of the technique, starting at the pre-operative visit and continuing up to and during the procedure, along with adequate sedation, will significantly increase the patient´s satisfaction with the technique, as well as their confidence in the anesthesiologist.

A blood analysis including blood counts and basic clotting biochemistry must be performed, particularly for more invasive surgical procedures such as prosthetic glenohumeral joint or proximal humerus fractures. Arthroscopic procedures themselves do not involve bleeding. A severe impairment of clotting is an absolute contraindication for performing the regional block technique, although it can be partially permissive if taking into account the benefit/risk in those patient at the limits of normality, and particularly when ultrasound-guided block is performed by an expert. We also investigate factors or conditions that potentially increase the risk of post-operative nausea and vomiting in the patient, which may require prophylactic drugs or adaptation of the anesthetic technique.

the patient must be informed of the pain they may experience after the surgical procedure, as well as of the various analgesic strategies available. of and understand the information provided during the pre-anesthesia visit, including the possible associated complications and setbacks, and they must provide informed consent for the anesthetic techniques that may be employed.

4. General considerations during surgery

Whether in the operating theatre or in an alternative location approved to perform the peripheral nerve block, access is required to a peripheral vein in the arm contralateral to the surgery at least. Where premedication with benzodiazepines or other hypnotics is required, it is desirable to provide the patient with a supplementary source of oxygen in the form of a low flow nasal cannula or face mask (11). Shoulder As shoulder arthroscopy does not involve a large degree of fluid loss, a small venous line will suffice (a 20G needle should be adequate). However, fluid deficits due to pre-operative fasting should be calculated.

Basic patient monitoring principles should be applied, including circulatory parameters such as heart rate and non-invasive blood pressure, partial oxygen saturation, continuous electrocardiogram leads II (for better evaluation of rhythm disturbances) and V5 (for better assessment of ST segment changes and repolarization). In cases where the patient receives mechanical ventilation or spontaneous ventilation through a supraglottic airway device, FiO_2 and fractional exhaled CO_2 should be continuously monitored, along with basic ventilation parameters (tidal volume, respiratory rate, index I:E, airway pressure and PEEP if applicable). The patient´s temperature should also be controlled systematically, given the considerable loss of heat that can occur during surgery.

position of the patient during arthroscopic examination is fundamental and poor positioning will affect the surgeon's movements, dexterity and maneuverability of the instruments, and traction vector placement. The position of the patient will depend on the type of surgery, the personal preferences of the surgeon and the specific workplace in question. Correct initial placement of the patient avoids subsequent postural adjustments during surgery, which can increase both surgical and recovery times.

5. Lateral decubitus

Proposed This method was first proposed by Wiley and Older (12), whereby the patient is positioned with a lateral tilt, leaving the arm exposed. No traction should be used, and the position of flexion and adduction of the arm should allow easy penetration of the shoulder joint.

In order to obtain greater diastasis of the joint, Andrews and Carson (13) positioned the arm at about 70° of abduction and 15° of flexion, with adequate longitudinal tension, although this may lead to overstretching the neurovascular structures (Figure 1). Different drivelines can be applied to the upper limb but the weight applied to traction should under no circumstances exceed 4-6 kg. Moreover, as the drive can induce ischemic stroke, traction for more than 2 hours should be avoided. Paulos (14) reported 30% transitional neuroapraxia after shoulder arthroscopy. Before traction, the upper limb should be slightly rotated internally at the elbow to reduce the tension on glenohumeral ligaments, thereby augmenting the joint space. In preparing the operating room is important to place the anesthesia machine beside the surgical bed to provide the surgeon with sufficient room to move and operate (Table 1).

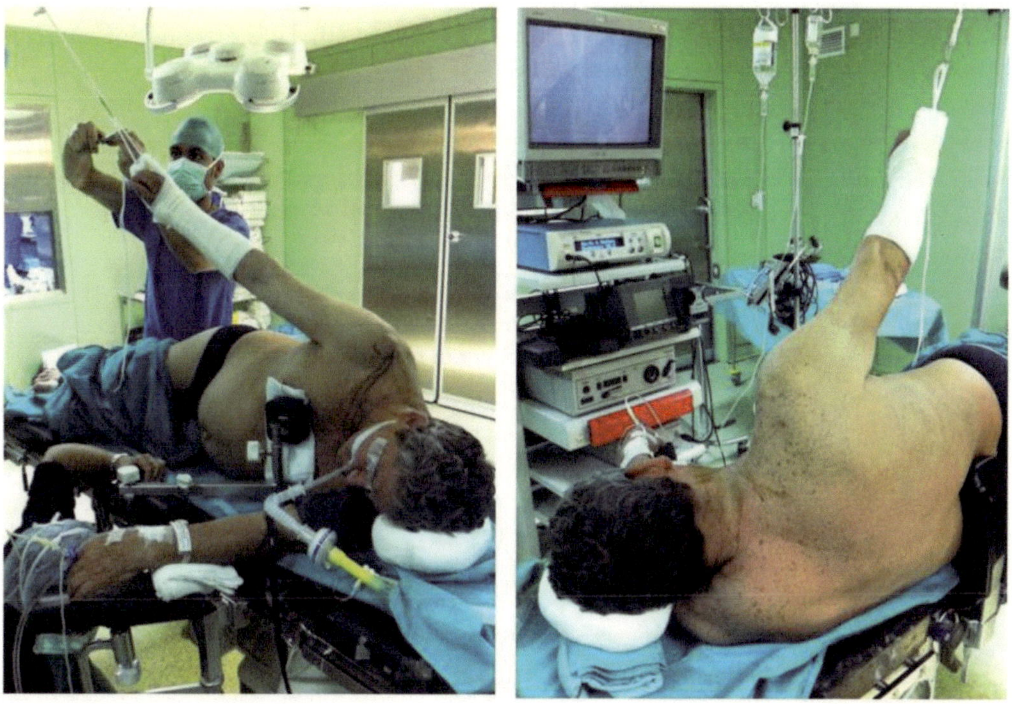

Fig. 1. Lateral decubitus position.

Lateral benefits	Disadvantages
Better view of the joint space with traction device	Difficulty of penetrating the joint due to the slope
More space for front and rear access	The conversion of arthroscopy to open surgery is uncomfortable
	Risk of excessive traction on the brachial plexus
	Poorly tolerated with only local anesthesia

Table 1. Patient position

6. Sedestatión beach chair position

Described This was described in 1988 by Skyhar, whereby the patient sits on the operating table with the help of specially designed brackets, with the trunk flexed 60-80° to the horizontal. The hemithorax on the affected side must be free in the dorsal region to situate the posterior shoulder portal. The head and neck are supported by a specific device, with the head in slight flexion and extension, avoiding extreme rotation that could have a detrimental effect by overdistending the brachial plexus (Figure 2). This position also reduces the risk of brachial plexus injuries when compared with the lateral position, and it is better tolerated with only local anesthesia (Table 2).

Advantages	Disadvantages
Better tolerated with local anesthesia	Poor display without pulling the joint and the axillary recess
Reduced patient installation time	Difficulty moving the lens if the position is not maintained
Upper limb mobility	Increased associated risk of hypotension
No need for traction	
Reduce Reduced risk of neuroapraxia	
Facilitates eventual conversion to open surgery	

Table 2. Characteristics of the Beach Chair Position

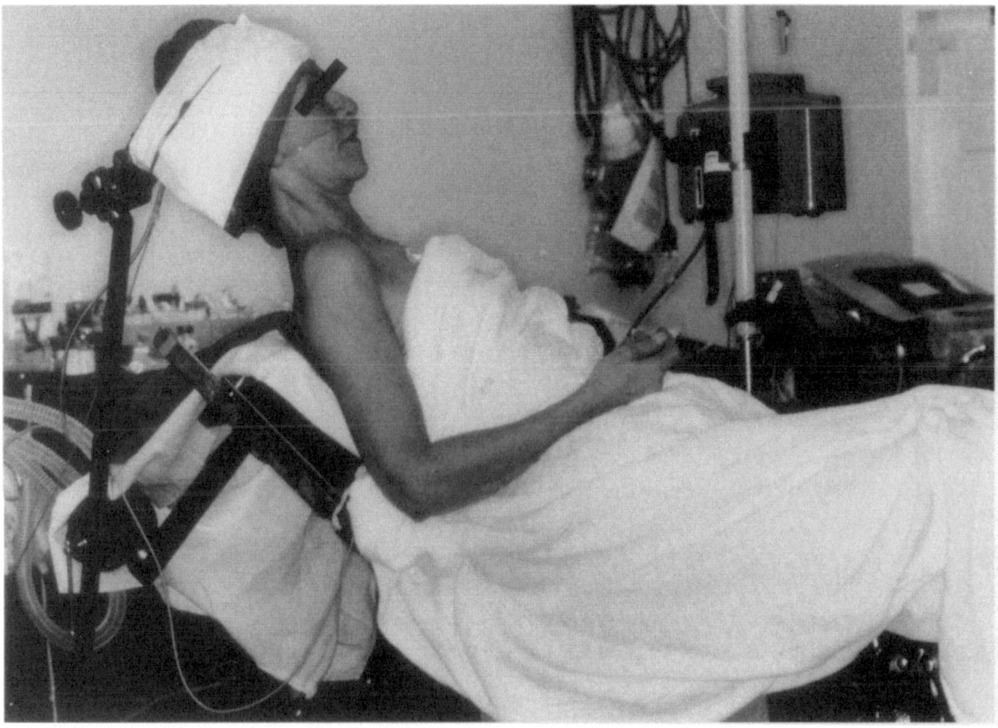

Fig. 2. Representation of the Beach chair position

The mMaintaining normothermia and preventing heat loss by the patient during surgery is essential due to the large amount of fluid infused into the joint. Hypothermia slows patient recovery. Indeed, shivering increases tissue oxygen demand and decreases cardiac output, thereby hindering proper oxygen and nutrient exchange to tissues, leading to acidosis. After surgery, the material that covers the patient is usually wet and cool, which also makes the patient cool. Using waterproof materials is effective, as is good continued aspiration of the instilled fluid. Furthermore, mechanical ventilation lowers the temperature by using a cold gas. Fluid heating systems and convection heating elements are usually effective in this kind of surgery for prophylaxis of hypothermia.

The interscalene and supraclavicular approaches to the brachial plexus (above the clavicle or proximal), have proven effective and safe for anesthesia and post-operative analgesia in arthroscopic shoulder surgery. Recently, a new safe and effective approach to arthroscopic shoulder surgery was advocated, blocking the suprascapular nerve and axillary nerve, although this is a preliminary study (15). The parascalene approach is also thought to offer safe and effective anesthesia for these procedures, as well as a unique benefits in the treatment of acute postoperative pain (16).

The intercostobrachial nerve comes from the thoracic nerve roots T1-T2 and it is responsible for the sensitivity of the anteromedial aspect of the arm. Since some techniques do not block the supraclavicular nerve, this is achieved with a subcutaneous wheel and 3-5 ml of local axillary anesthetic, superficial to the area of palpation of the axillary artery (Figure 3).

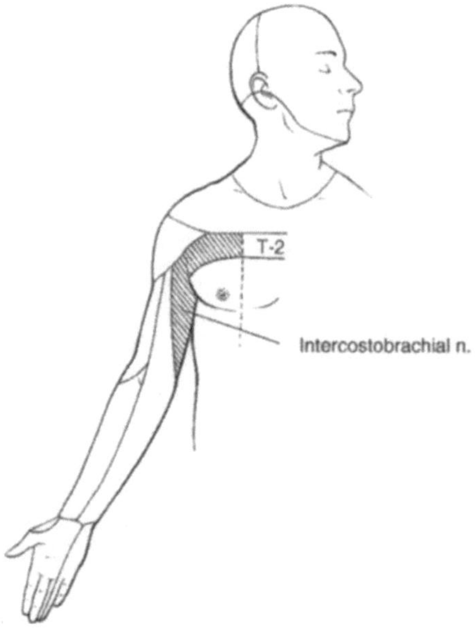

Fig. 3. Schematic representation of the sensitive area of the intercostobrachialis nerve.

7. Interscalenic approach to the brachial plexus

In blocking the brachial plexus in the proximal interscalene space, the anesthesia is applied to the roots or nerve trunks to achieve a metameric distribution of the anesthesia. The plexus is formed by the anterior divisions of the C5 to T1 nerves, with regular contributions from C4 and T2. When the nerve roots exit through the intervertebral foramina, they head down towards the first rib surrounded by a fascia or aponeurotic sheath. This sheath extends into the upper arm by forming partitions, which hinders the diffusion of the anesthetic. Just before you reach the first rib (interscalene space), the roots above are fused together to give three trunks, referred to as the superior (C5-C6), middle (C7) and lower (C8-T1) in a craniocaudal direction. Both the plexus and the scalene muscles are located within a limited anatomical region defined by the outer edge of the sternocleidomastoid muscle, the upper edge of the middle third clavicular and anterior border of the trapezius muscle. This area is located external to the jugular vein, which must be born in mind to avoid puncture.

In the interscalene groove, roots that form the brachial plexus begin to coalesce to give rise to the upper, middle and bottom trunk. At this site, the brachial plexus is located at an approximate distance of about 1 cm from the skin and therefore, it is advisable to use high-frequency (10-15 MHz) and low penetration (3 - 4 cm) probes for exploration.

8. Classic cross-cutting approach

To perform the block, the patient is placed in a supine position with the head rotated slightly to the side contralateral to the blockade. In the classical approach we use a probe situated transversely direction, putting it in the midline of the neck and starting at the level of the cricoid cartilage (Figure 4).

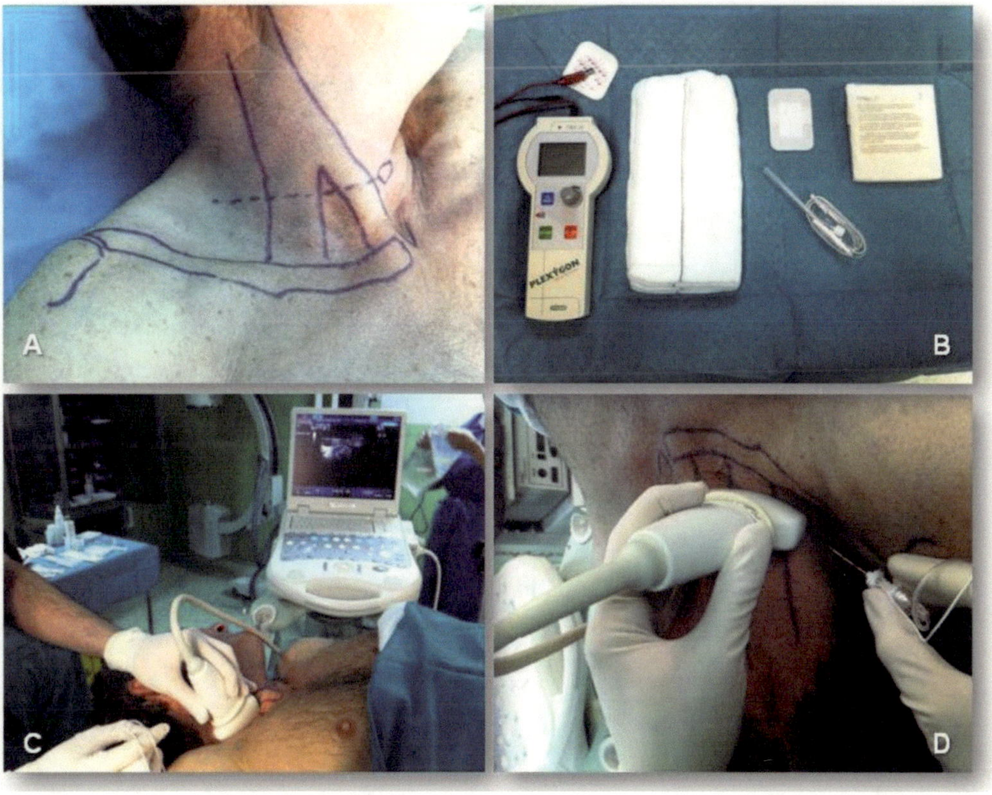

Fig. 4. A. Representation of the most relevant references in the neck skin to the perform an interscalene block. B. Material for blockade by neurostimulation. C. Plexus Neurolocalization by ultrasound. D. Plexus approach using ultrasound with needle insertion "flat" from the side.

In the resulting image and for educational purposes, three areas can be identified when using this approach. A superficial area (located in the upper area of the ultrasound screen) occupied mainly by muscle structures, most of them more shallow than the sternocleidomastoid muscle. A middle zone located immediately under the muscle plane described above in which the tracheal lumen and cricoid cartilage lie, and lateral to the tracheal lumen the homogeneous texture of the thyroid lobe can be observed (Figure 5a), together with two vascular structures: a) the most inner and rounded one going up to the pulsating carotid artery; and b) the outer triangular one that readily collapses on applying pressure with the scanning probe corresponds to the internal jugular vein (Figure 5b). A deep zone (located in the lower area of the ultrasound screen) the lower limit of which marks the vertebral transverse process, which at this level corresponds to C6. Once these structures have been identified, the probe can be moved laterally and by maintaining the same angle, interscalene scan plane is reached (Figure 5c).

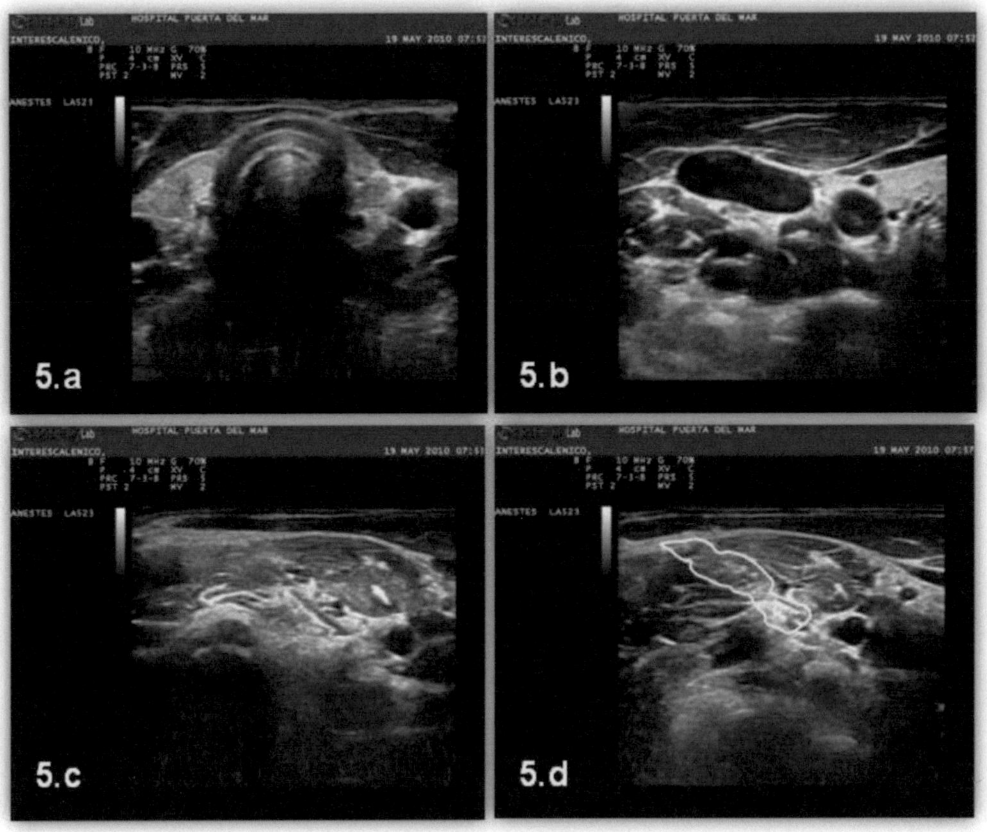

Fig. 5. Cervical screening ultrasound images left of the cricoid cartilage (C6), from medial to lateral. Figure 5b, the interscalene space can be seen just after the deposit of the local anesthetic (area designated).

Medium zone. Beneath the sternocleidomastoid muscle, the anterior scalene (located more medially) and middle scalene (located more laterally) muscles can be seen, and between the two muscles the roots of interscalene brachial plexus groove are located. Their images appear as oval or round, hypoechoic (dark image), hyperechoic rim (white) and often with a dot inside (Figure 5c).

Inferior zone. Located immediately under the scalene muscles, the longus colli can be identified lateral to the vertebral artery a round, hypoechoic and pulsating image crossing medially to laterally. It is important to differentiate the nervous structures (well rounded and hypoechoic but not pulsating) that are often in line but below them in the picture. If in doubt, the scan mode used color Doppler to show the pulsatile flow of the artery, which is not seen if the nerve roots are being explored.

9. "Alternative" cross-cutting approach

In an alternative approach described by Jack Vander Beek, the ultrasound scan is performed in the caudocraneal sense instead of the medio-lateral sweep of the "classic" technique. This approach is especially useful in patients with previous anatomical changes in the neck (surgery, radiotherapy, lean muscle bellies, etc.). Whichever approach is chosen, it is advisable to make subtle and rapid caudocraneal movements that will help visualize the nerve roots. It is advisable to define the scalene and focus on finding the nerves.

10. Implementation of the blockade

Having identified the brachial plexus in the interscalene space, the needle is inserted lateral to the transducer (flat) and with a local anesthetic bolus (remember the plexus is located about 1 cm from the skin), the needle is advanced while directly visualization the plane with the transducer until it enters the interscalene groove and is located adjacent to a nerve root. It is preferable to situate the needle at the deepest roots so that when we start to infuse the local anesthetic, it pushes us toward superficial plexus, improving the success rate. After gentle aspiration, we proceed to inject the local anesthetic, confirming the spread of local anesthetic into the interscalene groove by direct visualisation.

11. Indications

- Primarily for analgesia and anesthesia of shoulder and proximal arm.
- In cases of long-term surgery or intention analgesia, it may be appropriate to implant a catheter.

12. Complications

- Perimedulla Dissemination: which would produce a spinal block and require ventilation support. This can be prevented by aspiration prior to injection and checking there is no CSF fluid.
- Systemic toxicity: direct intravascular injection (perform test prior to aspiration) or by absorption of the anesthetic.
- Vasovagal syncope: due to a Bezold-Jarisch reaction (hypotension and bradycardia, possibly with extreme apnea). Cervical sympathetic blockage occurs and venous return becomes difficult due to the surgical position (sitting). It usually occurs 30-60 min after blockade. Treat with ephedrine or atropine if needed, and vascular fluid filling.
- Ipsilateral phrenic nerve palsy: is constant in the interscalene block. Translate a cephalic spread over C6.
- Changes in phonation, hoarseness if recurrent involvement (rare), superior laryngeal nerve block anesthesia of hemipharynx (more common). If phonation disturbance persists, consider anatomical nerve involvement and monitoring.
- Horner's syndrome: produced by affecting the stellate ganglion. If it persists, suspect anatomical node involvement such as hematoma.
- Pneumothorax.
- Delayed neurological dysfunction: usually transient.

Other considerations and peculiarities:

- Do not hold bilateral blocks in patients with respiratory disease.
- It is not entirely clear whether alterations can be made in hemostasis.
- May require superficial Superficial cervical plexus block may be required (sensitive innervations of the skin over the shoulder on top and above). This can be achieved by infiltrating 5-10 ml of anesthetic in a fan at the posterior lateral edge of the sternocleidomastoid muscle from the midpoint of an imaginary line between the mastoid and the clavicle.

13. Supraclavicular approach of brachial plexus

The supraclavicular fossa is limited by the outer edge of the sternocleidomastoid muscle, the middle third clavicular and the anterior border of trapezius. When the trunks of the brachial plexus abandon the interscalene space, they form 6 divisions, 3 above and 3 below. The brachial plexus is directed from the corresponding interscalene space to the axilla, passing over the 1st rib between the attachments of the anterior and middle scalene muscles, and below the collarbone. When the plexus lies between the first rib and the clavicle, it remains surrounded by a fascial sheath, maintaining a close relationship to the subclavian artery, although extending above and remaining external to it. The subclavian vein is located above the 1st rib and enters into the anterior scalene muscle.

For ultrasound imaging of the brachial plexus, the supraclavicular ultrasound probe should be placed in the supraclavicular fossa, parallel to the clavicle and the edge, touching its inside while at an angle to the chest. This represents the "guide" to locate the subclavian artery. It is desirable that this approach is made at a level that includes the artery in the center of the image, clearly positioned on the first rib, leaving the farthest edge of the pleura on each side. In that way, the nerves will be situated in a superior position external to the artery. It is sometimes possible to observe a cross-section of the subclavian vein, which appears as a hypoechoic round structure that does not pulsate, with internal strings of images that correspond to valvular structures. Anatomically, it is situated before the insertion of anterior scalenus muscle, and thus medial to the muscle in the image, and in most cases it is obscured by the clavicle.

14. Performing the technique

To achieve the supraclavicular block, the patient is placed in a prone position with the head turned slightly to the side contralateral to the blockade and with their arm parallel against their body. The probe is placed just above the collarbone, parallel to it, and the map obtained is the oblique coronal plane, that offers a cross section of the subclavian artery. In At this site, the brachial plexus is located approximately 1 cm from the skin and therefore, it is advisable to use high-frequency (10-15 MHz) and low penetration (3-4 cm) probes for exploration (Figure 6).

The needle is inserted through the lateral end of the probe, moving at an angle of about 20° to the skin and parallel to the transducer. After inserting the needle tip into the plexus and gentle aspiring, the local anesthetic solution is slowly injected. A sign of good distribution of the local anesthesia is the peripheral displacement of the divisions/trunks that form the plexus at this level, and the strengthening of their hyperechoic rim. It is recommended that the needle be replaced if the local anesthetic is distributed asymmetrically.

an even distribution of the local anesthetic will produce blockade in all the territories dependent on the brachial plexus nerve in > 80% of cases. To achieve uniform distribution of the anesthetic, a slow injection is paramount, along with high resolution ultrasound to directly observe its distribution.

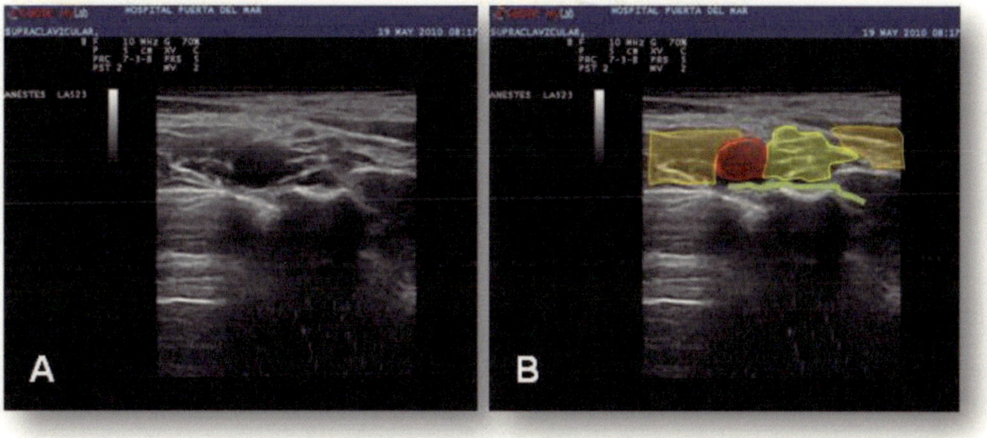

Fig. 6. A. Ultrasound anatomy of the supraclavicular brachial plexus. B. Schematic representation of the scalene muscles (orange), subclavian artery (red), first rib (white) and brachial plexus (Yellow)

The Brachial plexus blockage via the supraclavicular approach has some notable advantages:

- In the supraclavicular block, a single, uniformly distributes injection of local anesthetic may achieve a total blockage of all forearm and arm nerve territories, including the medial cutaneous nerves of the arm, the musculocutaneous forearm nerves and the axillary nerve.
- Compared with infraclavicular blockage, supraclavicular access is more effective in terms of radial blockade of the territory using a single puncture technique.

15. Complications

- Pneumothorax: classically described as late onset, although direct visualization of the pleura during blockade should reduce this potential complication.
- Systemic toxicity: direct intravascular injection (test by prior aspiration) or by absorption of the anesthetic.
- subclavian Subclaviar arterial puncture.
- ipsilateral Ipsilateral phrenic nerve palsy.
- Changes in phonation: hoarseness if the recurrent nerve is involvement (rare).
- Horner's syndrome: due to blocking the stellate ganglion.

- delayed Delayed neurological dysfunction: usually transient.

Other considerations and peculiarities:

- Given the possible occurrence of pneumothorax in the hours after the blockade, this may not be a good option for outpatient surgery.
- Contraindicated for use in patients with respiratory disease, contralateral recurrent paralysis and impaired hemostasis.
- It may be necessary to perform a concomitant intercostobrachial nerve block if there is prolonged use of a tourniquet. This nerve root emerges from D2-D3 and it is responsible for part of the sensitivity in the inside of the arm, lying over the artery in the subcutaneous tissue of the axilla.

16. Postoperative analgesic management

Proper management of acute post-operative pain after arthroscopic shoulder surgery enables patients to be discharged earlier, reducing the rate of rehospitalization, and facilitating early rehabilitation and recovery. Optimal pain control also includes evaluating the patient's physical and psychological situation, altered as a result of the surgery. As indicated, pain management should commence in the pre-operative period, while the use of neuromodulator drugs, such as gabapentin/pregabaline, can reduce post-operative pain and the need for analgesics after arthroscopic surgery for ruptured rotator cuff (17). In the intra-operative period, pain can be controlled by administering the appropriate analgesic anesthetic technique, both in terms of the type of approach and the local anesthetics used, as well as the intra-articular drugs administered (18). Post-operative management includes oral/IV analgesics, heated iv fluid and if necessary, the use of narcotics or continuous perineural infusion techniques (19).

Multiple studies have compared different Different therapeutic strategies have often been compared, including single dose perineural infiltration and continuous infusion techniques (20), technical perineural analgesia versus intravenous patient controlled analgesia, perineural versus intra-articular analgesia (21,22), etc. The pPain is usually worst during the first 48h and it is influenced by many factors apart from the surgery (23). In our experience, paracetamol administration in association with continuous intravenous infusion of NSAIDs scheduled during the first 48h successfully reduces post-operative pain, without provoking any serious side effects. Open shoulder surgery or failure in the regional block can require post-operative treatment with morphine by patient-controlled analgesia (PCA). The control and monitoring of these patients by the acute in-patient Pain Unit, or through telephone follow-up for out-patients, is very important to ensure adequate pain control and to optimize the needs of these patients. Different protocols can be used to adapt the therapy to the patient’s specific characteristics, and to diagnose and treat the different potential side effects.

Particular attention should be paid to patient ventilation, which can be compromised by previous handling of the airways or by diffusion of the liquid infused into the neck joint if the lateral decubitus position was used. Check the temperature of the patient as it may fall, ensure that the patient is maintained warm and that warm fluids are infused. It is possible that post-operartive nausea and vomiting may occur, especially when the blockade is associated with general anesthesia. Although rare, we can not forget the possibility of delayed onset neurotoxicity or cardiotoxicity, especially in elderly patients.

17. References

[1] Crile GW: Anesthesia of nerve roots with cocaine. Cleve Med J, 1897; 2: 355.

[2] Hirschel G: Die Anaesthesierung des Plexus Brachialis fuer die Operationen der oberen Extremitaet. Muenchen Med Wochenschr, 1911; 58: 1555.

[3] Kulenkampff D: Die Anaesthesierung des Plexus Brachialis. Zentralbl Chir, 1911; 38: 1337.

[4] Barash P: Die Anesthesia. Philadelphia Lippincott, 1989: page 13.

[5] Winnie A: Plexus Anesthesia; Vol 1: Perivascular techniques of brachial plexus blocks. Philadelphia, WB Saunders Co, 1984.

[6] Salcedo E, Shay P, Berrigan M: The pre-emptive analgesic effect of interscalene block prior to shoulder surgery (scientific poster). Reg Anesth 1996;21:107.

[7] Seltzer J, Greek R, Maurer P: The preemptive analgesic effect of regional anesthesia for shoulder surgery. Anesthesiology 1993;79:A815.

[8] D'Alessio J, Rosenblum M, Shea K: A retrospective comparison of interscalene block and general anesthesia for ambulatory surgery shoulder arthroscopy. Reg Anesth 1995;20:62-68

[9] Maurer P, Greek R, Torjman M: Is regional anesthesia more time efficient than general anesthesia for shoulder surgery. Anesthesiology 1993; 79:A897

[10] Greenberg C, Brown A: Cost containment--Utilization of techniques, personnel, equipment and supplies, in White P (ed): Ambulatory Anesthesia and Surgery, London, UK, Saunders, 1997, pp 635-647.

[11] Glenn M. et al. Cerebral Oxygen desaturation events assessed by near-infrared spectroscopy during shoulder arthroscopy in the beach chair and lateral decubitus position. Anest. Analg.2010; 111, 2: 496-505.

[12] Wiley AM, Older MW. Shoulder arthroscopy: Investigations with a fibrooptic instrument. Am J Sports Med 1980; 8:31

[13] Andrews JR, Carson WG, Ortega K. Arthroscopy of the shoulder: Technique and normal anatomy. Am J Sports Med 1984;12:1.

[14] Paulos LE, Franklin JL. Arthroscopy Shoulder Decompression: Development and application: a five years of experience. Am J Sports Med, 1990; 18: 235.

[15] Checcucci G. et al. A new technique for regional anesthesia for arthrorscopy shoulder surgery based on a suprascapular nerve block and an axillary nerve block: an evaluation of the first results. Arthroscopy 2008; 24: 689-696.

[16] Reig R, Sole J, Rauly E. Bloqueo paraescalénico para cirugía artroscópica de hombro. Rev. Esp. Anestesiol. Reanim. 2004; 51: 247-252.

[17] Yu S, Kim T: Can gabapentine help reduce postoperative pain in arthroscopic rotator cuff repair?A prospective, randomized, double-blind study. Arthroscopy 2010; 26:106-11.

[18] Ballieul RJ, et al. The peri-operative use of intra-articular local anesthetics: a review. Acta Anaesthesiol Belg 2009;60:101-8.

[19] Ruiz-Suarez M, Barber FA: Postoperative pain control after shoulder arthroscopy. Orthopedics 2008; 31: 1130-5.

[20] Young S, Cawley P: Postoperative pain managementfor arthroscopic shoulder surgery: interescalene block versus patient-controlled infusion of 0.25% bupivacaine. Am J Orthop 2006; 35: 231-4.

[21] Contreras-Dominguez V, et al. Eficacia del bloqueo interescalénico continuo en comparación a la analgesia intra-articular para el tratamiento del dolor postoperatorio en acromioplastias artroscópicas. Rev Esp Anestesiol Reanim 2008;55: 475-480.
[22] Ciccone W. et al. Assesment of pain relief provided by interescalene regional block and infusion pump after arthroscopic shoulder surgery. Arthroscopy, 2008;l 24: 14-19, .
[23] Anthony R. Brown. Regional anesthesia for shoulder surgery. Techniques in Regional Anesthesia and Pain Management, 1999; 3:64-78.

4

Arthroscopic Treatment of Distal Radius Fractures

Yukio Abe and Yasuhiro Tominaga
Saiseikai Shimonoseki General Hospital
Japan

1. Introduction

Distal radius fracture (DRF) is one of the most common traumatic events for the hand surgeon to treat. Numerous surgical procedures have been described for this fracture (Ruch et al., 2004); however, the ideal method of surgical management is still controversial. The latest development of a volar locking plate fixation markedly changed the treatment of DRF (Chen & Jupiter, 2007; Chung et al., 2006). Volar locking plate fixation creates a more rigid mechanical construct and allows early rehabilitation that can be initiated with the goal of an improved functional outcome; therefore, volar locking plate fixation currently has widespread popularity, even for dorsally displaced intraarticular fracture (Orbay & Fernandez, 2002; Willis et al., 2006).

The functional outcome of the treatment of DRF is considered to be affected by extraarticular alignment, anatomical reduction of the articular surface, intraarticular soft tissue injuries and postoperative complications. Wrist arthroscopy is currently recognized as an important adjunctive procedure in the management of DRF (Doi et al., 1999; Freeland & Geissler, 2000; Ruch et al., 2004). This is because arthroscopically assisted reduction and internal fixation of DRF cause minimal surgical intervention and provide not only excellent visualization of the joint surface for anatomical restoration of articular fragments but evaluate and treat intraarticular soft tissue injuries. Although it is better used in conjunction with percutaneous pinning and external fixation, wrist arthroscopy becomes problematic when plate fixation is performed because vertical traction has to be both applied and released during surgery; therefore, a plate presetting arthroscopic reduction technique (PART) using a volar locking plate has been developed, that can simplify the combination of plating and arthroscopy (Abe et al., 2008). PART can also be performed with minimal skin incision and is less invasive. This chapter will describe the procedure of PART and its effectiveness for the treatment of DRF.

2. Technique

All patients with DRF were managed initially with closed reduction and casting at the first visit to our clinic. Consecutive patients with inadequate reduction or re-displacement underwent arthroscopic reduction and volar locking plate fixation. Our surgical indications regarding radiological assessment included less than -10 degrees or over 20 degrees of palmar tilt, and over 2 mm of ulnar plus variance compared to the normal side.

Between July 2005 and May 2011, PART was performed in 155 wrists of 153 consecutive DRF patients. Thirty men and 123 women ranged in age from 18 to 84 years old (average age 62 years old). Besides the standard anteroposterior and lateral radiographs, internal and external rotation of the wrist radiographs, computerized tomography (CT), and 3-dimensional reconstruction CT are valuable in deciding a strategy for the reduction of DRF. Intraarticular fractures of the DRF were routinely investigated using these oblique views of radiographs and CT. Contralateral wrist radiographs must be taken with the goal of reducing the fracture for all patients. All the fractures were classified using the AO/ASIF classification system. The fractures consisted of 37 extra-articular (A2: 7, A3: 30) and 118 intra-articular (B3: 6, C1: 40, C2: 18, C3: 54) fractures. For restoration of the articular surface and treatment of soft tissue injury of intracarpal lesions, we consider that wrist arthroscopy may be indicated for all DRF. For this reason, even if it is an extraarticular fracture, arthroscopy was performed to evaluate intraarticular soft tissue injury. Contraindications include severe soft-tissue injury with an open fracture, multiple systemic fractures and compartment syndrome. The locking plates consisted of 106 Acu-Loc plates (Acumed, Hillsboro, Oregon), 39 DRV locking plates (Mizuho, Tokyo, Japan), and 10 other locking plates. The injuries of the scapholunate interosseous ligament (SLIL) and lunotriquetral interosseous ligament (LTIL) were evaluated according to Geissler's classification (Geissler et al., 1996), and triangular fibrocartilage complex (TFCC) tear was evaluated with Palmer's classification (Palmer, 1989).

2.1 Surgical technique

While carrying out PART, intraarticular fragments are almost reduced by manipulation before presetting the plate in AO type B, C1 and C2 of intraarticular fractures; in those cases, a small step-off or separation can easily be reduced arthroscopically; however, in the C3 type, central depression fragments or multifragments, in particular, are hardly reduced by manipulation, and reduction techniques, such as the joy-stick maneuver, tenaculum cramping, or pushing up the fragment from the intramedullary canal, are essential for arthroscopic reduction after presetting the plate (Fig.1).

The patient is positioned supine on the operating table, with the arm draped free on a hand table. A tourniquet is routinely applied to the upper arm and inflated. A longitudinal incision is made between the flexor carpi radialis tendon and the radial artery. The length of the skin incision can change by the severity of comminution at the volar cortex. The shortest one is 2.5cm for a simple metaphyseal fracture (Fig. 2A). The radial artery is identified and retracted radially. The median nerve is retracted ulnarly with the flexor digitorum profundus tendons. Care must be taken throughout the procedure to minimize excessive retraction of the median, palmar cutaneous, and radial sensory nerves. Retracting the flexor pollicis longus muscle ulnarly exposes the pronator quadratus muscle, which is not split but is elevated from the subperiosteum or split distal just one third to expose and reduce the fracture (Fig. 2B).

The fracture is reduced by manipulating the fragments using a periosteal elevator or by intrafocal pinning. Generally, the volar cortex of the radius is less comminuted, reduction of the volar cortex is an indicator of anatomical reduction. Anatomical reduction is confirmed under a fluoroscopy including the joint surface, and the temporary fixation is held with 3 smooth 1.5mm Kirschner wires (K-wires) inserted radially and dorsally. Placement of these wires should not interfere with the placement of the volar locking plate. Four or more K-wires are often necessary for osteoporotic patients. After temporary fixation, the volar locking plate is preset on the volar surface of the radius (Fig. 3). Subchondral support wires are inserted into the distal fragment through the distal hole of the plate, and a screw is inserted into the proximal fragment using the dynamic hole of the plate barrel as a temporary fixation. This screw is inserted in the center of the dynamic hole to slightly regulate the placement of the plate at the secure fixation. Because of a small skin incision, wrist has to be flexed to facilitate inserting this screw.

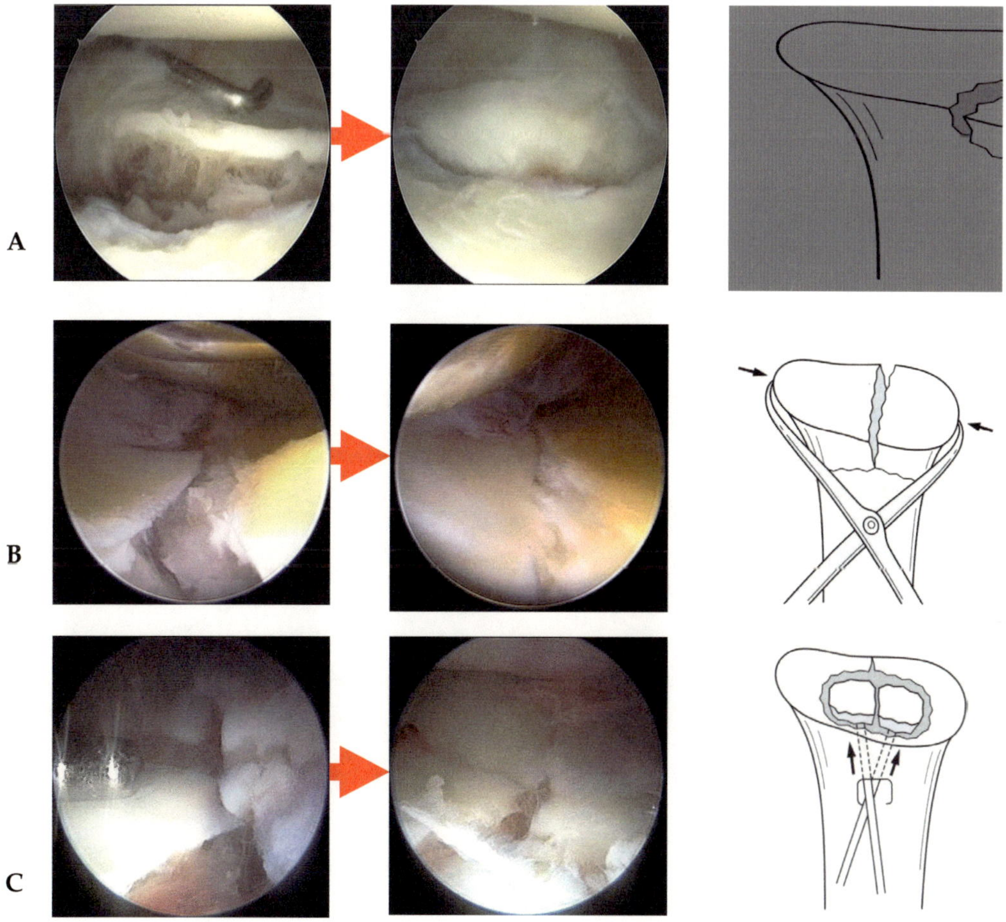

Fig. 1. Reduction techniques for intraarticular fragments. A: joy-stick maneuver, B: tenaculum cramping, C: pushing up from the intramedullary canal.

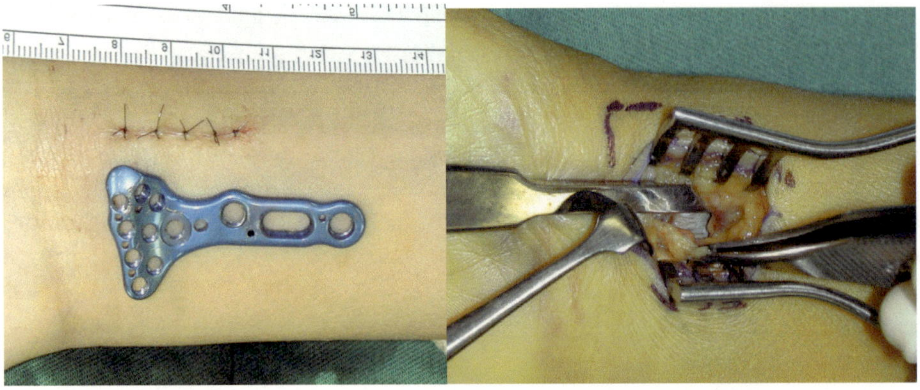

A B

Fig. 2. Minimally invasive technique in PART. The length of the skin incision is usually from 2.5cm to 3.0cm (A). The pronator quadratus muscle is not split but is elevated from the subperiosteum to protect the muscle belly (B).

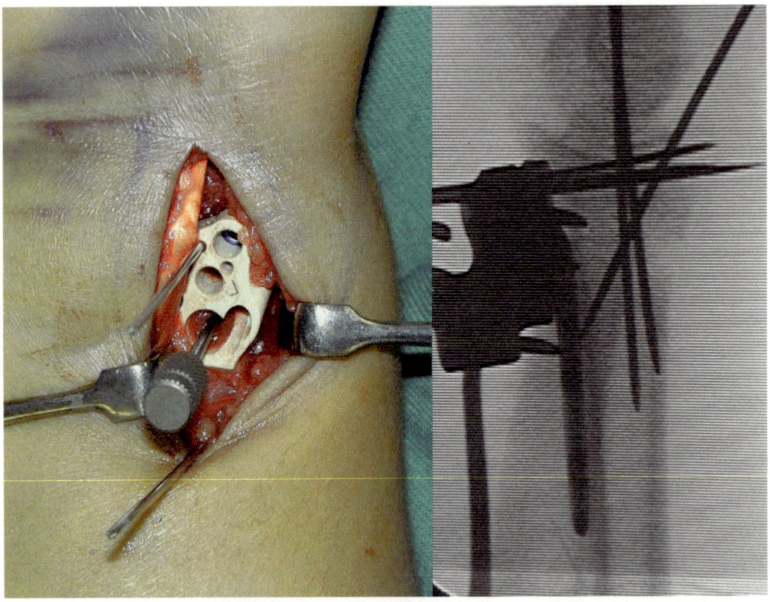

Fig. 3. A volar locking plate was preset on the radius

After the plate is preset, the wrist is suspended in vertical traction, and arthroscopy is performed. We generally use 3 arthroscopic portals to totally evaluate and treat the intraarticular fragments and soft tissue injuries (Fig. 4). Two dorsal portals are 3-4 portal (between the extensor pollicis longus tendon and the extensor digitorum communis tendons) and 4-5 portals (between the extensor digitorum communis tendons and the extensor digiti minimi tendon) that are well known and popularly used. Another portal is the volar radial portal (between the flexor carpi radialis tendon and the radial artery). Through this portal, we can adequately visualize the dorsal fragment of the intraarticular fracture and volar segment tear of the SLIL and LTIL (Abe et al., 2003; Abe et al., 2003). Because the volar side of the skin is already open, and the tendons, nerves, and artery are retracted, the volar portal can be safely accessed.

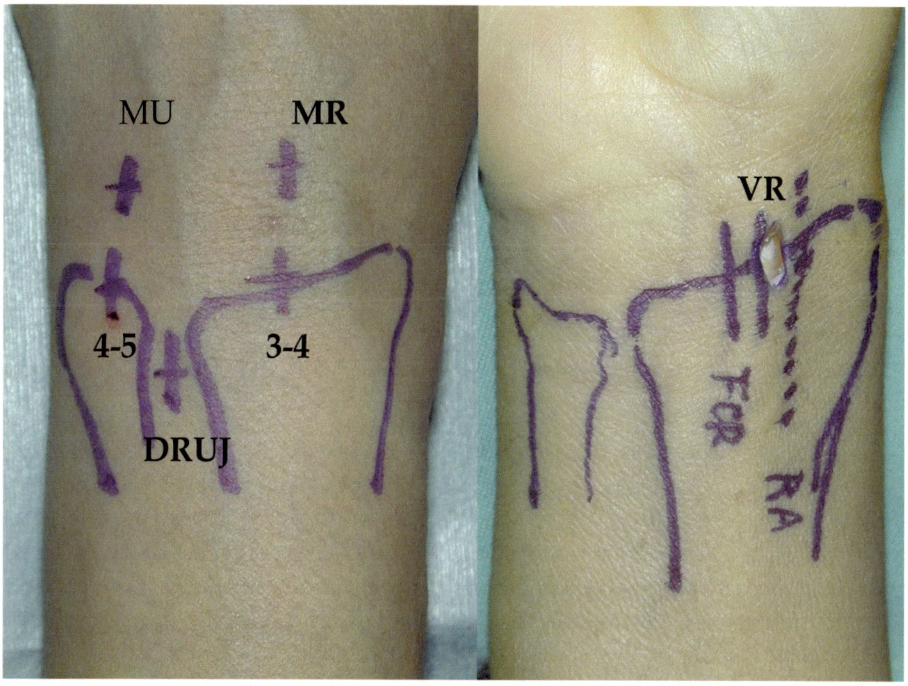

Fig. 4. Arthroscopic portals. MR (radial midcarpal portal) and MU (ulnar midcarpal portal) are used to evaluate the instability between scaphoid and lunate, lunate and triquetrum. DRUJ portal is used to investigate the foveal tear of the TFCC. VR: volar radial portal.

A 2.3-mm arthroscope with a 30-degree field of vision is introduced through the volar portal. The remaining hematoma in the joint is removed using a shaver inserted through the dorsal portal. The degree of dislocation of the dorsal fragments is evaluated initially from the volar portal. The volar side of the SLIL and the LTIL are also evaluated. An arthroscope is subsequently inserted from the dorsal portal, and total intraarticular fragments, including on the volar side, must be evaluated. The volar fragment is already reduced on initial manipulation, an intraarticular volar fragment may be an indicator of arthroscopic reduction. The subchondral K-wire that prevents reduction of the fragment then has to be removed. Central depression is reduced by pushing up from the intramedullary canal using a probe inserted at the dorsal fracture site. Radial and dorsal fragments are reduced using a joy-stick maneuver (Fig. 5). The K-wire, inserted initially to maintain the reduction, is often used as a joy-stick. The separate fragments are well reduced by a tenaculum cramping on the outside of the skin. After achieving reduction of the fragments, the subchondral K-wire is reinserted to maintain reduction. The major dorsal fragment is often fixed with a screw or a small plate independently.

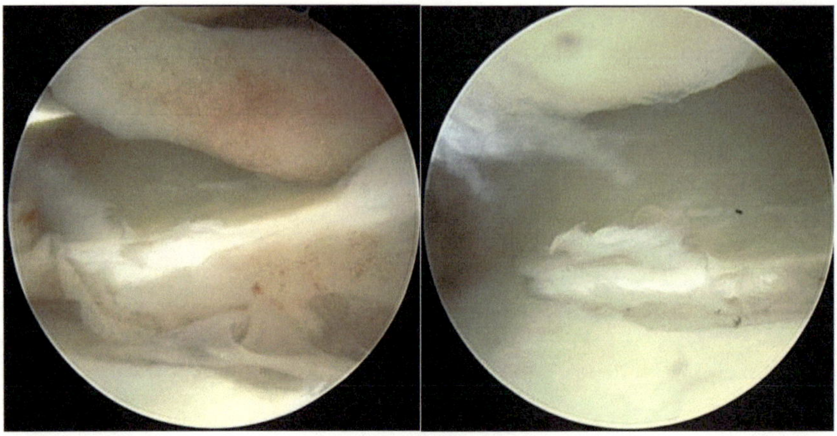

A B

Fig. 5. Arthroscopic reduction for the intraarticular fragments. A: pre-reduction, B: post-reduction. Dorsal fragment was elevated using joy-stick maneuver.

After reduction of the intraarticular fragments arthroscopically, associated cartilage and soft tissue injuries should be evaluated and treated. Our strategy for the treatment of SLIL injury is percutaneous pinning for grade III instability (Fig. 6), pinning, repair of the dorsal part of SLIL, and augmentation using a dorsal intercarpal ligament for grade IV instability in active patients. For TFCC injury, debridement is indicated for traumatic disk tears. Peripheral tear is repaired arthroscopically (Fig. 7). Both procedures are also indicated for active patients.

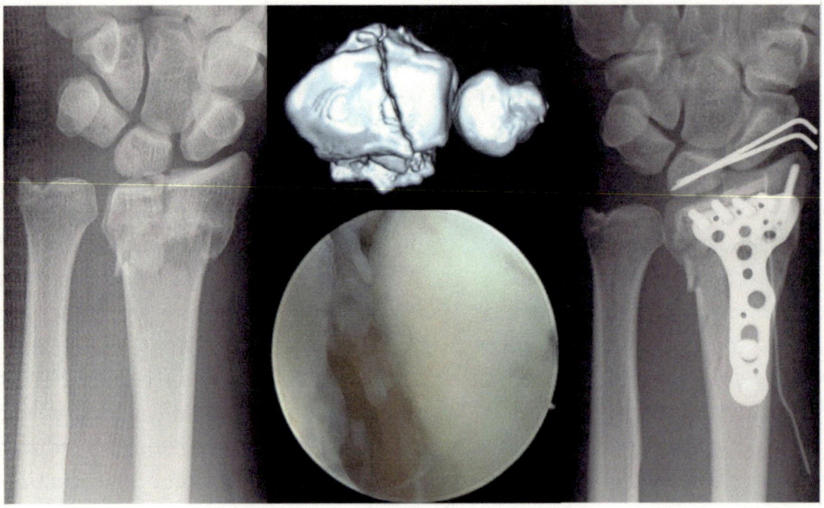

A B/C D

Fig. 6. This is a 47 y.o. male, C2 fracture (A, B) associated with grade III SLIL tear confirmed with midcarpal arthroscopy (C). Scapholunate joint was fixed with K-wires (D).

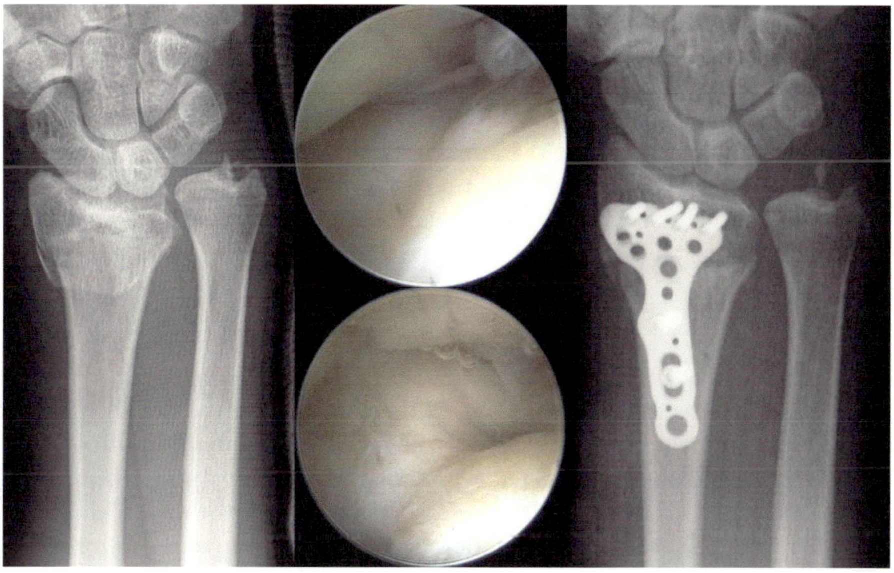

A **B / C** **D**

Fig. 7. This is a 53 y.o. male, A3 fracture (A) with TFCC ulnar styloid tear (B). Fracture was fixed with a volar locking plate (D), TFCC tear was repaired arthroscopically (C).

Intraarticular fragments and soft tissue injuries are treated, then vertical traction is removed, and the volar locking plate is subsequently and securely fixed to the distal radius (Fig. 8). After introducing the volar locking plate, we rarely perform bone grafting for dorsal bone defect. The wound is irrigated, a drain is inserted, and the overlying skin is closed.

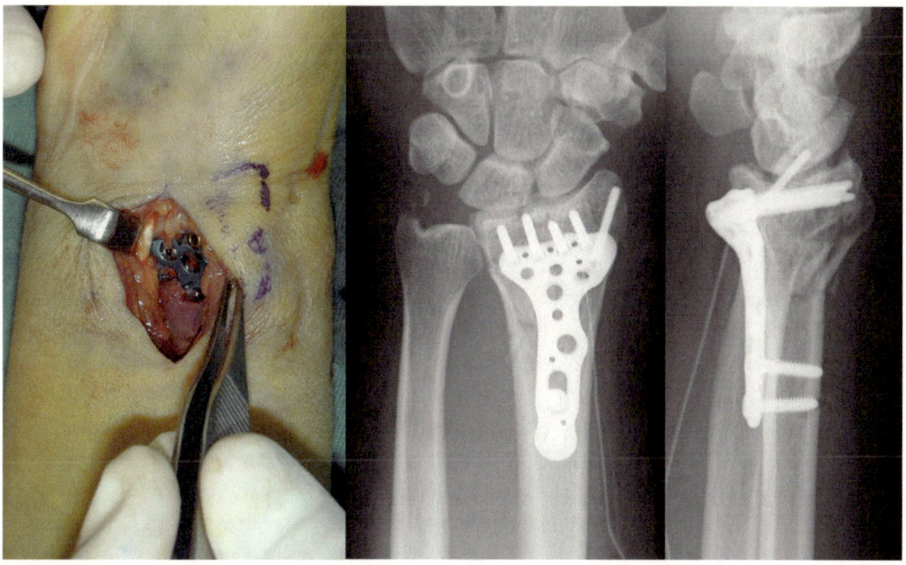

Fig. 8. Final fixation. The pronator quadratus muscle was preserved.

2.2 Postoperative management

Since the volar locking plate provides rigid fixation, early rehabilitation can be allowed. A dorsal splint is applied just after surgery, the splint is then removed during the daytime, and active wrist motion is started on the first day after surgery. From the second day, passive motion and grasping exercises are started with a therapist. The night splint is removed within 7 days after surgery. Forearm rotation exercises are prohibited in patients who have ulnar side injuries, such as distal ulna fracture, ulnar styloid fracture and TFCC repair until 3 weeks after surgery.

3. Outcomes

Final evaluation was obtained from the radiological outcome, measurements of wrist and forearm motion, grip strength, the Mayo modified wrist score (Cooney et al., 1994) and the Disabilities of the Arm, Shoulder and Hand (DASH) questionnaire. Wrist flexion-extension was assessed with a goniometer. Forearm supination and pronation were assessed with the elbow flexed 90 degrees at the patient's side. Grip strength was measured with a calibrated Jamar dynamometer. The average of three trials for both hands was recorded for all strength measurements. We could recognize several advantages of arthroscopic surgery for DRF. During PART, anatomical reduction of the articular surface was achieved with fluoroscopy initially, and reduction was re-confirmed with arthroscopy. In this process, we can recognize the dissociation between fluoroscopic and arthroscopic reduction, and this dissociation was assessed. The frequency and severity of intraarticular soft tissue injury could also be evaluated using arthroscopy.

Surgical time ranged from 38 to 150 minutes (average 82 minutes). The case that needed 150 minutes included SLIL repair and TFCC debridement. One-hundred ten wrists were followed up for over 1 year so far (by May 2011). The follow-up period ranged from 12 to 48 months (average 18 months). At final follow-up, the mean palmar tilt was 5.6 degrees (-10 to 16 degrees), radial inclination 26.1 degrees (18 to 31 degrees), and ulnar variance 0.1mm (-2mm to 5mm). The mean active extension of the wrist was 62.5 degrees (45 to 80 degrees, 92% on the uninjured side), and the mean flexion was 60.1 degrees (45 to 80 degrees, 88% on the uninjured side). The mean pronation of the forearm was 83.1 degrees (70 to 90 degrees, 96% on the uninjured side), and the mean supination was 86.5 degrees (75 to 95 degrees, 97% on the uninjured side). The mean grip strength was 88.2% (38% to 110% on the uninjured side).

In 118 wrists of intraarticular fractures, 108 wrists seemed to achieve reduction with fluoroscopy; however, there remained a gap or step-off of over 2mm in 38 cases (35.2%), confirmed arthroscopically. Among 155 wrists, SLIL injury was recognized in 44 wrists (28.9 %). According to Geissler's classification, 24 wrists were grade I, 4 were grade II, 13 were grade III and 3 were grade IV. Debridement for a torn ligament was performed in 4 wrists (grade I: 2, grade III: 2), scapholunate pinning was performed for 3 wrists of grade III, and 1 wrist of grade IV underwent reconstruction. LTIL injury was recognized in 23 wrists (14.8%). Nineteen wrists were grade I, 2 were grade II, 1 was grade III, and 1 was grade IV. Only 2 wrists of grade I were debrided for the torn ligament hung down. TFCC injury was recognized in 98 wrists (63.2%). Sixty-seven wrists were 1A tear, 5 were 1B, 1 was 1D, 7 were 1A+1B, 1 wrist was a foveal tear and 17 wrists were degenerative tear. Debridement was performed for 53 wrists (1A: 50, 1A+1B: 3), debridement and repair were performed in 1

wrist (1A+1B), repair was performed for one wrist of 1B tear and one foveal tear. Pinning was applied for one wrist of 1D tear.
The final results of 110 wrists according to the Mayo modified wrist score were 84 excellent, 24 good and 2 fair. The mean DASH score at final follow-up was 4.2 points (0 to 30). There were few complications: 3 re-dislocation of the distal fragment, 2 extensor pollicis longus rupture and 1 complex regional pain syndrome. The final results of these 6 cases were 4 good and 2 fair.

4. Summary

The theories of the treatment of peri- or intraarticular fractures are 1) recover alignment, 2) reduce intraarticular fragments, 3) treatment for intraarticular soft tissue injuries, 4) rigid fixation that allows early rehabilitation. Less invasive technique is recently advocated. Prognosis is generally less favorable for displaced, comminuted, intraarticular fractures. Treatment for DRF should also be performed according to these theories. Although various factors affect the prognosis of DRF, accurate reconstruction of the alignment of the radius with its carpal and ulnar articulations, articular surface and treatment of soft tissue injury of intracarpal lesions are the most important factors. Accurate reconstruction of the articular surface, with the goal of establishing anatomic congruency of that surface, is important to minimize the risk of late osteoarthritis. Knirk and Jupiter (1986) reported that displacement of 2 mm or more of the distal radial articular fragments resulted in traumatic osteoarthritis. Further investigation indicated that the critical tolerance for joint surface incongruity may be as little as 1mm (Fernandez & Geissler, 1991; Mehta et al., 2000; Trumble et al., 1994). We have experienced that reduction with a fluoroscopy is not always accurate compared to reduction with wrist arthroscopy. Dissociation between two reduction procedures was 35.2%. This rate is similar to other reports, such as 33% in Edwards (2001) and Lutsky's (2008).
If an associated carpal ligament or TFCC injury is suspected even in a nondisplaced DRF, adequate treatment is mandatory to prevent the development of carpal instability or ulnar side wrist pain. Geissler et al. (1996) demonstrated a considerable rate of soft tissue injuries associated with DRF. These soft tissue injuries have been thought to influence the functional outcome; however, the evaluations performed to date for intraarticular soft tissue injuries combined with DRF have not been sufficient. The causes of chronic wrist pain after DRF treatment were analyzed by Cheng et al. (2008): ulnocarpal abutment caused by mal-union, ulnar styloid non-union, intraarticular soft tissue injury and chondral lesion. Especially regarding the TFCC, some authors recommend acute arthroscopic repair of peripheral tear of TFCC in conjunction with distal radius fixation resulted in a highly satisfaction (Lindau et al., 2000; Ruch et al., 2003). Furthermore we have experienced over 10 cases of chronic wrist pain due to TFCC disk tear after healing of DRF with almost normal alignment. They were treated volar locking plate fixation without arthroscopic assessment or conservative treatment. For this reason, we consider that slit or flap tear of the disk should be debrided.
Wrist arthroscopy is an effective adjunct for this pathology; therefore, wrist arthroscopy may be indicated for all DRF. When volar plate fixation is indicated, the standard upright position makes it problematic to combine arthroscopy and plate fixation because traction has to be both applied and released; PART is able to solve this problem. An alternative is to use a traction table, which makes it possible to perform arthroscopy in a horizontal position (Culp & Osterman, 1995); however, this technique is sometimes more technically

demanding and, using a volar and dorsal approach simultaneously, may be difficult in this position. Slade et al. (2005) reported provisional K-wire fixation of the fracture fragments of the radius after arthroscopic reduction and volar locking plate fixation; however, several cases where re-displacement of the fragments occurred when performing arthroscopy in this sequence were experienced in our series.

The volar locking plate system has been shown a reliable and satisfactory result for the DRF without arthroscopy in some chapters. Chung et al. (2006) reported the results of 87 patients, mean age of 48.9 years old, including 65% of intraarticular fracture. One year after surgery, mean grip strength was 78.7% of the contralateral side, mean flexion was 58.0 degrees, extension was 60.5 degrees, pronation was 78.6 degrees and supination was 79.6 degrees. Lozano-Calderón et al. (2008) reported the results of 60 patients treated with a single, fixed angle volar plate. They were classified into 2 groups of early motion group (range of motion was started within 2 weeks) and late motion group (range of motion was started at 6 weeks). Early motion group that was similar with our series, demonstrated 68 degrees of flexion, 56 degrees of extension, 90 degrees of pronation and 88 degrees of supination at 6 months after surgery. Grip strength was 78% of contralateral side and DASH score was 8.5. The report of 54 patients with intraarticular DRF and a mean age of 63 years by Gruber et al. (2010) demonstrated 58 degrees of flexion, 57 degrees of extension, 83 degrees of pronation, 68 degrees of supination, grasping power was 71% of contralateral side at 6 years after surgery. DASH score was 5 points at 2 years follow up. Our results were superior to those of these reports. Our results were considered to be derived from the several advantages of PART. A volar locking plate that seems to offer the most stable construct (Osada et al., 2003) enables early range of motion and grasping exercises. PART is possible with a small skin incision and preserving the pronator quadratus muscle. Arthroscopic management is less harmful to soft tissue around the wrist joint; therefore, early rehabilitation can also be indicated. Irrigation to remove fracture hematoma and debris potentially reduces the inflammatory reaction and improves the range of motion. In addition, initial treatment for concomitant SLIL injury and TFCC tear may contribute these satisfactory results.

In conclusion, wrist arthroscopy is a feasible adjunct for the treatment of DRF, especially as it can evaluate the reduction of intraarticular fragments and soft tissue injury. In recent years, volar locking plate fixation has become popular, and simultaneous arthroscopic procedures for reduction have become problematic because vertical traction has to be applied and released during surgery. A PART can overcome these difficulties, and this technique can be performed with a small skin incision, preserving the pronator quadratus muscle, and simplifies the combination of plating and arthroscopy, and achieves good final result.

5. References

Abe Y, Doi K, Hattori Y, et al. A benefit of the volar approach for wrist arthroscopy. Arthroscopy. 2003; 19: 440-445.

Abe Y, Doi K, Hattori Y, et al. Arthroscopic assessment of the volar region of the scapholunate interosseous ligament through a volar portal. J Hand Surg. 2003; 28A: 69-73.

Abe Y, Tsubone T, Tominaga Y. Plate presetting arthroscopic reduction technique for the distal radius fractures. Tech Hand Up Extrem Surg. 2008; 12: 136-143.

Chen NC, Jupiter JB. Current concepts review. Management of distal radial fractures. J Bone Joint Surg. 2007; 89: 2051-2062.

Cheng HS, Hung LK, Ho PC et al.. An analysis of causes and treatment outcome of chronic wrist pain after distal radial fractures. 2008; 13: 1-10.

Chung KC, Watt AJ, Kotsis SV, et al. Treatment of unstable distal radial fractures with the volar locking plating system. J Bone Joint Surg. 2006; 88A: 2687-2694.

Cooney WP, Linscheid RL, Dobyns JH. Triangular fibrocartilage tears. J Hand Surg. 1994; 19A: 143-154.

Culp RW, Osterman AL. Arthroscopic reduction and internal fixation of distal radius fractures. Orthop Clin North Am. 1995; 26: 739-748.

Doi K, Hattori Y, Otsuka K, et al. Intra-articular fractures of the distal aspect of the radius: Arthroscopically assisted reduction compared with open reduction and internal fixation. J Bone Joint Surg. 1999; 81A:1093-1110.

Edwards CC II, Haraszti CJ, McGillivary GR, et al..Intra-articular distal radius fractures: Arthroscopic assessment of radiographically assisted reduction. J Hand Surg. 2001; 26: 1036-1041.

Fernandez DL, Geissler WB. Treatment of displaced articular fractures of the radius. J Hand Surg. 1991; 16A: 375-384.

Freeland AE, Geissler WB. The arthroscopic management of intra-articular distal radius fractures. Hand Surgery. 2000; 5: 93-102.

Geissler WB, Freeland AE, Savoie FH, et al. Intracarpal soft-tissue lesions associated with an intra-articular fracture of the distal end of the radius. J Bone Joint Surg. 1996; 78A: 357-365.

Gruber G, Zacherl M, Giessauf C et al. Quality of life after volar plate fixation of articular fractures of the distal part of the radius. J Bone Joint Surg. 2010; 92A: 1170-1178.

Knirk JL, Jupiter JB. Intra-articular fractures of the distal end of the radius in young adults. J Bone Joint Surg. 1986; 68A: 647-659.

Lindau T, Adlercruetz C, Aspenberg P. Peripheral tears of the triangular fibrocartilage complex cause distal radioulnar joint instability after distal radius fractures. J Hand Surg. 2000; 25A: 464-468.

Lozano-Calderon SA, Souer S, Mudgal C, et al. Wrist mobilization following volar plate fixation of fractures of the distal part of the radius. J Bone Joint Surg. 2008; 90A: 1297-1304.

Lutsky K, Boyer MI, Steffen JA et al.. Arthroscopic assessment of intra-articular distal radius fractures after open reduction and internal fixation from a volar approach. J Hand Surg. 2008; 33A: 476-484.

Mehta JA, Bain GI, Heptinstall RJ. Anatomical reduction of intra-articular fractures of the distal radius. J Bone Joint Surg. 2000; 82B: 79-86.

Orbay JL, Fernandez DL. Volar fixation for dorsally displaced fractures of the distal radius: a preliminary report. J Hand Surg. 2002; 27A: 205-215.

Osada D, Viegas SF, Shah MA, et al. Comparison of different distal radius dorsal and volar fracture fixation plates: a biomechanical study. J Hand Surg. 2003; 28: 94-104.

Palmer AK. Triangular fibrocartilage complex lesions; a classification. J Hand Surg. 1989; 14A: 594-606.

Ruch DS, Vallee J, Poehling GG, et al. Arthroscopic reduction versus fluoroscopic reduction in the management of intra-articular distal radius fractures. Arthroscopy. 2004; 20: 225-230.

Ruch DS, Weiland AJ, Wolf SW, et al. Current concepts in the treatment of distal radial fractures. Instr Course Lect. 2004; 53: 389-401.

Ruch DS, Yang CC, Smith BP. Results of acute arthroscopically repaired triangular fibrocartilage complex injuries associated with intra-articular distal radius fractures. Arthroscopy. 2003; 19: 511-516.

Slade JF, Taksali S, Safanda J. Combined fractures of the scaphoid and distal radius: a revised treatment rationale using percutaneous and arthroscopic techniques. Hand Clin. 2005; 21: 427-441.

Trumble TE, Schmitt SR, Vedder NB. Factors affecting functional outcome of displaced intra-articular distal radius fractures. J Hand Surg. 1994; 19A: 325-340.

Willis AA, Kutsumi K, Zobitz ME, et al. Internal fixation of dorsally displaced fractures of the distal part of the radius. J Bone Joint Surg. 2006; 88A: 2411-2417.

Part 3

Arthroscopy of the Hip

5

Arthroscopy after Total Hip Replacement Surgery

Cuéllar Ricardo[1], Ponte Juan[2], Esnal Edorta[3] and Tey Marc[4]
[1]University Hospital Donostia (San Sebastián)
[2]Quirón Hospital (San Sebastián)
[3]Alto Deba Hospital (Mondragón)
[4]Dexeus University Hospital (Barcelona)
Spain

1. Introduction

Hip arthroscopy has been available for some years. Although arthroscopy has not been as widely adopted in the hip joint as compared to its use in other joints, it is currently in a phase of rapid development.

This is mainly due to the description of femoroacetabular impingement syndrome, where hip arthroscopy has proven to be a precious diagnostic and therapeutic tool. The development and improvement of the technique together with the instrumentation has allowed broadening its indications.

The hip joint, is more difficult to access than other joints such as the knee and shoulder. This is due to its tight congruency, the degree of coverage of the ball and socket articular surfaces - the acetabulum extends beyond the equator of the femoral head - the powerful surrounding muscles and the proximity of important vessels and nerves.

These anatomical features restrict the manoeuvrability of the arthroscopic instruments making hip arthroscopy a more demanding technique.

With the techniques for the knee and shoulder joints already well established, we have witnessed the development of arthroscopy for the diagnosis and treatment of hip disorders over the last decade (Johnston et al., 2008; Kelly et al., 2003; Larson et al., 2009; Lubowitz & Poehling, 2006). Arthroscopic techniques have improved, increasing the surgical indications and achieving better outcomes (Byrd, 2006; Byrd & Jones, 2009; Larson & Giveans, 2009; Philippon, 2007a, 2007b). This procedure is performed in children and in adults for both diagnostic and therapeutic purposes, (Kocher et al., 2005; McCarthy & Lee, 2006; Parisien, 1988; Philippon et al., 2007b; Roy et al., 2009; Sampson, 2006), the most commonly treated disorder being femoroacetabular impingement syndrome (Philippon et al., 2007b).

The first publication concerning visualization of the hip joint was by Burman in 1931, who reported his experience in 20 hips using a 4-mm arthroscope and the use of water to achieve joint distension (Burman, 1931). He described the anterior peritrochanteric portal, concluding that this was the best option for visualizing the hip joint. He concluded that the hip joint was not suitable for arthroscopy due to the inability to access and visualize what nowadays is known as the central compartment. Although there were some other reports in the intervening years, it is considered that Gross, in 1977, was the first person to describe the

clinical application of this approach and its therapeutic effect in hip diseases in children (Legg-Calvé-Perthes disease, congenital dislocation and epiphysiolysis). He used a 2.2-mm arthroscope and manual distraction. The use of traction was first described by Eriksson who employed forces of between 300 to 400 Newtons to distract the hip (Eriksson et al., 1986). The first description of the use of traction in the supine position was made by Byrd 8Byrd, 1994); while Glick was the first to report the use of the lateral decubitus position (Glick et al., 1987). Monllau published results of a study demonstrating that hip arthroscopy required instruments with a minimum length of 16 cm (Monllau et al., 2003).
It is well known that following total hip replacement THR, pain disappears in approximately 95-98% of the cases, usually between 3 to 6 months up to a year after surgery. However, between 1 and 2% of patients refer persistence of pain. Although prosthesis components loosening is responsible for these complications in more than 90% of the cases, there are other potential causes of pain such as heterotopic ossification, muscle and tendon pain around the prosthesis, impingement and radiating back pain. In 1% of the cases the cause of pain remains unknown (Witvoët, 2001).
There is a clear similarity between the aforementioned sources of ongoing pain after hip replacement and those reported in relation to persistence of pain after knee replacement. Since 1989, several authors have reported the use of arthroscopy as a diagnostic and therapeutic tool in painful complications of knee implants, Wasilewski being the earliest (Bocell et al., 1991; Johnson et al., 1990; Lawrence & Kan, 1992; Lucas et al., 1999; Markel et al., 1996; Scranton, 2001; Tzagarakis et al., 2001; Wasilewski & Frankl, 1989a, 1989b). The use of arthroscopy in selected patients with hip implants represents a step forward in diagnosis and possible treatment of painful, apparently well implanted prostheses (Cuéllar et al., 2009; McCarthy et al., 2009; Bajwa & Villar, 2011). In our hospital environment we have established an arthroscopic protocol for hip implant monitoring, similar to the approach we use in knee replacement patients and indicate arthroscopic surgery in cases in which, despite the prosthesis being apparently well implanted, patients continue to experience pain (Cuéllar et al., 2009).

2. Differential diagnosis

The differential diagnosis of pain following THR is wide and includes intrinsic and extrinsic causes to the implant. Septic or aseptic loosening is the cause of intrinsic complications in more than 90% of cases, but there are other potential causes such as stress fractures, mechanical failure or elasticity of the implant itself, subluxation or impingement (Bozic & Rubash, 2004; Smith & Rorabeck, 1999). Additionally there are other extrinsic causes of pain including lumbar radicular pain, neurogenic or vascular claudication (Beck, 2009), heterotopic ossification, trochanteritis or trochanteric non-union (Brown & Callaghan, 2008), peripheral nerve lesions (Malik et al., 2007), tendon and muscle pain around the implant (adductor and iliopsoas tendinitis, arthrofibrosis) (Hyman et al., 1999), femoral or inguinal hernia, and, more rarely, concomitant malignant conditions (Merkel et al., 1985). Finally, in around 1% of cases the source of the pain is never found.
The protocol that we routinely use for differential diagnosis includes a detailed medical history and a thorough clinical examination, laboratory tests (FBC, ESR, and CRP), Radiology investigations (X-rays, CT scan, and scintigraphy) and diagnostic nerve blocks.
Of all the possible causes of pain (Bozic & Rubash, 2004; Smith & Rorabeck, 1999; Witvoët, 2001), we highlight those which we can be addressed using arthroscopy (Table 1): loosening (diagnostic value), tendon pain (iliopsoas, piriformis and plica syndromes or arthrofibrosis)

(Bajwa & Villar, 2011; Beck, 2009; Smith & Rorabeck, 1999), trochanteritis, subluxation and femoroacetabular impingement syndrome (Bajwa & Villar, 2011; Beck, 2009; Bozic & Rubash, 2004; Brown & Callaghan, 2008; Malik et al., 2007; Smith & Rorabeck, 1999), acute and sub-acute infection (Hyman et al., 1999; McCarthy et al., 2009), and pain of unknown origin (Bozic & Rubash, 2004; Witvoët, 2001).

1. Pain associated with the site of surgical approach	Neuralgia Calcification Trochanteritis
2. Pain due to the prosthesis itself	Septic or aseptic loosening "Tip effect"
3. Tendon and muscle pain	Piriformis syndrome Psoas syndrome Arthrofibrosis / plica
4. Neuropathic pain	Algodystrophy
5. Referred pain	Lumbar, vascular…
6. Femoroacetabular impingement	Cam, pincer
7. Acute infection in total hip prosthesis	Acute arthritis
8. Pain of unknown origin	Differential diagnosis

Table 1. **Causes of pain following total Hip Replacement and indications for arthroscopic surgery**. In blue font: Indications for diagnostic hip arthroscopy; in red font: Indications for diagnostic and therapeutic hip; and in black: those conditions which cannot be addressed using arthroscopic surgery

2.1 Prosthesis loosening

A battery of complementary tests is available for its diagnosis. These include blood tests (CRP and ESR), X-rays and particularly scintigraphy.

The combination of scintigraphy tests with Ga^{67}, Tc^{99}, and In^{111}- labelled leukocytes has high sensitivity and specificity for the diagnosis of implant loosening and for distinguishing between septic and aseptic inflammation (Merkel et al., 1985, 1986; Rushton et al., 1982).

We routinely perform arthocentesis and take samples of synovial tissue from three or four areas around the prosthetic joint, as a first stage at the beginning of the surgical procedure. Samples were sent to the Pathology Unit. None of the patients receive antibiotic therapy for at least 5 days prior to the intervention and prophylaxis is not initiated until after the samples were taken. The assessment of signs of loosening is completed by applying force with a blunt-ended instrument to all the prosthetic components in turn and carrying out movements causing leverage under arthroscopy and fluoroscopic control (Fig-1).

2.2 Tendon pain (iliopsoas tendonitis)

Tendon inflammation around the implant is one of the typical causes of pain after THR. Amongst these, iliopsoas tendonitis secondary to hip replacement has a prevalence of up to 4.3% according to several authors (Ala Eddine et al., 2001; Bricteaux et al., 2000; Dora et al., 2007). Various factors can be responsible for iliopsoas inflammation, but particular attention should be drawn to changes in the course of the tendon due to the resection of the femoral head in hip replacement surgery. This modifies the course of the tendon bringing it closer to the medial edge of the prosthetic acetabulum and femoral neck, increasing the probability of impingement (O'Sullivan et al., 2007).

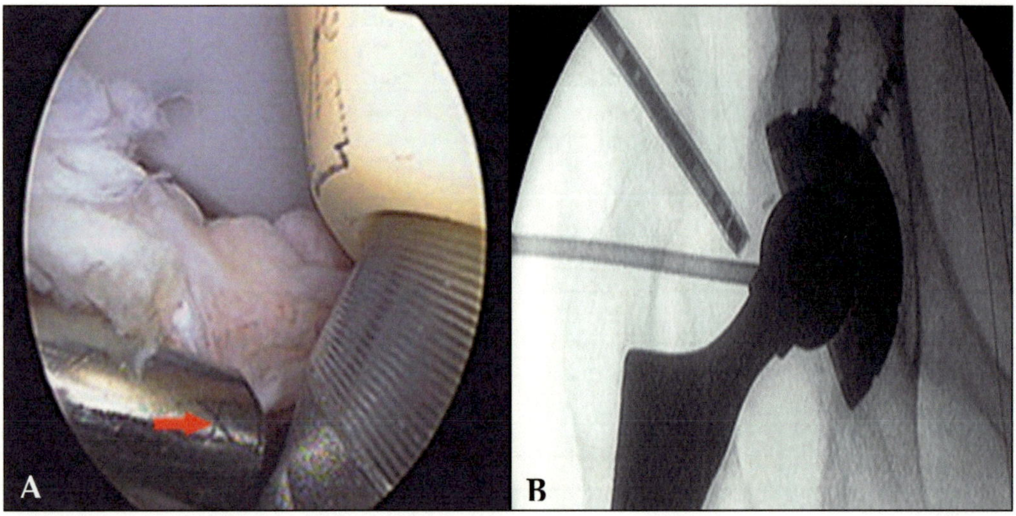

Fig. 1. Assessment of prosthetic component loosening under A) direct visualisation and B) fluoroscopic control.

A main cause of pain is related to the acetabular component being in the wrong position (retroversion and lateralisation) or being too large. Non-cemented hip prostheses tend to have a larger diameter than cemented polyethylene implants, and thus, are more often associated with tendonitis due to iliopsoas impingement (Ala Eddine et al., 2001; Bajwa & Villar, 2011; Bricteaux et al., 2000; Dora et al., 2007; O'Sullivan et al., 2007). Tendonitis may be also caused by extrusion of the cement or by the screw used being too large in relation to the course of the iliopsoas tendon (Jasani et al., 2002; O'Sullivan et al., 2007).

There are other causes which are less common and more difficult to demonstrate such as: impingement on the femoral neck due to the presence of residual anteromedial osteophytes; the shape of certain types of prostheses, which increases the risk of impingement in the transition area between the femoral head and the femoral neck; and increased femoral offset (O'Sullivan et al., 2007).

In a small percentage of cases it is not possible to identify the precise cause of the tendonitis. This may be due to anatomical factors as pointed out by Noble, whose study showed that the proximal femur is flatter in women than in men, a subtle difference that might favour impingement. This theory is supported by the sex ratio of 3:1 (Noble et al., 1995).

Tendonitis should be suspected in the presence of referred pain in the groin during activities requiring active flexion of the hip, especially climbing stairs and getting in and out of cars. In the physical examination, pain will be reproduced on performing movements that stretch the iliopsoas (hyperextension, external rotation) or resisted flexion, as well as internal rotation.

With regards to treatment options, the conservative approach is always considered first, injecting corticosteroids around the tendon under ultrasound guidance (Adler et al., 2005; Ala Eddine et al., 2001; Bricteaux et al., 2000; Dora et al., 2007; O'Sullivan et al., 2007; Wank et al., 2004). However, the degree of clinical improvement varies greatly and this procedure is often unsuccessful (Adler et al., 2005; Ala Eddine et al., 2001; Bricteaux et al., 2000; Cuéllar et al., 2009; Jasani et al., 2002; McCarthy et al., 2009; O'Sullivan et al., 2007). Other therapeutic options include iliopsoas tenotomy by conventional surgical techniques

techniques (Bricteaux et al., 2000; Della Valle et al., 2001; Heaton & Dorr, 2002; Taher & Power, 2003) and, more recently, using arthroscopic techniques (Cuéllar et al., 2009; McCarthy et al., 2009). Iliopsoas tendon lengthening has also been proposed (Trousdale et al., 1995). In some cases, the acetabular component needs to be revised.

2.3 Trochanteritis - Gluteal muscle tears

A frequent cause of pain following hip replacement surgery, commonly associated with Trendelenburg gait pattern. This is more common when a transgluteal approach has been used (Horwitz et al., 1993; Masonis & Bourne, 2002; Nolan et al., 1975; Obrant et al., 1989; Svensson et al., 1990). The pathological findings are very similar to those found in rotator cuff tendons in the shoulder, as has been previously described (Bunker et al., 1997; Kagan, 1999). These include bursitis, tendonitis and other tendon injuries, as well as muscle atrophy.

The diagnosis of these conditions can be reached using modified MRI techniques to minimise the artefacts generated by the implants and performing the imaging using frequency-encoding gradient parallel to the long axis of the prosthesis (Pfirrmann et al., 2005; Twair et al., 2003; White et al., 2000).

In most patients with hip implants some fluid accumulates around the trochanter. Pfirrmann Pfirrmann et al., 2005) reports in his paper that he found a volume than greater than 4 mls of fluid in those patients with pain and a limp. The same paper reports statistics concerning other complications in the trochanteric region related to hip replacement surgery: defects in the gluteus minimus and gluteus medius tendons were found in 56% and 62% symptomatic patients, respectively, compared to in just 8% and 16% of asymptomatic patients; while poor gait was associated with tears larger than 2.5 cm.

MRI allows assessing muscle atrophy and fatty degeneration. As in the shoulder, these signs are a poor prognostic factor. These findings are associated with a Trendelenburg gait and are almost exclusively seen in patients with painful hips (Pfirrmann et al., 2005). Another cause of this gait pattern is a lesion in the superior gluteal nerve, which may result from hip surgery, in particular, when the lateral approach is used. (Ramesh et al., 1996). The approaches that entail greater trochanter osteotomy may cause pain due to non union, failure to remove loose bone fragments or breakage of the wires used in the procedure. Treatment in such cases often requires surgical intervention, although it is possible to remove loose bone fragments and wires using bursoscopy. (Cuéllar et al., 2009).

The treatment of greater trochanter pain syndrome and trochanteric bursitis can also be achieved using bursoscopy (Weber & Berry, 2007). High-grade tears of gluteal tendons may need to be repaired by open surgery (Weber & Berry, 2007), but can also be addressed using arthroscopy.

2.4 Intra-articular adhesions: Arthrofibrosis

This is a common cause of pain following hip surgery (Beck, 2009; Krueger et al., 2007). Any adhesions within the joint capsule or around the femoral neck tend to cause impingement, producing pain and limiting mobility (Krueger et al., 2007). Indeed, such adhesions have been described as a potential cause of pain in relation to hip prostheses. (Bajwa & Villar, 2011; Cuéllar et al., 2009; McCarthy et al., 2009). We reported the presence of structured fibrous bands occupying the medial recess (Fig-2 A,B) (Cuéllar et al., 2009). We also found fibrous structures located between the acetabulum and the prosthetic neck and in wider areas across the new joint (Fig-3 A,B).

The symptoms are similar to those of iliopsoas tendonitis. Patients refer pain in the groin radiating down the inner thigh during activities involving flexion of the hip, such as climbing stairs, but also going down stairs and up or downhill, getting in and out of cars, and turning over in bed . (Beck, 2009; Krueger et al., 2007). There are usually no signs of iliopsoas tendonitis with ultrasound-guided injections, and the response to nerve block tends to be non conclusive or negative.

A definitive diagnosis can be obtained by arthroscopy. Treatment consists of debridement and removal of the adhesions, by the same arthroscopic portal (Cuéllar et al., 2009; Krueger et al., 2007; McCarthy et al., 2009).

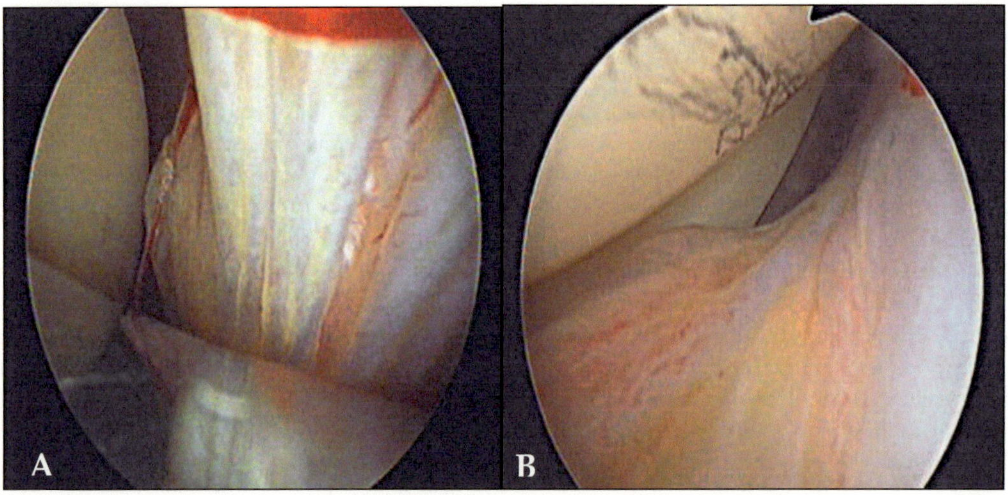

Fig. 2. Structured fibrous bands in the medial compartment: A) medial and B) infero-medial view (righ hip)

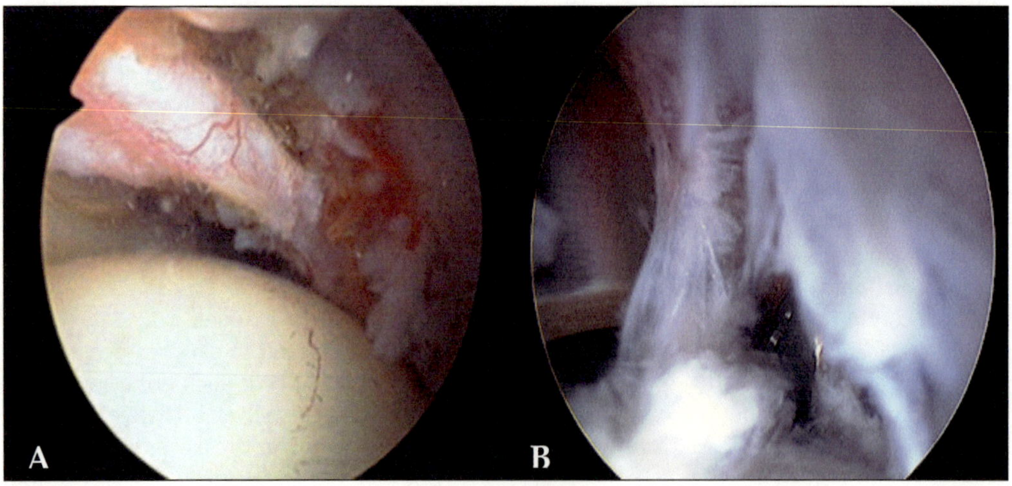

Fig. 3. Fibrosis: A) between the acetabulum and the prosthetic neck; and B) widespread arthrofibrosis

2.5 Femoro-acetabular impingement - Subluxation-Prosthesis dislocation

The principles of impingement in the prosthetic hip are similar to those described by Ganz for the normal hip (Ganz et al., 2003). A cam type impingement is found in implants with small femoral heads that are poorly differentiated from the femoral neck, Pincer type impingement is caused in those hips where there's been inadequate and insufficient removal of osteophytes. Finally, mixed cam-pincer impingement is caused by a combination of having a small femoral head, a ratio between head and neck of less than 2.0, over sizing of the acetabular component, and a polyethylene liner having sharp rather than rounded edges (Malik et al., 2007).

Certain anatomical conditions may increase the risk of prosthetic impingement. It has been reported that very flexible patients have a greater risk of impingement at the extremes of the range of motion (Beaulé et al., 2002; Geller et al., 2006). There is a difference in tilt of the pelvis when the patient is supine on the operating table, and when they are active in movement. This difference tends to lead to an overly horizontal positioning of the acetabular component, which makes impingement more likely (Malik et al., 2007; McCollum & Gray, 1990).

The short term clinical consequences of prosthetic impingement include pain, reduced mobility, instability, subluxation and frank dislocation (Barrack et al., 2001; Barrack, 2003; Brien et al., 1993; Brown & Callaghan, 2008; Cobb et al., 1996; Hedlundh & Carlsson, 1996; Malik et al., 2007; McCollum & Gray, 1990; Padgett et al., 2006). In the longer term, excessive friction between the prosthetic components results in the release of metallic particles and wear of metallic edges which may lead to metallosis and osteolysis. These make early loosening of the implant more likely.

It is not always easy to identify impingement on the basis of patient medical history, clinical examination or radiographic studies, given that it is a dynamic process. Patients with pain and subluxation require CT scans to identify the presence of osteophytes and the relative position and orientation of the components. (Cuéllar et al., 2009; Cuéllar et al., 2010; Pierchon et al, 1994). As we have indicated in previous studies (Cuéllar et al., 2009, 2010), the best way to demonstrate the existence of instability is by Examination Under Anesthesia (EUA) with X ray control (Fig- 4 A,B A,B).

Hip resurfacing implants, having larger femoral heads, offer a greater degree of mobility and stability but the ideal ratio between femoral head and neck is hard to achieve and, therefore, they involve a higher risk of impingement with associated instability (Fig-4 B). (Bajwa & Villar, 2011; Cuéllar et al., 2009; Cuéllar et al., 2010; Khanduja & Villar, 2008).

2.6 Pain of unknown origin - Other causes of pain

In around 1% of the cases the cause of pain remains unknown.

Lumbar spine and radicular pain should be ruled out because of the well known association between degenerative changes in the spine and hip joint. Pain in the gluteal area extending beyond the popliteal region also suggests that it has its origin in the lumbar spine (Bozic & Rubash, 2004; White, 1998). Patients with lumbar spine disorders may experience worsening of radicular pain after hip replacement surgery due to increase in mobility and physical activity (Bozic & Rubash, 2004; Bohl & Steffee, 1979).

Pain that begins when a patient starts walking is commonly associated with loosening, and iliopsoas tendonitis, but it can also be derived from lumbar spine disorders (Bozic & Rubash, 2004; Bohl & Steffee, 1979)

Pain radiating into the upper thigh is associated with loosening of the femoral component, while referred pain in the middle of the thigh is related to the tip of the femoral stem, pressuring the femur. This so called "tip effect" is caused by micro movements of the femoral stem pressuring its surrounding cortical bone bone (Bourne et al., 1994; Bullow et al., 1996; Robbins et al., 2002).

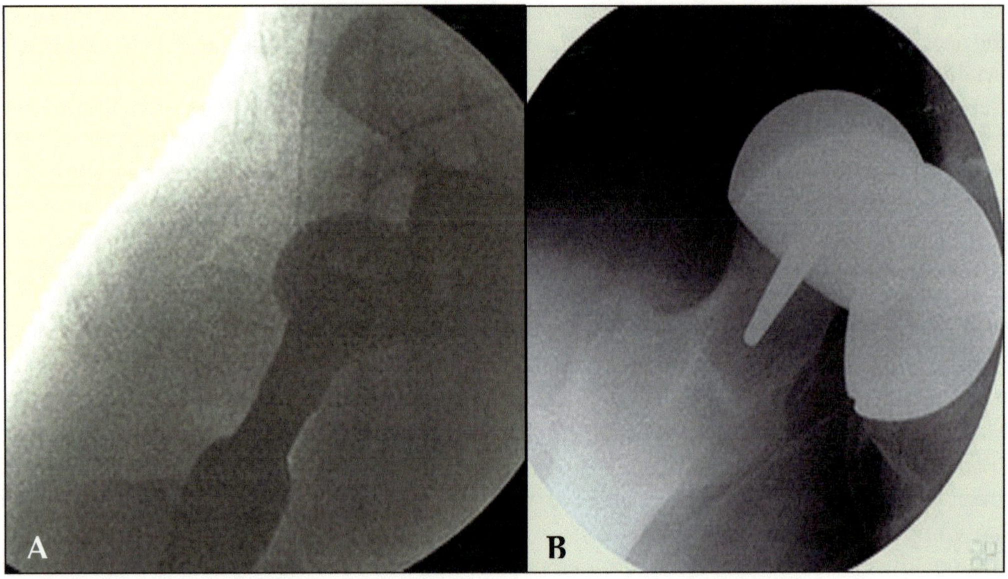

Fig. 4. EUA showing instability of: A) THR and B) in a resurfacing implant

On the other hand, pain in the inguinal or gluteal areas is associated with acetabular loosening, osteolysis and iliopsoas tendonitis. Other less common causes of inguinal pain are: inguinal hernia (Gaunt et al., 1992), inguinal lymphadenopathy, and psoas abscesses, as well as a range of gynaecological and genitourinary disorders (Smith & Rorabeck, 1999).
Continuous pain at rest or at night may also be due to a lumbar spine condition, but in such cases malignancy or sepsis should be ruled out (Bozic & Rubash, 2004; Evans & Cuckler, 1992).
Other factors that may trigger pain are trauma and systemic processes (Bozic & Rubash, 2004). A recent fall may have caused a fracture of the components (in particular, femoral heads and acetabular cups made of alumina) or loosening. The presence of pain after a systemic process, such as dental or gastrointestinal diagnostic or surgical procedures, should make us suspect arthritis (Robbins et al., 2002). Factors that increase the risk of prosthetic infection include obesity, diabetes, rheumatoid arthritis and immunosuppression (Canner et al., 1984).
A detailed history should provide us information and enable a more accurate diagnosis (Bozic & Rubash, 2004).

3. Method of treatment

Patients are referred to our Arthroscopy Unit due to persistence of pain, lack of a clear diagnosis, failure of conservative treatment (physiotherapy, NSAIDs, and psoas ultrasound guided injections) or instability.

In all cases, we complete a diagnostic protocol including a full clinical history, blood tests (FBC, ESR, CRP); imaging tests (X-rays, CT and MRI scans); scintigraphy (Tc, Ga, In labeled leukocytes); and ultrasound-guided psoas injections. In some cases scintigraphy and CT scans are repeated after a period of at least 3 months to rule out implant loosening.
We perform arthroscopic surgery before indicating revision total hip replacement surgery in all cases of persistent pain where the cause of this has not been clearly identified.
Patients fulfil an informed consent form.

3.1 Surgical procedure

The procedure lasts between 60 and 90 minutes.
The anaesthetist selects the most appropriate anaesthetic technique in each case: spinal anaesthesia, general anaesthesia or a combination of both.
The patient lies supine on a traction table, as this facilitates fluoroscopic control of the procedure. In all cases, the procedure is preceded by examination under anaesthesia to assess instability and the presence of "snapping".
Joint distraction is required only in a few cases.
We favour the anterolateral and the anterior arthroscopic portals. Depending on therequirements in each case, the posterior peritrochanteric or another distal anterior portal may be additionally used
To gain access, progressive larger dilatators are slid into position through a nitinol guidewire previously inserted under fluoroscopic control (Fig. 5 A, B).
We routinely follow a three steps protocol 1) collection of samples for culture 2) assessment of the degree of loosening of the components; and 3) assessment and treatment of the condition itself.

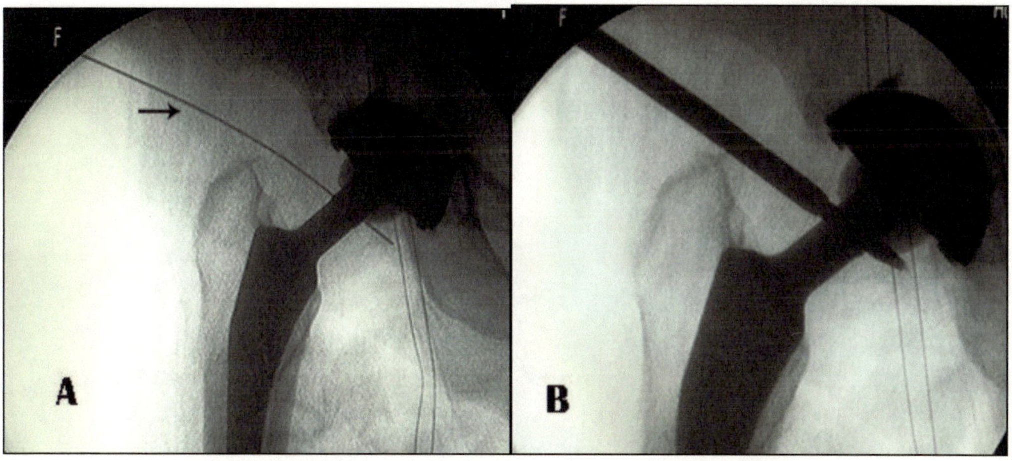

Fig. 5. Introduction of a "nitinol" guide wire under fluoroscopic control (A) Progresive larger dilators are slide into position (B).

3.2 Specific surgical procedures

3.2.1 Psoas tenotomy

The indications for psoas tenotomy are tendonitis or painful internal snapping hip syndrome that have not improved with conservative treatment, in particular with ultrasound-guided steroid injections. We use the same concept and technique as those applied in cases of iliopsoas tendonitis in patients that have not had total hip replacement surgery. As standardised by Ilizaliturri, there are two ways to perform tenotomy (Ilizaliturri et al., 2009): 1) at its site of insertion on the lesser trochanter, and 2) along its course close to the joint. In the latter, the tendon can be partially seen behind the articular capsule or can be directly observed through an orifice that communicates the joint with the iliopectinea bursa.

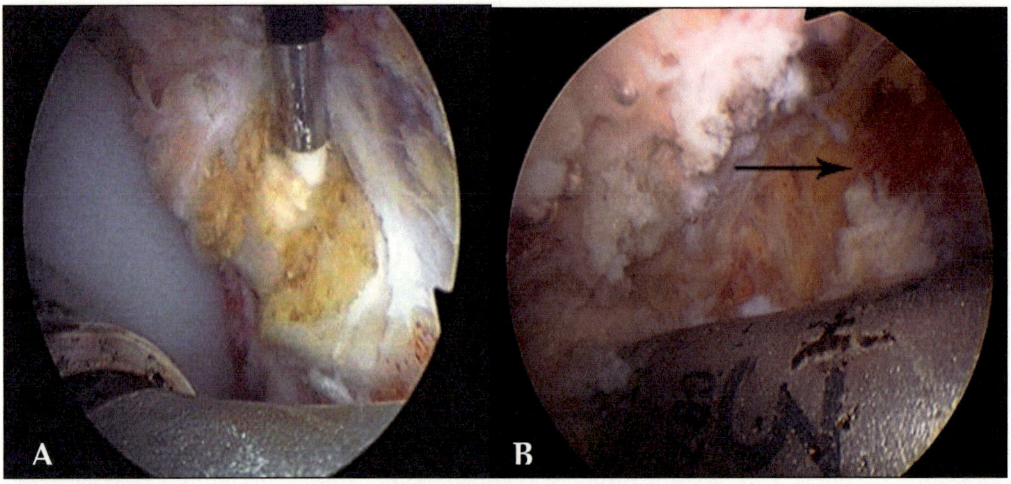

Fig. 6. Psoas tenotomy: Tenotomy at the level of the acetabular rim (A). Release of the tendinous fibres up to the level of the muscle fibres (B)

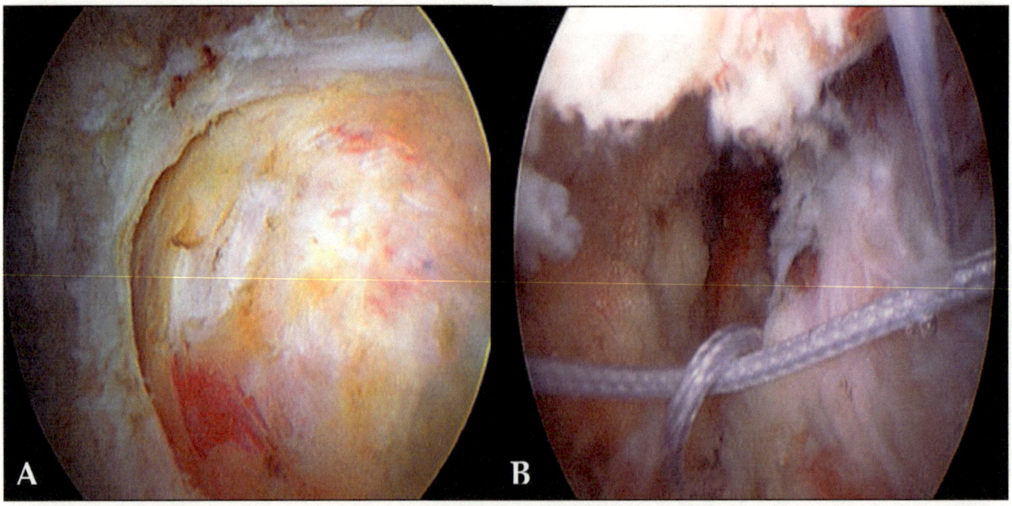

Fig. 7. Gluteal muscle tears in a right hip, seen through the distal peritrochanteric portal: A) similarity to rotator cuff ttears, B) repair with suture anchors

The psoas tendon is divided close to the acetabular component in the cases in which there is evident acetabular involvement (Fig. 6 A, B A, B). If this is not clear, the tenotomy is performed near the lesser trochanter. In any case, only the tendinous fibres are releasd , stopping the intervention when the muscular fibres are reached (Fig. 6 B).

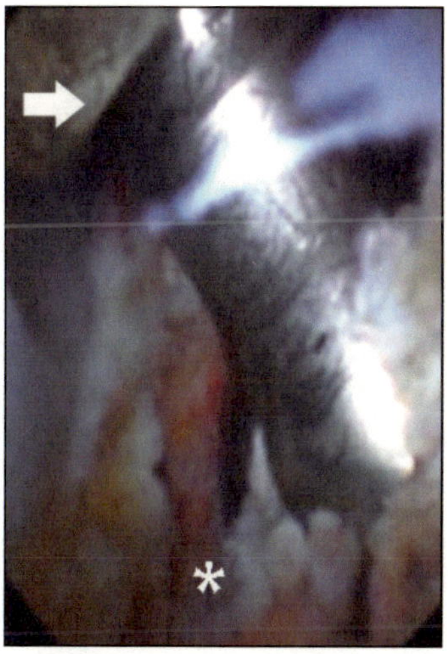

Fig. 8. Impingement of the acetabular rim of the implant on the lesser trochanter (white asterisk) leading to dislocation of this right hip (white arrow)

3.2.2 Trochanterplasty - Gluteal muscle repair

Hip Bursitis and trochanteritis are treated by debridement in the same way as in non prosthetic hips. An early description of a bursectomy using bursoscopy was given by Bradley (Bradley & Dillingham, 1998). Problems related to the peritrochanteric space can be approached from the peripheral compartment or using the inside-outside technique, described by Ilizaliturri. We perform bursoscopy at a second stage following the arthroscopic examinatiooon of the hip joint. For this reason we tend to perform the technique from the peripheral compartment, reorienting the peritrochanteric portal. Aditionaly we use one or two portals, one distal and one proximal to the tip of the trochanter.

A wide range of techniques can be used. These include debridement, trochanteric abrasion, z-tenotomy of the fascia lata and suture using anchors, depending on the condition to be treated. There is a great similarity between gluteus medius and minimus tears with shoulder rotator cuff injuries (Fig. 7 A), It is suspected that that their prevalence is higher than believed to date and that this condition may be responsible for many cases of pain in the trochanter region after hip replacement surgery. Treatment is similar and involves repair by placement of suture anchors (Cuéllar et al., 2010). (Fig. 7 B).

3.2.3 Plica resection for arthrofibrosis

Fibrous structures are a potential cause of pain related to hip replacement surgery (Bajwa & Villar, 2011; Cuéllar et al. 2009; McCarthy et al., 2009). The symptoms in such cases are similar to those of iliopsoas tendonitis: inguinal pain radiating down the inner thigh and pain during activities involving flexion of the hip like climbing stairs and slopes, getting in and out of cars, and turning over in bed among others (Beck, 2009; Krueger et al., 2007).

Often large longitudinal fan shaped fibrous adhesions, occupying the medial recess can be found (Cuéllar et al., 2009). (Fig-2). In these cases, mechanical debridement and thermo coagulation are performed, and any scar tissue around the joint the synovial plica is resected.

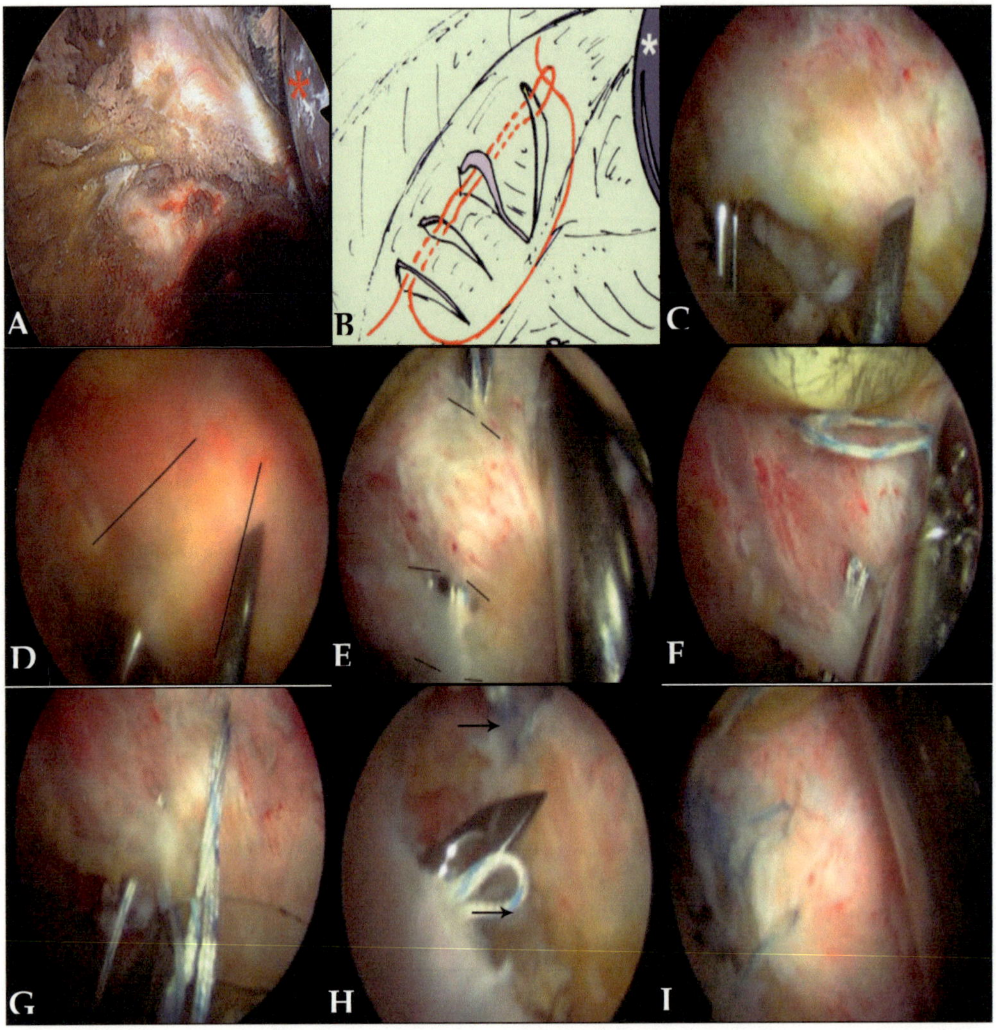

Fig. 9. Capsular plicature technique: A) Redundant capsular tissue in a case of an unstable THR; B) illustration of the technique used in cases of instability, by threading a double no. 2 suture through parallel incisions secured with a loop knot; C) Dissection of the capsular plane from the underlying muscle using a blunt dissector; D) once the capsular plane has been freed; E) two or three parallel incisions are made in the redundant capsule. A double no. 2 suture is threaded in and out through alternate incisions using a bird-beak passer; F) An end loop is left; G) one end of the suture is brought through the end loop and the two ends of the suture are knotted; H) the procedure can be repeated; I) until sufficient reduction of the redundant capsular volume is achieved.

3.2.4 Abrasion for impingement

To date, we have only treated one case of impingement of the edge of the acetabular component on the lesser trochanter. This impingement caused dislocation of the prosthesis (Bajwa & Villar, 2011; Cuéllar et al., 2010). (Fig-8). Preoperative investigations (X-ray and CT scan) showed a short femoral neck leading to cam impingement with a head/neck ratio <2.
Arthroscopy-guided exploration confirmed the presence of impingement between the lesser trochanter and the inferior edge of the acetabulum in external rotation which caused prosthesis dislocation and left redundant capsular tissue in the anterior and lateral recesses. The bone across all the contact area between the lesser trochanter and the prosthetic acetabulum was shaved away until the impingement disappeared. This was combined with capsulorraphy, as described below.

3.2.5 Capsular plicature

In cases of instability, plication of redundant capsular tissue is performed. This is achieved by threading a double no. 2 suture through parallel incisions in the capsule secured with a loop knot, in a similar manner to the technique described for the treatment of instability of a non-prosthetic hip (Shindle et al., 2006; Tibor & Sekiya, 2008). (Fig. 9).
Surgery is indicated after failure of conservative treatment with Physiotherapy and muscle strength rehabilitation focussed in the trochanteric and pelvic region.
A CT scan should be carried out to confirm that there is no significant acetabular anteversion or retroversion nor signs of prosthetic components loosening.
Before proceeding with surgery, a EUA is carried out under X ray control looking for instability or snapping.
The main operative finding often is the presence of a large capsular recess generally located in the lateral and posterior aspects of the hip joint (Fig. 9 A, B). Capsular plicature is preceded by dissecting the capsular plane from the underlying muscle (Fig. 9 C, D), using a blunt dissector. In the posterior recess, this is carried out through a posterior and lateral approach and supported in the muscular plane of the lateral rotator group of muscles (obturator externus, gemelli). The sciatic nerve runs laterally and is protected by this muscular plane. In the anterior plane, we dissect the capsular plane from the rectus femoris. Once the capsular plane to be plicated has been freed, we make two or three parallel incisions with a scalpel. Through these, we thread a double no. 2 suture in and out using a bird-beak passer leaving an end loop (Fig. 9 E). Subsequently, one end of the suture is brought through the end loop. Finally, the two ends of the suture are knotted, gathering up the redundant capsular volume, like a tobacco pouch" (Fig. 9 F, G). The procedure can be repeated in other regions of the capsule as many times as necessary to obtain sufficient reduction of the redundant capsular volume (Fig. 9 H, I). During this procedure laxity is checked until all signs of instability have disappeared.
In the postoperative period no orthosis is usually required. Patients are, however, given guidance concerning how to avoid movements that might cause new dislocations and instructed to perform exercises to strengthen the glutei muscles. Patients are discharged 24 to 48 hours after surgery

4. Clinical evidence

In our experience, it was possible to gain access to the prosthetic joint with the arthroscopic instruments in all cases. This was technically more demanding in cases of arthrofibrosis

where the fibrous bands make the cavity difficult to visualize and therefore more time is required to perform the debridement procedure.
At follow up, three months after surgery, patients that underwent psoas tenotomy had recovered the range of hip flexion to grade 4 and by 6 months all patients had regained grade 5 strength.
We have found that patients with lumbar spine disorders experience more back and radiating leg pain after having their painful prosthetic hips treated.
In all the cases of capsulorraphy the instability and the episodes of subluxation had disappeared. This was maintained at the 6-month and 1-year follow-ups. None of the patients had to undergo further surgery in relation to their hip replacement. They were given instructions to avoid hip flexion of more than 100°, especially together with external rotation and adduction.
We have not observed any neurovascular complications.

5. Discussion

In 1% of the cases the reason for the persistence of pain following hip replacement surgery remains unknown (Witvoët, 2001). Despite this, the cause of pain should always be investigated and we should not rush in carrying out revision surgery (Witvoët, 2001). This is where arthroscopy plays an important role enabling a progress in the diagnosis and a potential treatment in certain patients whose prostheses, although apparently properly implanted, continue to cause pain (McCarthy et al., 2009). This is already being used as a diagnostic and therapeutic tool in some painful complications associated with total knee replacements (Bocell et al., 1991; Johnson et al., 1990; Lawrence & Kan, 1992; Lucas et al., 1999; Markel et al., 1996; Scranton, 2001; Tzagarakis et al., 2001; Wasilewski & Frankl, 1989a, 1989b).
Access can be gained to the prosthetic joint using the arthroscopic technique and instruments. It is possible to apply this to resurfacing type prostheses, as indicated in the only paper that we found on this topic (Khanduja & Villar, 2008).
We favour capsular plication using sutures rather than thermal methods.
Regarding the use of ultrasound-guided steroid injections into the psoas (Adler et al., 2005; Ala Eddine et al., 2001; Bricteaux et al., 2000; Dora et al., 2007; O'Sullivan et al., 2007; Wank et al., 2004), we believe that this technique has few advantages: it is not easy to perform; and in our opinion doesn´t provide much information, even in cases in which it was clear intraoperatively that there was tendon involvement. The outcomes reported in the literature are very variable and it is often not successful (Adler et al., 2005; Ala Eddine et al., 2001; Bricteaux et al., 2000; Cuéllar et al., 2009; Jasani et al., 2002; McCarthy et al., 2009; O'Sullivan et al., 2007; Witvoët, 2001). For this reason, we recommend that this technique is not used systematically, but rather only in selected cases.
It is possible to perform endoscopy-guided trochanteric bursoscopy and fasciotomy. Additionally, if necessary, gluteal muscle repair can be performed.
To date we have not treated any patients with acute or subacute arthritis, but we believe that the arthroscopy technique could be used in such cases, similarly to when indicated in infected total knee replacements (Hyman et al., 1999; McCarthy et al., 2009).
To avoid prosthetic dislocation in the immediate postoperative period, unnecessary wide capsulotomies should not be done, and the patents should be given clear instructions about postural training (Cuéllar et al., 2009).

6. Conclusions

Arthroscopy can be successfully applied to the diagnosis and treatment of pain of unknown origin after hip replacement surgery. This very often associated with lumbar spine disorders, other medical conditions and old age. This association makes the differential diagnosis difficult.

The technique has proven to be especially useful in the treatment of instability, muscular and tendon pain and arthrofibrosis.

On the other hand, the technique has not been found to be reliable for identifying cases of loosening of prosthetic components.

7. References

Adler, R.S.; Buly, R.; Ambrose, R. & Sculco, T. (2005). Diagnostic and therapeutic use of ultrasound-guided psoas peritendinous injections. *American Journal of Roentgenology*, Vol. 185, (2005), pp. (940-943), DOI:10.2214 AJR.04.1207.

Ala Eddine, T.; Remy, F.; Chantelot, C.; Giraud, F.; Migaud, H. & Duquennoy, A. (2001). Anterior iliopsoas impingement alter total hip arthroplasty: diagnosis and conservative treatment in 9 cases. *Revue de Chirurgie Orthopédique et Reparatrice de L'Appareil Moteur*, Vol.87, (2001), pp. (815-819), ISSN 0035-1040.

Bajwa, A.R. & Villar, S.N. (2011). Arthroscopy of the hip in patients following joint replacement. *Journal of Bone and Joint Surgery Br*, Vol.93, No.4, (2011), pp. (890-896), DOI 10.1302/0301-620X.93B7.24902.

Barrack, R.L., Butler, R.A. Laster, D.R. & Andrews, P. (2001). Stem desing and dislocation after revision total hip arthroplasty: clinical results and computer modeling. *The Journal of Arthroplasty*, Vol. 16, No. 8 SI, (2001), pp. (S8-S12), DOI 10.1054/ARTH 2001.28359

Barrack, R.L. (2003). Dislocation after total hip arthroplasty: implant design and orientation. *Journal of American Academy of Orthopaedic Surgeons*, Vol. 11, N° 2, (2003), pp. (89-99), PMID 12670135.

Beaulé, P.E.; Schmalzriued, T.P.; Udomkiat, P. & Amstutz, H.C. (2002). Jumbo femoral head for the treatment of recurrent dislocation following total hip replacement. *Journal of Bone and Joint Surgery Am*, Vol. 84, N° 2, (2002), pp. (256-263), PMID 11861732.

Beck, M. (2009). Groin pain alter open FAI surgery. *Clinical Orthopaedics and Related Research*, No.467, (2009), pp. (769-774), ISSN 0009-921X.

Bohl, W. & Steffee, A. (1979). Lumbar spinal stenosis: a cause of continued pain and disability in patients after total hip arthroplasty. *Spine*, Vol. 4, N° 2, (1979), pp. (168-173), ISSN 0362-2436.

Bourne, R.B.; Rorabeck, C.H., Ghazal, M.E. & Lee, M.H. (1994). Pain in the thigh following total hip replacement with a porous-coated anatomic prosthesis for osteoarthrosis. *Journal of Bone and Joint Surgery Am*, Vol. 76, N° 10, (1994), pp. (1464-1470), PMID 7929493.ñ¡.

Bocell, J.R.; Thorpe, C.D. & Tullos, H.S. (1991). Arthroscopic treatment of symptomatic total knee arthroplasty. *Clinical Orthopaedics and Related Research*, No.271, (October 1991), pp. (125-134), ISSN 0009-921X.

Bozic, K.J. & Rubash, H.E. (2004). The painful total hip replacement. *Clinical Orthopaedics and Related Research*, No.420, (2004), pp. (18-25), ISSN 0009-921X.

Bradley, D.M. & Dillingham, M.F. (1998). Bursoscopy of the trochanteric bursa. *The Journal of Arthroscopy and Related Surgery*, Vol. 14, N° 8, (1998), pp. (884-887), ISSN 0749-8063/98/1408-1810.

Bricteaux, S.; Seutin, B.; Beguin, L.; Farizon, F. & Fessy, M.-H. (2000). Arthroplastie totale de hanche doloreuse; rechercher les conflicts avec le psoas: A propos de 10 cas. *Revue de Chirurgie Orthopédique et Reparatrice de L'Appareil Moteur*, Vol.86 (S-II), (2000), pp. (SII 84-85), ISSN 0035-1040.

Brien, W.W., Salvati, E.A.; Wright, T.M. & Burstein, A.H. (1993). Dislocation following THA: comparison of two acetabular component designs. *Orthopedics*, Vol. 16, N° 8, (1993), pp. (869-872), PMID 8415270.

Brown, T. & Callaghan, J.J. (2008). Impingement in total hip replacement: mechanism and consequences. *Current Orthopaedics*, Vol.22, No.6, (December 2008), pp. (376-391), DOI:10.1016.

Bullow, J.U.;.Scheller, G.; Arnold, P.; Synastchke, M. & Jani, L. (1996). Uncemented total hip replacement and thigh pain. *International Orthopaedics*, Vol. 20, N° 2, (1996), pp. (56-69) PMID 8739695.

Bunker, T.D.; Esler, C.N. & Leach, W.J. (1997). Rotator-cuff tear of the hip. *Journal of Bone and Joint Surgery Br*, Vol.79, No.4, (1997), pp. (618-620), ISSN 0301-620X/97/47033.

Burman, M.S. (1931). Arthroscopy or the direct visualization of joints. *Journal of Bone and Joint Surgery*, Vol.4, (1931), pp. (669-695).

Byrd, J.W.T. (1994). Hip arthroscopy utilizing the supine position. *The Journal of Arthroscopy and Related Surgery*, Vol.10, No.3, (June 1994), pp. (275-280), ISNN 0749-8063.

Byrd, J.W.T. (2006). Hip arthroscopy: Surgical indications. *The Journal of Arthroscopy and Related Surgery*, Vol.22, No.12, (December 2006), pp. (1260-1262), ISSN 0749-8063-062212-6404.

Byrd, J.W.T. & Jones, K.S. (2009). Hip arthroscopy for labral pathology: Prospective analysis with 10-year follow-up. *The Journal of Arthroscopy and Related Surgery*, Vol.25, No.4, (April 2009), pp. (365-368), ISSN 0749-8063-09.

Canner, G.C.; Steinberg, M.E.; Heppenstall, R.B. & Balderston, R. (1984). The infected hip after total hip arthroplasty. *Journal of Bone and Joint Surgery Am*, Vol. 66, N° 9, (1984), pp. (1393-1399), ISSN 0021-9355.

Cuéllar, R.; Aguinaga, I.; Corcuera, I. & Baguer, A. (2009). Artroscopia en prótesis de cadera: resultados preliminares (en español original). *Cuadernos de Artroscopia*, Vol.16, No.2, (October 2009), pp. (35-42), ISNN 1134-7872.

Cuéllar, R., Aguinaga, I., Corcuera, I.; Ponte, J. & Usabiaga, J. (2010). Arthroscopic treatment of unstable Total Hip Replacement. *The Journal of Arthroscopy and Related Surgery*, Vol.26, No.6, (June 2010), pp. (861-865), ISNN 0749-8063-9564, DOI 10.1016.

Cobb, T.K.; Morrey, B.F. & Ilstrup, D.M. (1996). The elevated-rim acetabular liner in total hip arthroplasty: relationship to postoperative dislocation. *Journal of Bone and Joint Surgery Am*, Vol. 78, N° 1, (1996), pp. (80-86), ISSN 0021-9355.

Della Valle, C.J.; Rafii, M. & Jaffe, W.L. (2001). Iliopsoas tendonitis after total hip arthroplasty. *The Journal of Arthroplasty*, Vol.16, No.7, (2001), pp. (923-926), PMID 11607911.

Dora, C.; Houweling, M.; Koch, P. & Sierra, R.J. (2007). Iliopsoas impingement alter total hip replacement. The resuilts of non-operative Management, tenotomy or acetabular revision. *Journal of Bone and Joint Surgery Br*, Vol.89, No.8, (2007), pp. (1031-1035), ISSN 0301-620X.

Erikson, E.; Arvidsson, I. & Arvidsson, H. (1986). Diagnostic and operative arthroscopy of the hip. *Orthopedics*, Vol.9, No.2, (1986), pp. (169-176), PMID 3960759.

Evans, B.G. & Cuckler, J.M. (1992). Evaluation of the painful total hip arthroplasty. *The Orthopedic Clinics of North America*, Vol. 23, N° 2, (1992), pp. (303-311), PMID 1570142.

Ganz, R.; Parvizi, J.; Beck, M., Leunig, M.; Notzil, H. & Siebenrock, K.A. (2003). Acetabular impingement: a cause for osteoarthritis of the hip. *Clinical Orthopaedics and Related Research*, No.417, (2003), pp. (112-120), ISSN 0009-921X..

Gaunt, M.; Tan, S. & Dias, J. (1992). Strangulated obturator hernia masquerading as pain from a total hip rcplacement. *Journal of Bone and Joint Surgery Br*, Vol.74, N° 5, (1992), pp. (782-783), ISSN 0301-620X/92/5R61.

Geller, J.A.; Malchau, H.; Bragdon, C.; Greene, M. et al. (2006). Large diameter femoral heads on highly cross-linked poyethilene: minimum 3-year results. *Clinical Orthopaedics and Related Research*, No.447, (2006), pp. (53-59), ISSN 0009-921X.2006.

Glick, J.M.; Sampson, T.G.; Gordon, R.B.; Behr, J.T. & Schmidt, E. (1987). Hip arthroscopy by the lateral approach. *The Journal of Arthroscopy and Related Surgery*, Vol.3, (1987), pp. (4-12), ISNN 0749-8063.

Gross, R.H. (1977). Arthroscopy in hip disorders in children. *Orthopaedic Review*, Vol.6, (1977), pp. (43-49).

Heaton, K. & Dorr, L.D. (2002). Surgical release of iliopsoas tendon for groin pain after total hip arthroplasty. *The Journal of Arthroplasty*, Vol.17, No.6, (2002), pp. (779-781), DOI 10.1054/ARTH.2002.33570.

Hedlundh,U. & Carlsson, A.S. (1996). Increased risk of dislocation with collar reinforced modular heads of the Lubinus SP-2 hip prosthesis. *Acta Orthopaedica Scandinavica*, Vol. 67, N° 2, (1996) pp. (204-205), PMID 8623583.

Horwitz, B.R.; Rockowitz, N.L.; Goll, S.R.; Booth, R.E. Jr.; Balderston, R.A.; Rothman, R.H. & Cohn, J.C. (1993). A prospective randomized comparison of two surgical approaches to total hip arthroplasty. *Clinical Orthopaedics and Related Research*, No.291, (1993), pp. (154-163), ISSN 0009-921X.

Hyman, J.L., Salvati, E.A., Laurencin, C.T.; Rogers, D.E.; Maynard, M. & Brause, B.D. (1999). The arthroscopic drainage, irrigation, and débridement of late, acute total hip arthroplasty infections. *Journal of Arthroplasty*; Vol.14, No.8, (December 1999), pp. (903-910), PMID 10614878.

Jasani, V.; Richards, P. & Wynn-Jones, C. (2002). Pain related to the psoas muscle after total hip replacement. *Journal of Bone and Joint Surgery Am*, Vol.84, No.8, (2002), pp. (991-993), ISSN 00219355.

Johnson, D.R.; Friedman, R.J.; McGinty, J.B.; Mason, J.L. & St Mary, E.W. (1990). The role of arthroscopy in the problema total knee replacement. *The Journal of Arthroscopy and Related Surgery,* Vol.6, No.1, (March 1990), pp. (31-32), ISNN 0749-8063.

Johnston, T.L.; Schenker, M.L.; Briggs, K.K. & Philippon, M.J. (2008). Relationship between offset angle alpha and hip chondral injury in femoroacetabular impingement. *The Journal of Arthroscopy and Related Surgery,* Vol.24, No.6, (June 2008), pp. (669-675), ISSN 0749-8063-08-2406-7302.

Kagan, A. (1999). 2nd rotator cuff tears of the hip. *Clinical Orthopaedics and Related Research,* No.368, (1999), pp. (135-140), ISSN 0009-921X.

Khanduja, V. & Villar, R.N. (2008). The role of arthroscopy in resurfacing arthroplasty of the hip. *The Journal of Arthroscopy and Related Surgery,* Vol.24, No.1, (January 2008), pp. (122e1), ISNN 0749-8063-08-2401-6501.

Kelly, B.T.; Williams, R.J. III & Philippon, M.J (2003). Hip Arthroscopy: Current Indications, Treatment Options, and Management Issues. *The American Journal of Sports Medicine,* Vol.31, No.6, (November/December 2003), pp. (1020-1037), ISSN 0363-5465-103-3131-1020.

Kocher, M.S.; Kim, Y.J.; Millis, M.B.; Mandiga, R.; Siparsky, P.; Micheli, L.J. & Kasser, J.R. (2005). Hip arthroscopy in children and adolescents. *Journal of Pediatric Orthopaedics,* Vol.25, No.5, (2005), pp. (680-686), PMID 16199955.

Krueger,A.; Leunig, M.; Siebenrock, K.A. & Beck, M. (2007). Hip arthroscopy after previous surgical hip dislocation for femoroacetabular impingement. *The Journal of Arthroscopy and Related Surgery;* Vol. 23, N° 12, (2007), pp. (1285-1289), ISSN 0749-8063/07/2312-6610.

Ilizaliturri, V.M.; Chaidez, C.; Villegas, P.; Briceño, A. & Camacho-Galindo, J. (2009). Prospective randomized study of 2 different techniques for endoscopio iliopsoas tendon release in the treatment of internal snapping hip síndrome. *The Journal of Arthroscopy and Related Surgery,* Vol. 25, N° 2, (2009), pp. (159-163), ISSN 0749-8063/09/2502-8171.

Ilizaliturri, V.M.; Martínez-Escalante, F.A.; Chaidez, P.A. & Camacho-Galindo, J. (2006). Endoscopio iliotibial band release for externa snapping hip síndrome. *The Journal of Arthroscopy and Related Surgery,* Vol. 22, N° 5, (2006), pp. (505-510), ISSN 0749-8063/06/2205-5156.

Larson, C.M.; Guanche, C.A.; Kelly, B.T.; Clohisy, J.C. & Ranawat, A.S. (2009). Advanced techniques in hip arthroscopy. *Journal of American Academy of Orthopaedic Surgeons, Instructional Course Lecture,* Vol. 58, (2009), pp. (423-436), PMID 19385552.

Larson, C.M. & Giveans, M.R. (2009), Arthroscopic debridement versus refixation of the acetabular labrum associated with femoroacetabular impingement. *The Journal of Arthroscopy and Related Surgery,* Vol.25, No.4, (April 2009), pp. (369-376), ISSN 0749-8063-09-2504-8590.

Lawrence, S.J. & Kan, R.O. (1992). Arthroscopic lysis of adhesions after New Jersey LCS total knee arthroplasty. *Orthopedics,* Vol.15, No.8, (August 1992), pp. (943-944), PMID 1508769.

Lubowitz, J.H. & Poehling, G.G. (2006). Hip Arthroscopy: An Emerging Gold Standard. *The Journal of Arthroscopy and Related Surgery,* Vol. 22, No.12, (December 2006), pp. (1257-1259), ISSN 0749-8063-06-2212-1780.

Lucas, T.S.; DeLuca, P.F.; Nazarian, D.G.; Bartolozzi, A.R. & Booth, R.E. Jr (1999). Arthoscopic treatment of patellar clunk. *Clinical Orthopaedics and Related Research*, No.367, (1999), pp. (226-229), ISSN 0009-921X.

Malik, A.; Maheshwari, A. & Dorr, L.D. (2007). Impingement with total hip replacement. *Journal of Bone and Joint Surgery Am*, Vol.89, No.8, (2007), pp. (1832-1842), ISSN 00219355.

Markel, D.C.; Luessenhop, C.P.; Windsor, R.E. & Sulco, T.A. (1996). Arthroscopic treatment of peripatellar fibrosis alter total knee arthroplasty. *Journal of Arthroplasty*, Vol.11, No.3, (April 1996), pp. (293-297), PMID 8713909.

Masonis, J.L. & Bourne, R.B. (2002). Surgical approach, abductor function, and total hip arthroplasty dislocation. *Clinical Orthopaedics and Related Research*, No.405, (2002), pp. (46-53), ISSN 0009-921X.

McCarthy, J.C., Jibodh, S.R. & Lee, J.A. (2009). The role of arthroscopy in evaluation of painful hip arthroplasty. *Clinical Orthopaedics and Related Research*, No.467, (2009), pp. (174-180), ISSN 0009-921X.

McCollum, D.E. & Gray, W.J. (1990). Dislocation after total hip arthroplasty. Causes and prevention. *Clinical Orthopaedics and Related Research*, No.261, (1990), pp. (159-170), ISSN 0009-921X.

Merkel, K.D.; Brown, M.L.; Dewanjee, M.K. & Jr Fitzgerald, R.H. (1985). Comparison of indium-labeled-leucocyte imaging with sequential technetium-gallium sacanning in the diagnosis of low-grade musculkoskeletal sepsis: A prospective study. *Journal of Bone and Joint Surgery Am*, Vol.67, No.3, (1985), pp. (465-476), ISSN 00219355.

Merkel, K.D.; Brown, M.L. & Jr Fitzgerald, R.H. (1986). Sequential technetium99m HMDP-gallium-67 citrate imaging for the evaluation of infection in the painful prosthesis. *Journal of Nuclear Medicine*, Vol. 27,(1986), pp. (1413-1417).McCarthy, J.C. & Lee, J.A. (2006). Hip arthroscopy: indications, outcomes and complications. *American Academy of Orthopaedic Surgeons, Instructional Course Lecture*, Vol.55, (2006), pp. (301-308), PMID16958465.

Monllau, J.C.; Solano, A.; León, A.; Hinarejos, P. & Ballester, J. (2003). Tomographic study of the arthroscopic approaches to the hip joint. *The Journal of Arthroscopy and Related Surgery*, Vol.19, No.4, (April 2003), pp. (368-372), ISNN 0749-8063-03-1904-3152.

Noble, Ph.C.; Box, G.; Kamaric, E.; Fink, M.J.; Alexander, J.W. & Tullos, H.S. (1995). The effect of aging on the shape of th proximal femur. *Clinical Orthopaedics and Related Research*, No.316, (1995), pp. (31-44), ISSN 0009-921X.

Nolan, D.R.; Fitzgerald, R.H.; Jr. Beckenbaugh, R.D. & Coventry, M.B. (1975). Complications of total hip arthroplasty treated by reoperation. *Journal of Bone and Joint Surgery Am*, Vol.57, (1975), pp. (977-981), ISSN 00219355.

Obrant, K.J., Ringsberg, K. & Sanzen, L. (1989). Decreased abduction strength after Charnley hip replacement without trochanteric osteotomy. *Acta Orthopaedica Scandinavica*, Vol. 60, N° 3, pp. (305-307), PMID 2750505.

O'Sullivan,M.; Chin Tai, Ch.; Richards, S.; Skyrme, A.D.; Walter, W.L. & Walter W.K. (2007). Iliopsoas Tendonitis: A complication after total hip arthrosplasty. *The Journal of Arthroplasty*, Vol.22, No.2, (2007), pp. (166-170), ISSN 0883-5403-07-1906-0004.

Padgett, D.E.; Lipman, J., Robie, B. & Nestor, B.J. (2006). Influence of total hip design on dislocation: a computer model and clinical analysis. *Clinical Orthopaedics and Related Research*, No.447, (2006), pp. (48-52), ISSN 0009-921X.

Parisien, J.S. (1988). Arthroscopy Surgery of the hip, In: *Arthroscopic Surgery*, Parisien, J.S. (Ed.), pp. (283-292), McGraw-Hill, Inc., ISBN 0-07-048474-0, U.S.A..

Pfirrmann, Ch.W.A.; Notzli, H.P.; Dora, C.; Hodler, J. & Zanetti, M. (2005). Abductor tendons and muscles assessed at MR imaging after total hip arthroplasty in asymptomatic and symptomatic patients. *Radiology*, Vol.235, (2005), pp. (969-976), DOI 10.1148/radiol.2353040403.

Philippon, M.J.; Stubbs, A.J.; Schenker, M.L.; Maxwell, R.B.; Ganz, R. & Leunig, M. (2007). Arthroscopic management of femoroacetabular impingement: Osteoplasty technique and literature review. *The American Journal of Sports Medicine*, Vol. 35, No.9, (November/December 2007), pp. (1571-1580), ISNN 10-1177-0363546507300258.

Philippon, M.J.; Schenker, M.L.; Briggs, K. & Kuppersmith, D. (2007) Femoroacetabular impingement in 45 professional athletes: Associated pathologies and return to sport following arthroscopic decompresion. *Knee Surgery, Sports Traumatology, Arthroscopy*, Vol.15, No.7, (May 2007), pp. (908-914), DOI 10.1007/s00167-007-0332-x.

Pierchon, F.; Pasquier, G.; Cotton, A.; Fontaine, C. Clarisse, J. & Duquennoy, A. (1994). Causes of dislocation of total hip arthroplasty. CT study of component alignment. *Journal of Bone and Joint Surgery Br*, Vol.76, N° 1, (1994), pp. (45-48), ISSN 0301-620X.

Ramesh, M., O'Byme, J.M.; McCarty, N.; Jarvis, A.; Mahalingham, K. & Cashman, W.F. (1996). Damage to the superior gluteal nerve after the Hardinge approach to the hip. *Journal of Bone and Joint Surgery Br*, Vol.78, No.6, (1996), pp. (903-906), ISSN 0301-620X/96/61289903-906.

Robbins, G.M., Masra, B.A.; Garbuz, D.S. & Duncan, C.P. (2002). Evaluation of pain in patients with apparently solidly fixed total hip arthroplasty components. *Journal of American Academy of Orthopaedic Surgeons*, Vol. 10, N° 2, (2002), pp. (86-94), PMID 11929203.

Roy, D.R. (2009). Arthroscopy of the hip in children and adolescents. *Journal of Children´s Orthopaedic*, Vol.3, No.2, (April 2009), pp. (89-100), DOI 10.1007/s11832-008-0143-8.

Rushton, N.; Coakley, A.J.; Tudor, J. & Wraight, E. (1982). The value of technetium and gallium scanning in assessing pain alter total hip replacement. *Journal of Bone and Joint Surgery Br*, Vol.64, No.3, (1982), pp. (313-318), ISSN 0301-620X-82-3068-0313.

Sampson, T.G. (2006). Arthroscopic treatment of femoroacetabular impingement: a proposed technique with clinical experience. *American Academy of Orthopaedic Surgeons, Instructional Course Lecture*, Vol.55, (2006), pp. (337-346), PMID 16958469.

Scranton, P.E. Jr (2001). Management of knee pain after total knee arthroplasty. *Journal of Arthroplasty*; Vol.16, No.4, (June 2001), pp. (428-435), PMID 11402404.

Shifrin, L.Z. & Reis, N.D. (1980). Arthroscopy of a dislocated hip replacement: a case report. *Clinical Orthopaedics and Related Research*, No.146, (1980), pp. (213-214), ISSN 0009-921X.

Shindle, M.K., Ranawat, A.S. & Kelly, D.T. (2006). Diagnosis and Management of traumatic and atraumatic instability the hip in the athletic patient. *Clinics in Sports Medicine*, Vol. 25, N° 2, (2006), pp. (309-326), PMID 16638494.

Smart, L.R.; Oetgen, M.; Noonan, B. & Medvecky, M. (2007). Beginning hip arthroscopy: indications, positioning, portals, basic techniques and complications. *The Journal of Arthroscopy and Related Surgery*, Vol.23, No.12, (December 2007), pp. (1348-1353), ISSN 0749-8063-07-2312-7252.

Smith, P. & Rorabeck, C. (1999). Clinical evaluation of the symptomatic Total hip Arthrosplasty. In: *Revision Total hip Arthroplasty*, Steinberg, M. & Garino, J. (Eds.), pp. (109-120), Lippincott Williams & Wilkins, Philadelphia.

Svensson, O.; Skold, S. & Blomgren, G. (1990). Integrity of the gluteus medius after the transgluteal approach in total hip arthroplasty. *The Journal of Arthroplasty*, Vol.5, No.1, (1990), pp. (57-60), PMID 2319249.

Taher, R.T. & Power, R.A. (2003). Iliopsoas tendon dysfunction as a cause of pain after total hip arthroplasty relieved by surgical release. *The Journal of Arthroplasty*, Vol.18, No.3, (2003), pp. (387-388), PMID 12728436.

Tibor, L.M. & Sekiya, J.K. (2008). Differential diagnosis of pain around the hip joint. *The Journal of Arthroscopy and Related Surgery*; Vol. 24, N° 12, (2008), pp. (1407-1421), ISSN 0749-8063/08/2412-8249.

Trousdale, R.T.; Cabanela, M.E. & Berry, D.J. (1995). Anterior iliopsoas impingement after total hip arthroplasty. *The Journal of Arthroplasty*, Vol.10, No.4, (1995), pp. (546-549), PMID 8523018.

Twair, A.; Ryan, M.; O'Connell, M.; Powel, T.; O'Byrne, J. & Eustace, S. (2003) MRI of failed total hip replacement caused by abductor mule avulsion. *American Journal of Roentgenology*; Vol. 181, (2003), pp. (1547-1550), DOI 10.2214.

Tzagarakis, G.P.; Papagelopoulos, P.J.; Kaseta, M.A.; Vlamis, J.A.; Makestas, M.A. & Nikolopoulos, K.E. (2001). The role of arthroscopic intervention for symtomatic total knee arthroplasty. *Orthopedics*, Vol.24, No.11, (November 2001), pp. (1090-1997), PMID 11727813.

Vernace, J.V.; Rothman, R.H.; Booth, R.E. Jr & Balderston, R.A. (1989). Arthroscopic Management of the patellar clunk syndrome following posterior stabilized total knee arthroplasty. *Journal of Arthroplasty*; Vol.4, (1989), pp. (179-182), PMID 2746250.

Wank, R.; Miller, T.T. & Shapito, J.F. (2004). Sonographically guided injection of anesthetic for iliopsoas tendinopathy after total hip arthroplasty. *Journal of Clinical Ultrasound*, Vol. 32, N° 3, (2004), pp. (354-357), PMID 15293303.

Wasilewski, S.A. & Frankl, U. (1989). Arthroscopy of the painful dysfunctional total knee replacement. *The Journal of Arthroscopy and Related Surgery*, Vol.5, No.4, (December 1989), pp. (294-297), ISNN 0749-8063.

Wasilewski, S.A. & Frankl, U. (1989). Fracture of polyethylene of patellar component in total knee arthroplasty, diagnosed by arthroscopy. *Journal of Arthroplasty*, Vol.4(S), (1989), pp. (S19-S22), PMID 2584983.

Weber, M. & Berry, D.J. (2007) Abductor avulsion after primary total hip arthroplasty: results of the repair. *The Journal of Arthroplasty*, Vol.22, No.2, (2007), pp. (166-170)1997;12:202-206.

White, R. (1998). Evaluation of the painful total hip arthroplasty. In: *The adult hip*, Callagan, J.; Rosenberg, A. & Rubash, H. (Eds.), pp. (1377-1385), Lippincott-Raven Publishers, Philadelphia.

White, L.M.; Kim, J.K.; Mehta, M., Merchant, N.; Scheweitzer, M.E.; Hutchinson, C.R. & Gross, A.E. (2000). Complications of total hip arthroplasty: MR imaging-Initial experience. *Radiology*, Vol. 215, Nº 1, (2000), pp. (254-262), PMID 10751496.

Witvoët, J. (2001). Diagnostic et conduite à tenir devant une prosthèse totale de hanche douloureuse. In: *Encyclopedie Medico Chirurgica*, Appareil locomoteur, Editions Scientifiques et Médicales, pp. (14-316-A-10). Elsevier SAS, París.

Part 4

Arthroscopy of the Knee

6

Management of Knee Articular Cartilage Injuries

Joshua D. Harris and David C. Flanigan
The Ohio State University Sports Medicine Center and Cartilage Restoration Program
USA

1. Introduction

Articular cartilage is a unique, biologically active tissue. In the knee, it serves as the end-bearing surface for the distal femur and proximal tibia, forming a diarthrodial synovial joint capable of enduring years of impact loading. Made of hyaline cartilage, the near-frictionless surface distributes load throughout motion across 6 degrees of freedom, reducing stress transmission to the underlying subchondral bone. This permits weight-bearing during both activities of daily living and high-impact athletics. In fact, forces in the knee joint may approach 8-times body weight during deep knee bends(Reilly and Martens 1972) and pressures up to 12 MPa during maximal quadriceps contraction(Huberti and Hayes 1984) (a pressure equivalent to being ¾ mile under water). These biomechanical properties rely on compression and deformation, a direct result of the biphasic nature of articular cartilage consisting primarily of water and extracellular matrix. Variation in this tissue's thickness and the joint's radii of curvature further influence biomechanics because of compartmental-specific loading profiles within the tibiofemoral and patellofemoral "joints" of the knee.

Arthroscopic appearance of articular cartilage in the knee (Figure 1a) should display a glistening, smooth, white surface that is firm to manual or instrumented palpation. Any disruption in the smooth surface or the tactile feel is abnormal. The loss of articular cartilage is the *sine qua non* of osteoarthritis. Histologic examination reveals relatively hypocellular tissue that lacks a vascular supply, neural input and output, and lymphatic drainage. These features contribute to the minimal innate healing response of isolated chondral damage and also illustrate the difficulty in making a clinical diagnosis of an isolated chondral defect (Figure 1b). Further, the role of the subchondral bone and its complex interaction with the overlying layered structure of cartilage has been emphasized in recent literature, not only in defect creation and progression, but also in surgical treatments. At the current time, these surgical procedures, cartilage repair and restoration, are designed to prevent and/or delay the initiation and/or progression of osteoarthritis.

2. Anatomy and biomechanics

The knee joint is the largest in the human body. It is a modified hinge allowing motion in the flexion / extension (sagittal), varus / valgus (coronal), and internal / external rotation planes (axial). These motions have both osteocartilaginous and soft tissue ligamentous constraints. The patella articulates with the femoral trochlea and the medial and lateral femoral condyles articulate with the medial and lateral menisci and tibial plateaus. The collateral (medial and lateral collateral, MCL and LCL) and cruciate (anterior and posterior cruciate, ACL and PCL) ligaments are restraints to abnormal motion in one or more planes.

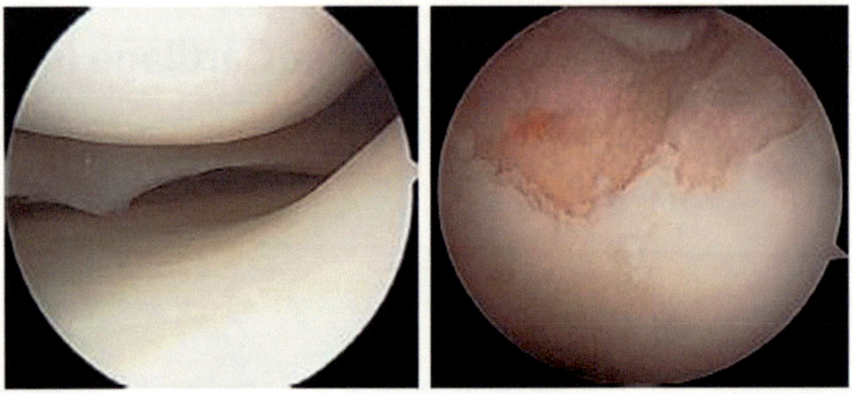

Fig. 1. 1a) Arthroscopic photograph of normal knee articular cartilage demonstrating smooth, white, glistening surface; 1b) Arthroscopic photograph of isolated, full-thickness chondral defect of femoral trochlea.

2.1 Tibiofemoral compartments

Articular cartilage in the tibiofemoral joint articulates with both meniscus and opposing surface articular cartilage. The menisci increase surface contact area, thus reducing stress transmission to the under- or over-lying articular cartilage. Both anatomy and kinematics are significantly different within each of the tibiofemoral compartments(Iwaki, Pinskerova et al. 2000). This asymmetry is reflected in that the lateral compartment tends to axially rotate around a relatively stationary medial compartment with knee flexion.

Kinematically, the medial compartment of the knee operates like a ball (femoral condyle) and socket (tibial plateau and meniscus)(Scott 2005). In the sagittal plane, the medial femoral condyle is composed of two arcs of different radii of curvature and the medial tibial plateau of two angled flat surfaces(Iwaki, Pinskerova et al. 2000). The more anterior surface (extension radius / facet) of the femur has a larger radius than that of the posterior surface (flexion radius / facet). The tibia's angled flats, together with the firmly-attached medial meniscus, create a concavity in which the femoral condyles contact.

Contrary to the medial side, the lateral compartment of the knee has a convex-to-convex articulation in the sagittal plane (Figure 2). Without a lateral meniscus, the lateral compartment operates via nearly point-on-point contact. With a single radius of curvature, the femoral condyle tends to roll back on the tibial plateau, which supports a more loosely-attached lateral meniscus, with knee flexion(Iwaki, Pinskerova et al. 2000). The fixed axis medially combined with greater mobility laterally supports the "screw-home mechanism" of tibial internal rotation with increasing knee flexion(Blankevoort, Huiskes et al. 1988).

Similar to the anatomic asymmetry between the medial and lateral compartments, the biomechanical loading profiles are also unique. In a normal knee, the lateral meniscus covers a greater surface area (~80%) of the plateau than the medial (~60%)(Clark and Ogden 1983), thus transmitting a larger proportion of the axial load while weight-bearing (50% medially versus 70% laterally)(Fukubayashi and Kurosawa 1980; Ahmed and Burke 1983). Following meniscectomy, all load is transmitted through the articular cartilage and the femur - tibia geometrical asymmetry medially versus laterally plays a greater role. This is reflected by the nearly 300% increase in contact stress laterally versus 100% increase medially after total meniscectomy(Kettelkamp and Jacobs 1972; Fukubayashi and Kurosawa 1980). These findings clearly illustrate the chondroprotective role of the menisci in the knee (Figures 3a, 3b).

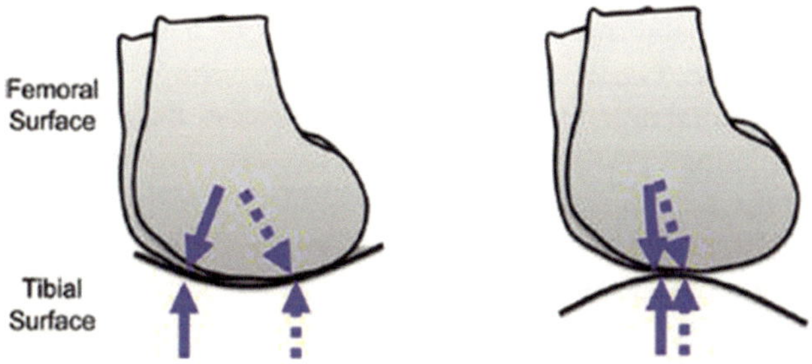

Fig. 2. The "ball-in-socket" schematic of the medial compartment articulation (left); the less congruent, convex-on-convex articulation of the lateral compartment (right) (reproduced with permission from Koo S, Rylander J, Andriacchi T: Knee joint kinematics during walking influences the spatial cartilage thickness distribution in the knee, in *Journal of* Biomechanics 2011; 44(7): 1408. Publisher Elsevier).

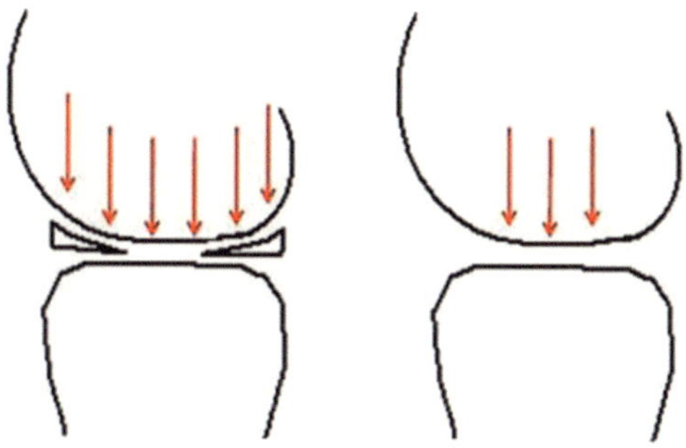

Fig. 3. 3a) Sagittal profile of knee with normal menisci. Axial load distributed across surfaces of menisci and articular cartilage; 3b) Sagittal profile of knee without meniscus. Axial load distributed over articular cartilage only. With same force and smaller area of articulation, increased stress transmitted to articular cartilage.

2.2 Patellofemoral compartments

The patellofemoral articulation consists of the patella, the largest sesamoid in the human body, and the trochlea, a groove located on the anterior distal femur. The patella normally sits within a suprapatellar pouch in full extension and begins to engage the trochlea around 20 to 30 degrees of knee flexion. A vertically-oriented ridge on the articular surface of the patella separates the patella into medial and lateral facets. The superior 75% of the patella is articular cartilage, while the inferior 25% is non-articulating bone. The thickness of the articular cartilage in the patella can be the thickest in the human body, up to 5- or 6-mm (Scott 2005). This portends the ability to withstand high joint reactive forces seen in the patellofemoral articulation. The trochlea is separated into medial and lateral facets by a vertically-oriented trough that continues inferiorly into the intercondylar notch. The lateral facet of the trochlea extends anteriorly slightly more than that of the medial facet, providing a lateral buttress to patellar instability. The bony articular congruity attained by the patella and trochlea provides inherent static stability to the patellofemoral articulation.

The biomechanics of the patellofemoral joint are dependent upon both bony and soft tissue constraints. The patella engages the trochlea at approximately 20 degrees of knee flexion. At this position, the medial patellofemoral ligament functions as a primary restraint to lateral patellar translation(Conlan, Garth et al. 1993). With increasing flexion, the patella contacts the trochlea via a horizontal area of contact. Near extension, the inferior articular surface of the patella is "articulating." With increasing flexion, the horizontal contact area moves further proximal on the patella until this area is divided into two separate areas of contact on the medial and lateral femoral condyles at around 120 degrees of flexion. Contact pressure in the patellofemoral joint is greatest between 60 and 90 degrees of flexion, with maximum pressures of up to 12 MPa attained during forceful extensor mechanism quadriceps contractions(Huberti and Hayes 1984).

2.3 Microscopic anatomy

The microscopic composition of articular cartilage appears as a highly-organized, layered system of cells and extracellular matrix (ECM). The chondrocyte is the only cell present in articular cartilage and occupies only 5% of its total volume(Lieberman 2009). Thus, this cell is exclusively responsible for maintenance of the ECM. It receives its nutrition from synovial fluid diffusion from the interior of the joint. Embedded within the ECM, the chondrocyte is relatively immunoprivileged. This isolation also accompanies a lack of vascular or nerve connections, or lymphatic drainage. Thus, cartilage has a limited innate healing capacity.

Articular cartilage can be broadly grouped into two separate layers of uncalcified and calcified cartilage (Figure 4). More superficially, the uncalcified region may be divided into three zones: Superficial (tangential), transitional (or intermediate / middle), and deep (or radial). The superficial zone contains thin, elongated chondrocytes and collagen fibrils that parallel the articular surface. The primary function of this layer is tensile strength. An acellular clear film composed of collagen fibrils, the lamina splendens, is the articulating surface of the superficial zone visible upon gross or arthroscopic inspection. Given its proximity to the joint surface, the water content in the superficial zone is not surprisingly the highest amongst the layers (~80%). Proteoglycan content is lowest in this zone.

The transitional zone occupies approximately 50% of the thickness of uncalcified cartilage. This intermediate layer demonstrates thicker, more obliquely oriented collagen fibers. Compared to the superficial zone, the transitional zone has less water and collagen and greater proteoglycan content. Further, chondrocytes in this zone are more round with higher metabolic activity, evidenced by increasing numbers of intracellular organelles like mitochondria, endoplasmic reticulum, and Golgi membranes(Scott 2005).

The deep zone has the lowest water content (65%) of the uncalcified cartilage layers, reflecting its distance from the articular surface. Although the collagen content is lowest, the fiber diameter is greatest in this zone. The fibers are oriented perpendicular to the joint surface, anchoring the uncalcified cartilage layers to the calcified cartilage zone beneath across the undulating tidemark, the threshold of vascular penetration of the underlying subchondral bone. Proteoglycan content is highest in the deep zone. Chondrocytes are round and arranged in vertical columns.

The calcified cartilage zone is a vascularized layer deep to the tidemark. This zone has a high calcium mineral content and low proteoglycan content. Although most of the collagen in articular cartilage is Type II (90% - 95%), there is a small amount of Type X collagen found in this zone, as it is associated with hypertrophic chondrocytes and calcification of cartilage. Beneath the calcified cartilage layer, separated by a thin cement line, is the subchondral bone, consisting of a lamellar cortical bony endplate and underlying cancellous trabeculae(Madry, van Dijk et al. 2010).

Chondrocytes produce the entirety of the content of the ECM, including proteoglycans, collagen, and non-collagenous proteins. Although proteoglycans represent only approximately 10% of the dry weight of articular cartilage, they give it most of its compressive strength(Ulrich-Vinther, Maloney et al. 2003). Glycosaminoglycans (GAGs), chondroitin sulfate (CS) and keratan sulfate (KS) bind to core protein which, in turn, binds to hyaluronic acid (HA) via link protein, forming an aggrecan proteoglycan molecule (Figure 5a). The negative charge associated with GAGs in aggrecan attracts water, thus attempting to increase tissue swelling. However, the collagen fiber network interconnections prevent swelling and tissue pressure increases (Figure 5b). This property is unique and gives articular cartilage its resilience to compression and deformation.

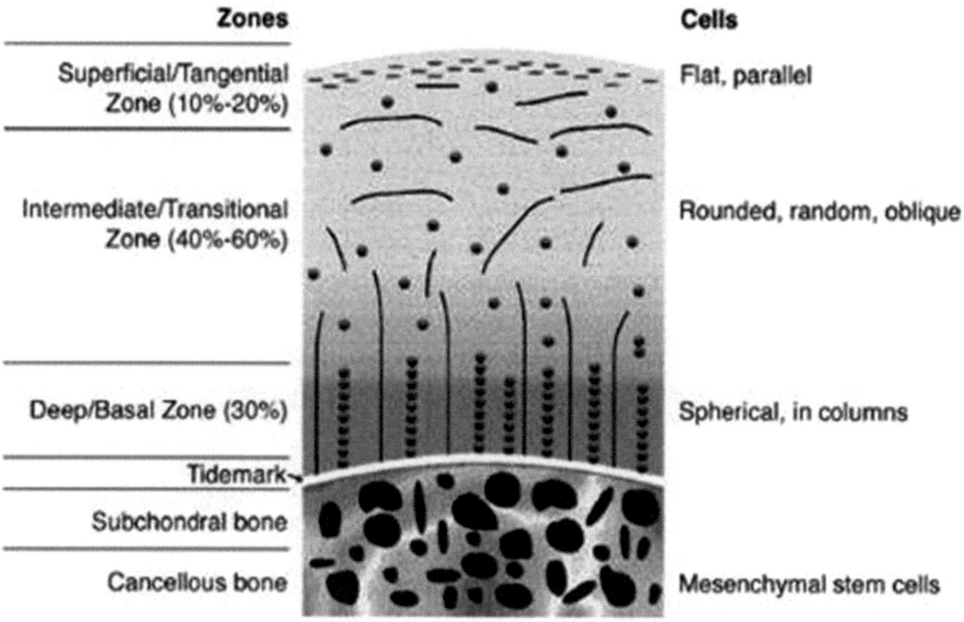

Fig. 4. 4) Schematic depiction of chondrocyte and collagen fibril distribution within the layers of articular cartilage (reproduced with permission from Ulrich-Vinther M, et al: Articular cartilage biology, in *Journal of the American Academy of Orthopaedic Surgeons* 2003; 11: 422. Publisher AAOS)

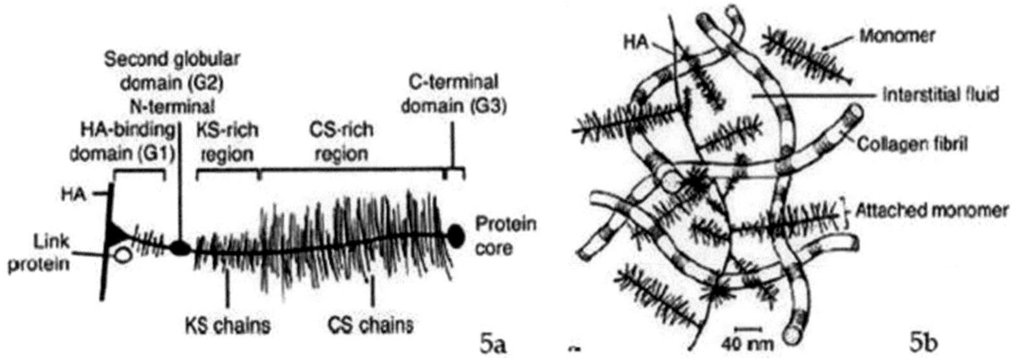

Fig. 5. 5a) Proteoglycan aggrecan molecule composed of chondroitin (CS) and keratan sulfate (KS) glycosaminoglycans, a protein core, and link protein attached to hyaluronic acid (HA) chain; 5b) ECM structure of collagen fibrils intertwined in aggrecan molecules (reproduced with permission from Ulrich-Vinther M, et al: Articular cartilage biology, in *Journal of the American Academy of Orthopaedic Surgeons* 2003; 11: 423. Publisher AAOS)

3. Focal articular cartilage injury

3.1 Prevalence and natural history

Chondral defects in the knee may be seen in up to 63% of knee arthroscopies(Curl, Krome et al. 1997). The prevalence of arthroscopically-detected full-thickness defects is 16%(Flanigan, Harris et al. 2010). Full-thickness focal lesions with an area of 1 cm^2 to 2 cm^2 are seen in approximately 5% of all knee arthroscopies in patients less than 40 years of age(Hjelle, Solheim et al. 2002; Aroen, Loken et al. 2004; Widuchowski, Widuchowski et al. 2007). In an exclusively athletic population, chondral pathology is more common than in the general population. The overall prevalence of full-thickness defects in this population is 36%(Flanigan, Harris et al. 2010). Further, the prevalence of full-thickness lesions is 59% in an asymptomatic group of professional basketball players and runners. The reasons for the increased prevalence in the athlete are multifactorial. Compared with the general population, athletes are 12 times more likely to develop osteoarthritis of the knee(Roos 1998; Drawer and Fuller 2001).

The natural history of the isolated chondral defect and to what degree the isolated defect may become symptomatic is incompletely understood(Buckwalter 1998). Full-thickness lesions may progress due to biomechanical overload with stress concentration around the rim of a defect(Guettler, Demetropoulos et al. 2004), subchondral bone structural changes(Minas and Nehrer 1997), and intra-articular inflammatory cytokine concentration elevations(Fraser, Fearon et al. 2003). Full-thickness defects obviate the shock-absorbing and load-transmitting function of articular cartilage(Minas 1999). The subchondral bone eventually bears the load (Figure 6). Subchondral bone overgrowth has been observed in patients undergoing autologous chondrocyte implantation (ACI), especially in more chronic, larger defects on the lateral femoral condyle(Henderson and LaValette 2005). The subchondral plate becomes sclerotic with vascular congestion and periarteriolar nociceptive fiber stimulation(Minas, Gomoll et al. 2009). The stiffer subchondral plate alters the biomechanical properties of the subchondral bone-articular cartilage interface, which increases shear forces with weight-bearing. Further, subchondral plate thickening and sclerosis due to tidemark advancement is a component of osteoarthritis(Radin and Rose

1986; Burr and Radin 2003). With increasing defect size, these osteocartilaginous changes can only be more greatly accelerated(Flanigan, Harris et al. 2010).

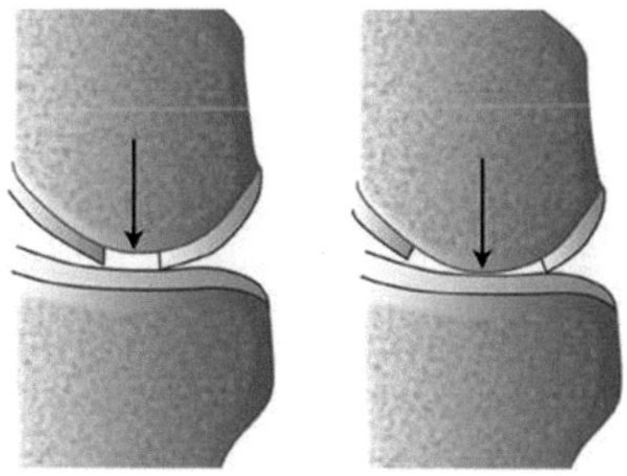

Fig. 6. Well-shouldered, small full-thickness chondral defect with no contact on underlying subchondral bone (left); larger full-thickness defect exhibits subchondral bone contact by the opposing surface (reproduced with permission from The American Academy of Orthopaedic Surgeons in: Jones D and Peterson L: Autologous chondrocyte implantation, Lecture in *Journal of Bone and Joint Surgery, American* 2006; 88A(11): 2503. Publisher AAOS)

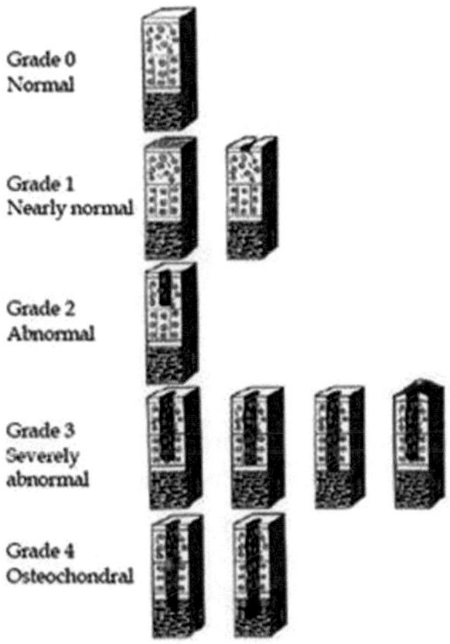

Fig. 7. International Cartilage Repair Society (ICRS) cartilage injury classification (reproduced from the ICRS Cartilage Injury Evaluation Package [www.cartilage.org], with permission from the ICRS).

3.2 Classification systems

The two most commonly used classification systems for arthroscopic analysis of chondral defects in the knee are the Outerbridge system and the International Cartilage Repair Society (ICRS) system (Figure 7). The Outerbridge system grades defects I - IV(Outerbridge 1961). Grade 1 lesions exhibited softening or swelling of cartilage; Grades 2 and 3 both exhibit fragmentation and fissuring of cartilage, with Grade 2 being less than ½ inch and Grade 3 being greater than ½ inch diameter; Grade 4 defects exhibit subchondral bone exposure. The newer ICRS system(Brittberg and Winalski 2003) is advantageous as it accounts not only for lesion area (cm^2), but also depth, while Outerbridge does not. Osteochondritis dissecans lesions can also be classified according to a similar ICRS-OCD system(Brittberg and Winalski 2003). This classification is based on lesion stability.

3.3 Clinical presentation

Patients with focal chondral defects of the knee may be asymptomatic. Articular cartilage is an aneural tissue. Thus, the presence of a defect does not necessarily produce pain. However, patients with full-thickness chondral defects may demonstrate major limitations in pain and function, according to the Knee Injury and Osteoarthritis Outcomes Score (KOOS)(Heir, Nerhus et al. 2010). In fact, the KOOS quality of life subscore for patients with focal cartilage defects were not significantly different from those patients with OA enrolled for knee osteotomy or arthroplasty. Further, patients with cartilage defects had significantly worse overall KOOS and all KOOS subscores versus patients with anterior cruciate ligament (ACL) deficiency. Patients with chondral defects may also have other concurrent extra- and intra-articular confounders, which make the diagnosis of chondral pathology difficult. Nevertheless, patients with symptomatic chondral defects generally complain of activity-related pain located in a region that correlates with the intra-articular location of the defect for tibiofemoral defects. Patellofemoral lesions generally cause anterior knee pain, worse with prolonged knee flexion or stair climbing. The exact mechanism to account for pain due to pathology in an aneural tissue is not completely understood. However, stimulation of nociceptive fibers in the subchondral bone is one current accepted theory(Mach, Rogers et al. 2002). Further, inflammatory cartilage breakdown products may cause joint effusion with capsular distension in conjunction with synovitis, both leading to joint pain. Patients with chondral flaps may also present with mechanical symptoms such as catching or clicking. Clearly, diagnosis of chondral pathology is complex and requires a thorough history and physical examination, with imaging and arthroscopic examination often required.

4. Articular cartilage imaging

Advances in technology have allowed improved imaging of articular cartilage. These include more sensitive and specific magnetic resonance imaging (MRI) sequences. Further, the ability to both directly and indirectly analyze cartilage qualitatively and quantitatively and its biochemical composition has been enhanced with MRI techniques like dGEMRIC (delayed gadolinium-enhanced MRI of cartilage), T1-rho, T2 mapping, sodium imaging, and diffusion-weighted imaging.

4.1 X-ray

Standard radiographs should always be included in the workup of articular cartilage pathology. Generally speaking, the presence of diffuse arthritic change precludes most cartilage repair or restoration procedures. The 45 degree weight-bearing posteroanterior x-ray (Rosenberg view) (Figure 8) is the most accurate, sensitive and specific for detection of major degenerative changes in the tibiofemoral joint(Rosenberg, Paulos et al. 1988). However, x-ray is extremely important in analysis of the weight-bearing mechanical axis (Figure 8) of the lower extremity for those patients that are enrolled for cartilage surgery.

Articular cartilage defects in the medial compartment are at higher risk for progression if varus malalignment exists (and lateral compartment for valgus, as well)(Linden 1977; Hughston, Hergenroeder et al. 1984; Messner and Maletius 1996; Sharma, Song et al. 2001).

Therefore, surgical correction of tibiofemoral malalignment to neutral or overcorrection is recommended in conjunction with most cartilage surgery (Figure 8). Thus, in addition to standard radiographic workup (extension standing anteroposterior [AP], Rosenberg view, lateral, and Mercer Merchant views), the full-length bilateral hip-to-ankle x-ray allows calculation of mechanical axis of the limb and the necessary alignment correction.

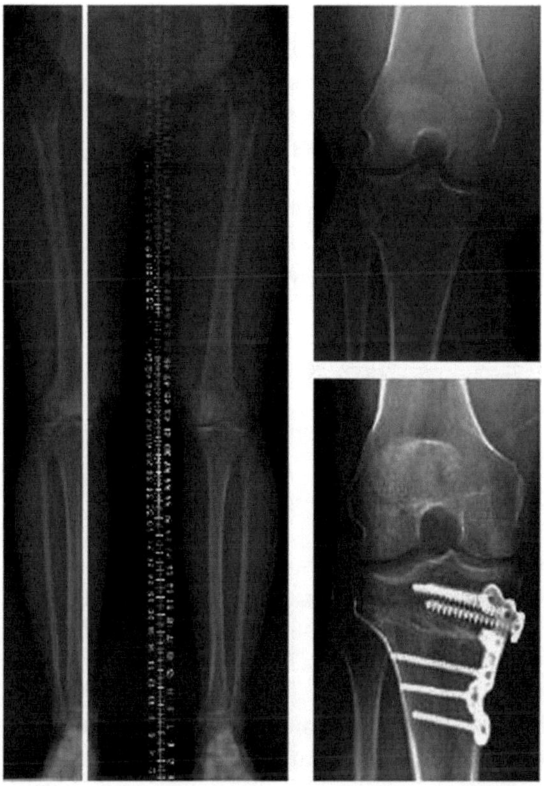

Fig. 8. Left) Standing hip-to-ankle x-ray demonstrating mechanical axis of lower extremity (in medial compartment); Right upper) Rosenberg view (no evidence of OA); Right lower) Rosenberg view after high tibial osteotomy.

4.2 Magnetic resonance imaging (MRI)

MRI is highly advantageous in imaging articular cartilage. This non-invasive modality avoids ionizing radiation, has superior sensitivity and specificity for articular cartilage, and allows for high contrast with proximate structures. Standard MRI sequences in imaging cartilage include conventional spin-echo (SE) and gradient-recalled echo (GRE), and fast SE sequences. The morphologic features of cartilage, evaluated with these standard techniques, can be semi-quantitatively analyzed with the WORMS (whole-organ MRI score)(Peterfy, Guermazi et al. 2004). Also, the MOCART (magnetic resonance observation of cartilage repair tissue) has been demonstrated to be accurate, reliable, and reproducible in post-ACI assessment of cartilage restoration tissue(Marlovits, Singer et al. 2006). Fast SE sequences are included in the ICRS cartilage repair evaluation package for non-invasive assessment of cartilage following surgery. Fat-suppression techniques increase the contrast between articular cartilage and the underlying subchondral bone. Short-tau inversion recovery (STIR) sequences are an example of a fat-suppression technique used for imaging cartilage defects.

T1-weighted series illustrate anatomic features of articular cartilage well, but have poor contrast between it and synovial fluid. T2-weighted series demonstrate better contrast between cartilage and joint fluid. Proton-density-weighted series are an intermediate, providing high contrast and excellent intra-cartilaginous structure.

The biphasic extracellular matrix of articular cartilage includes both fluid and a collagen-aggrecan network. The negatively-charged GAGs of aggrecan molecules allow for ions like gadolinium diethylenetriaminepentaacetic acid $(Gd\text{-}DTPA)^{-2}$ and sodium (Na^{+}) to interact to quantitatively measure proteoglycan content(Crema, Roemer et al. 2011). dGEMRIC utilizes $Gd\text{-}DTPA^{-2}$ based on the fact that its negative charge allows it to cluster where the GAG content is relatively low. Thus, since $Gd\text{-}DTPA^{-2}$ concentration is measured via T1, T1 mapping after intravenous (IV) $Gd\text{-}DTPA^{-2}$ allows for quantitative assessment of GAG concentration(Crema, Roemer et al. 2011). Higher $Gd\text{-}DTPA^{-2}$ indicates lower GAG content, while lower $Gd\text{-}DTPA^{-2}$ indicates higher GAG content.

While standard T2-weighted series provide a qualitative assessment of extracellular matrix of cartilage, T2 mapping quantitatively describes variations in relaxation time of cartilage via collagen network-water interaction. Higher T2 is seen in early stages of degenerative osteoarthritis(Dunn, Lu et al. 2004). Although T2 maps do not demonstrate any relationship between T2 and grade of defect or arthritic change (marker of severity of disease)(Koff, Amrami et al. 2007), they have demonstrated the ability to longitudinally assess cartilage repair or restoration tissue following surgery(Welsch, Mamisch et al. 2008).

Just as dGEMRIC may measure proteoglycan content, T1-rho values can also be used to assess extracellular matrix composition. The loss of articular cartilage early in osteoarthritis displays a higher T1-rho value than normal cartilage(Stahl, Luke et al. 2009). T1-rho measures not only proteoglycan content, but also collagen and other non-collagen proteins within the matrix(Mlynarik, Trattnig et al. 1999). This increased sensitivity makes it useful for detection of early arthritic change.

Sodium is a positively-charged ion that must equilibrate exactly with the negative charge imparted by GAGs in ECM of articular cartilage. Thus, normal hyaline articular cartilage exhibits high sodium content, while chondral defects and osteoarthritis exhibit lower sodium content due to loss of GAGs. This makes sodium imaging techniques attractive due to its ability to directly measure GAG content without the use of contrast material.

5. Articular cartilage surgery

Articular cartilage surgery can be broadly grouped into three categories: Palliative techniques that are, as the name implies, intended to relieve pain secondary to chondral pathology; repair techniques that invoke stimulation of the underlying subchondral bone marrow (MST), including microfracture, subchondral drilling, and abrasion arthroplasty; and restoration techniques that attempt to transfer or produce normal hyaline articular cartilage, including autologous chondrocyte implantation (ACI), osteochondral autograft / mosaicplasty, osteochondral allograft, and other cell-based surgical treatments.

5.1 Palliative techniques

Palliative techniques are minimally-invasive, arthroscopic surgeries intended to relieve pain due to articular cartilage disease. Debridement consists of removal of unstable, loose flaps or fronds of articular cartilage and loose bodies. This heterogeneous definition also encompasses lavage, which removes inflammatory joint fluid containing catabolic enzymes. All potentially mechanically-irritating pathology is removed and unstable, irregular edges of articular cartilage and meniscal tissue are smoothed.

Arthroscopic debridement may be indicated in certain groups of patients. The American Academy of Orthopaedic Surgeons (AAOS) Clinical Practice Guidelines (Level V evidence; Grade of Recommendation C)(Richmond, Hunter et al. 2009) recommend arthroscopic partial meniscectomy and / or loose body removal in patients with symptomatic osteoarthritis with primary complaints (mechanical symptoms) of torn meniscus or loose body. However, these guidelines do not recommend arthroscopic debridement or lavage in patients with symptomatic osteoarthritis without mechanical symptoms (Level I and II evidence; Grade of Recommendation A).

In patients with isolated chondral defects, the post-operative rehabilitation following certain cartilage repair or restoration techniques may preclude their use. Some athletes (professional or amateur) may not be willing to forego part of a competitive season or at least one full season due to concerns of scholarships, salaries, contracts, signing bonuses, other endorsements, public image, and career length. Further, many athletes are aware of certain surgical techniques and media coverage has instilled preconceived, irrational notions about their efficacy. Thus, arthroscopic debridement may be an effective, quick method to return an athlete to sport. Do not perform microfracture or other more advanced cartilage surgery if the patient has not consented or is unwilling to undergo the rehabilitation following surgery.

5.1.1 Surgical technique

Standard arthroscopic portals (working anteromedial and viewing anterolateral) are generally all that are required for this technique. Systematic diagnostic arthroscopy ensures that each location in the joint is inspected and no pathology left untreated. This includes the suprapatellar pouch, medial and lateral gutters, menisci, chondral surfaces, and cruciate ligaments within the notch. If access to the posterior compartments is indicated, the arthroscope may be placed through the notch and accessory posteromedial or posterolateral portals created to evaluate for loose bodies or posterior horn meniscal pathology. Some loose bodies may be removed with suction on an arthroscopic shaver, however others may require a grasper and either a separate incision or enlarging one of the standard portals. Degenerative chondral flaps and meniscal tears may be removed or trimmed to stable, smooth edges with a combination of arthroscopic biters, shavers, and curettes. Thorough palpation of all surfaces with a probe ensures no pathology is missed. If osteophytes are present, an arthroscopic burr may be required to contour this down as it may be a source of mechanical impingement and loss of motion.

5.1.2 Outcomes

Short- and mid-term outcomes of arthroscopic debridement are good to excellent (variably defined) in up to 75% of patients(Sprague 1981; Fond, Rodin et al. 2002). Patients whose primary symptom is mechanical generally have a better prognosis(Baumgaertner, Cannon et al. 1990; Ogilvie-Harris and Fitsialos 1991). Shorter duration of symptoms(Yang and Nisonson 1995; Fond, Rodin et al. 2002), normal coronal plane alignment(Baumgaertner, Cannon et al. 1990; Aaron, Skolnick et al. 2006), and no evidence of joint space narrowing(Jackson and Dieterichs 2003; Aaron, Skolnick et al. 2006) also are predictive of better outcomes.

5.2 Cartilage repair techniques

Cartilage repair techniques intend to stimulate the subchondral bone marrow (marrow-stimulation techniques, MST) to induce mesenchymal stem cell infiltration into a chondral defect with formation of a clot that may differentiate into repair tissue. This tissue is generally fibrocartilage, with a ratio of Type II to I collagen that is less than that of normal hyaline articular cartilage. The biomechanical properties and durability of fibrocartilage are inferior to that of hyaline cartilage. Microfracture, subchondral bone drilling, and abrasion arthroplasty are MSTs.

5.2.1 Surgical technique

Standard diagnostic arthroscopy is performed prior to assessment of a lesion amenable to microfracture. The use of a tourniquet is not recommended as this precludes assessment of depth of penetration of arthroscopic awl with egress of marrow fat or blood. The defect is prepared by creation of vertical walls with stable rims with a full radius resector or curette and removal of the calcified cartilage zone with a curette. Thus, poorly-shouldered lesions are not well-suited for this treatment. A stable subchondral plate is desired, so caution is warranted when debriding the calcified cartilage zone so that the plate is not compromised. Arthroscopic awls of variable angles (0°, 30°, 45°, 60°, and 90°) may be used to create multiple holes, the microfractures, perpendicular to the surface penetrated. The sequence of hole creation should be centripetal, from the periphery inward, approximately 3-4 mm apart and 3-4 mm deep (Figure 9). Do not place holes so close as to converge upon one another. Once complete, reduce arthroscopic pump pressure to visualize marrow contents from each of the holes. Do not use an intra-articular drain post-operatively, as this will remove the desired clot formation within the defect. Steadman has stressed the importance of post-operative rehabilitation following microfracture. Immediate continuous passive motion (CPM) is indicated for at least 8 hours per day for at least 8 weeks. Return to competitive sports is not allowed prior to 6 to 9 months.

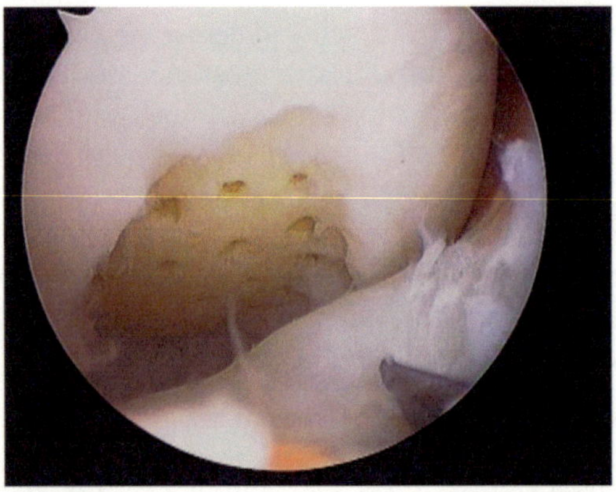

Fig. 9. Arthroscopic photograph of microfracture of medial femoral condyle defect.

5.2.2 Outcomes

In horse and human studies, microfracture has been consistently shown to produce a greater quantity of repair tissue versus no treatment of an isolated chondral defect(Frisbie, Trotter et al. 1999; Mithoefer, McAdams et al. 2009). Better outcomes have been demonstrated with the creation of smooth, vertical walls of the defect and removal of the calcified cartilage layer directly beneath the tidemark(Frisbie, Morisset et al. 2006).

Microfracture is generally indicated for a full-thickness, chondral defect (after debridement of the defect to stable rims with exposed bone) of the femoral condyles, trochlea, patella, or tibial plateau. The pioneer of microfracture (Steadman) has successfully utilized microfracture in degenerative arthritis(Miller, Steadman et al. 2004). Although microfracture has been used in high-performance athletes (NFL) with excellent outcomes and return-to-play(Steadman, Miller et al. 2003), other studies have shown less success in high-performance professional athletes, with low rates of return-to-sport and decreased performance if able to return(Cerynik, Lewullis et al. 2009; Namdari, Baldwin et al. 2009).

Outcomes of microfracture are mixed. Long-term outcomes have been successful (mean 11 years, range 7 to 17 years) in patients less than 45 years age, without malalignment or meniscal or ligamentous pathology, graded by both subjective and objective outcome measures(Steadman, Briggs et al. 2003). Recent systematic reviews have shown excellent short-term clinical outcomes following microfracture(Mithoefer, McAdams et al. 2009; Harris, Siston et al. 2010). However, after 18 to 24 months, outcomes tend to deteriorate, especially in patients with defects larger than 2 to 4 cm^2, longer pre-operative duration of symptoms, prior surgeries to the knee, and older age (Mithoefer, McAdams et al. 2009; Harris, Brophy et al. 2010; Harris, Siston et al. 2010). Further, microfracture may compromise future outcomes following ACI. A three times greater risk of failure after ACI has been shown in those patients with previous microfracture versus those without(Minas, Gomoll et al. 2009). In general, it appears that microfracture is best suited for younger patients with small defects who have normal alignment and a short pre-operative duration of symptoms and are willing to comply with post-operative rehabilitation.

5.3 Cartilage restoration techniques

Cartilage restoration techniques either transfer (mosaicplasty, osteochondral autograft and allograft) or attempt to produce (cell-based treatments such as ACI) normal hyaline articular cartilage.

5.3.1 Osteochondral autograft / mosaicplasty

Osteochondral autograft (OAT) and mosaicplasty are two similar techniques that harvest an osteochondral plug(s) from a "less weight-bearing" part of the knee and transplant them to a defect on a more weight-bearing, articulating location. Given the three-dimensional complexity of the articular surfaces of the knee, one can anticipate that stable congruity of the transplanted plug is paramount to the procedure's technical success. This procedure (Figure 10) can place one or many plugs of variable sizes to fill a defect. If one plug is used and is flush with surrounding cartilage, no fibrocartilaginous tissue from the underlying subchondral bone will be formed. If more than one plug is used, however, the intervening areas fill with fibrocartilage. Since this is an osteochondral transplant, chondral *and* osteochondral defects may be treated without the need for bone grafting (as opposed to other cartilage surgery). This technique, however, is limited by donor-site supply. This has prompted most authors to limit the size transplanted to no greater than 4 or 5 cm^2. Despite concerns for donor-site morbidity following harvest, long-term donor-site complaints (measured by Bandi score) are minor and present in small numbers of patients, including high-level athletes (3% - 5%)(Hangody, Vasarhelyi et al. 2008; Hangody, Dobos et al. 2010).

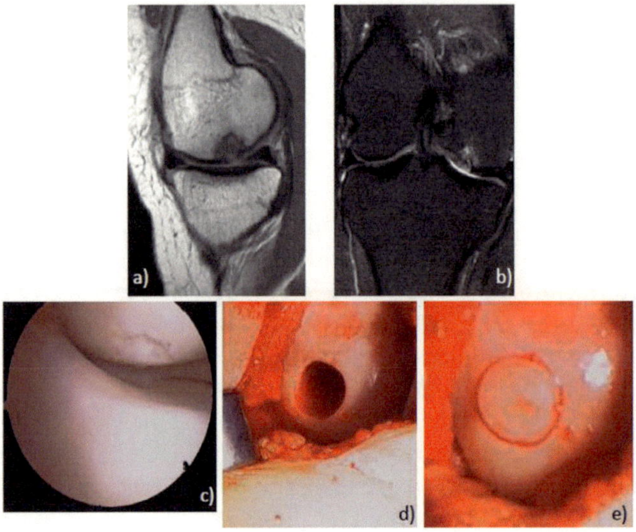

Fig. 10. 10a) Sagittal MRI demonstrating osteochondral defect of medial femoral condyle; 10b) Coronal MRI demonstrating same defect; 10c) Arthroscopic photograph of defect; 10d) Mini-arthrotomy image after recipient site preparation; 10e) Flush plug placed.

5.3.1.1 Surgical technique

Osteochondral autograft may be performed all-arthroscopically or via mini-arthrotomy. Either is acceptable, although arthroscopically may be technically more demanding. Standard diagnostic arthroscopy is performed initially. The defect is prepared by obtaining stable smooth edges with vertical walls. Once this is complete, the defect is then precisely measured and templated. There are several unique proprietary designs available to harvest and place plugs. However, the general principles of each are the same: A sharp cutting harvester, perpendicular to the surface, is impacted to a pre-determined depth and donor plug is harvested. The size of the harvester can be range from 2.5 to 10 mm in diameter. Donor sites include the intercondylar notch, and superomedial and superolateral borders of the femoral condyles. These donor sites should properly be described as "less weight-bearing" regions, rather than non-weight-bearing regions(Simonian, Sussmann et al. 1998; Ahmad, Cohen et al. 2001). The recipient site is prepared to accept the graft to the correct depth. The plug is then placed press-fit via instrumented manual impaction. Plugs should be placed flush circumferentially, as plugs placed proud demonstrate significantly greater contact pressure around the plug's rim and the opposing surface(Harris, Solak et al. 2011). Even plugs countersunk beneath the surrounding normal cartilage create significant pressure increases around the rim of the normal cartilage(Koh, Wirsing et al. 2004). It cannot be overemphasize that critical for this procedure's success is flush plug placement achieved via perpendicular plug harvest and transplantation.

5.3.1.2 Outcomes

Outcomes following osteochondral autograft / mosaicplasty have been largely good or excellent. In an exclusively athletic population of nearly 400 patients at nearly 10 year mean follow-up, good or excellent clinical outcomes were observed in 91% of femoral condyle OAT, 86% tibial, and 74% patellofemoral(Hangody, Dobos et al. 2010). The timing of return to sport after OAT is faster than that after microfracture or ACI(Harris, Brophy et al. 2010). Also, the rate of return to sport and overall clinical outcomes after OAT are better than that after microfracture(Harris, Brophy et al. 2010). Except for more rapid clinical improvement, no significant difference has been demonstrated between OAT and ACI with regard to clinical outcomes(Harris, Brophy et al. 2010; Harris, Siston et al. 2010).

5.3.2 Osteochondral allograft

Principles of osteochondral allograft are similar to those of autograft, with the difference being the source of the osteochondral plug. Although concern for disease transmission, cell viability, and host-graft immunogenicity exist, this technique is a very useful treatment for larger chondral and osteochondral defects (usually greater than 2 to 4 cm^2). There is no limitation to the size of graft used, as entire condyles may be transplanted. Given the size constraints imposed by the transplanted graft, most allografts are implanted via an arthrotomy, although some cases may allow all-arthroscopic placement, just as with OAT.

5.3.2.1 Surgical technique

Just as with OAT, the defect is prepared to stable smooth rims with vertical walls using a sharp curette or full-radius resector and then sized. The cylindrical dowel graft is then prepared to match the size of the defect. The dowel graft is then press-fit into its recipient socket via instrumented manual impaction. Supplemental fixation is generally not required. A shell graft technique is another viable option when the dowel technique is not possible because of defect location or size. The shell is prepared freehand and usually requires fixation. This technique is technically more demanding than the dowel.

5.3.2.2 Outcomes

Outcomes after osteochondral allograft demonstrate good to excellent outcomes in 72% to 94% of patients at long-term follow-up with 5 year Kaplan-Meier survivorship around 95%, 10 year survival around 80% - 85%, and 15 year survival around 65%(Garrett 1994; Shasha, Krywulak et al. 2003; Gross, Shasha et al. 2005; Emmerson, Gortz et al. 2007). Although technically demanding, osteochondral allograft has long-term proven success in patients with larger defects and bone loss that may have failed a prior cartilage surgery.

5.3.3 Autologous chondrocyte implantation (ACI)

ACI is a two-stage cartilage restoration technique indicated for lesions greater than 2 cm^2 on the femoral condyles, trochlea, or patella. Stage 1 involves arthroscopic assessment of the defect and a full-thickness cartilage biopsy. Stage 2 involves cell implantation via arthrotomy under a periosteal or collagen membrane patch or, more recently, outside the U.S., cell placement onto a three-dimensional scaffold that can potentially be placed all-arthroscopically. The premise behind ACI is that a biopsy and growth in culture of your own cells should theoretically produce normal hyaline articular cartilage upon implantation. However, dedifferentiation of chondrocytes when grown in monolayer culture and subsequent re-differentiation upon implantation has produced "hyaline-like" cartilage. This tissue has a Type II collagen and proteoglycan composition that is close, but not identical to that of normal hyaline articular cartilage.

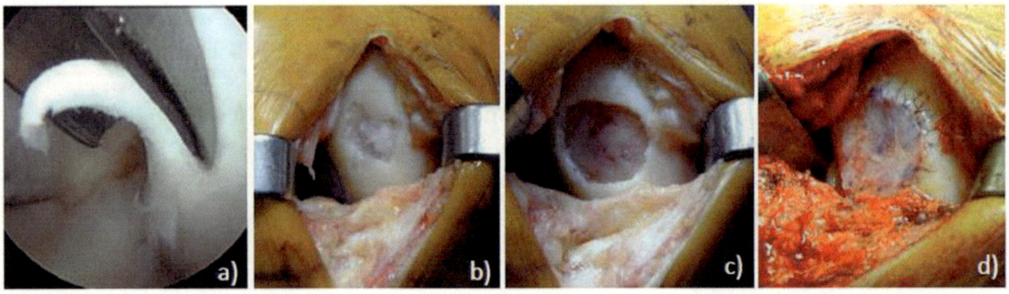

Fig. 11. 11a) Arthroscopic biopsy taken from intercondylar notch; 11b) Knee arthrotomy revealing full-thickness femoral condylar defect; 11c) Defect following debridement to stable rims; 11d) Following suture of periosteal patch and implantation of cultured autologous chondrocytes. (Reproduced with permission from Alford JW and Cole BJ: Cartilage restoration, Part 2: Techniques, outcomes, and future directions, in *American Journal of Sports Medicine* 2005; 33: 443-460. Publisher Sage Publications).

5.3.3.1 Surgical technique

ACI Stage 1 involves standard diagnostic arthroscopy with debridement of the defect and a full-thickness cartilage biopsy taken from the intercondylar notch (Figure 11a), or superomedial or superolateral edge of the medial or lateral femoral condyles, respectively. An arthroscopic ring curette or notchplasty gouge may be used to obtain two or three slivers of cartilage ~ 5 mm x 8 mm (~200 - 300 mg; 200,000 - 300,000 cells). Larger defects may warrant larger amount of tissue. The biopsy should contain a small sample of bone. Currently, the biopsy remains viable for implantation for two years after harvest. It is critical to determine the complete extent and size of the lesion by removing all loose, unstable, undermined, and unhealthy cartilage to well-shouldered, vertical walls. Healthy stable cartilage is required at the time of Stage 2. Upon implantation during Stage 2, removal of all cartilage in the bed is required down to, but not into, the subchondral bone. Any inadvertent penetration into the bone will generate undesirable bleeding. Epinephrine-soaked neuropatties may be used to achieve adequate hemostasis. With stable vertical walls (Figure 11c), the patch can be sutured (using lubricated 6-0 Vicryl suture on a P1 cutting needle) (Figure 11d) in with one small opening remaining at the most superior portion of the patch to allow for cell implantation. Sutures should be spaced 3 to 4 mm apart with a 3 mm bite onto normal cartilage and the knots tied on the patch side. Inject sterile saline under patch to test watertightness prior to inserting cell solution via 18-gauge angiocatheter. Apply fibrin glue as necessary to ensure watertight closure. Once cells are implanted, suture the remaining opening and fibrin glue as needed.

5.3.3.2 Variations in technique (ACI generations)

Currently, three generations of ACI exist. First-generation techniques involve cell implantation under a periosteal or collagen membrane patch via arthrotomy. Second-generation techniques utilize either arthrotomy or arthroscopy to implant cells via cell-seeded, three-dimensional bioabsorbable scaffolds. Third-generation technique uses either arthrotomy or arthroscopy to deliver in-vitro treated cells within chondro-inductive and chondro-conductive, three-dimensional matrices. Although clinical outcomes of first- and second-generation ACI are not significantly different, first-generation (especially with periosteal cover) has a significantly greater number of complications, failures, and unplanned re-operations than second-generation(Harris, Siston et al. 2011).

5.3.3.3 Outcomes

Outcomes after ACI are good to excellent in approximately 90% of patients at short- and mid-term follow-up(Peterson, Minas et al. 2000; Bentley, Biant et al. 2003; Mandelbaum, Browne et al. 2007). Long-term follow-up reveals 92% patient satisfaction with significant improvements in subjective and objective clinical outcome scores (224 patients at mean 13 year follow-up, range 12 to 20 years)(Peterson, Vasiliadis et al. 2010). Several recent systematic reviews have compared ACI to other cartilage surgeries and have indicated a trend toward improved clinical and tissue outcomes following ACI versus microfracture and OAT at mid- and short-term follow-up(Harris, Siston et al. 2010; Vavken and Samartzis 2010). The quality of evidence in the literature is methodologically poor(Jakobsen, Engebretsen et al. 2005; Harris, Siston et al. 2011) and only further higher quality randomized comparative clinical trials will be able to determine if one cartilage repair or restoration technique is superior.

6. Role of alignment in cartilage surgery

6.1 Role of mechanical axis of lower extremity

The mechanical axis of the lower extremity (straight line drawn from center of hip to center of ankle) normally lies just medial to the medial tibial spine. Varus malalignment brings this axis further inside the medial compartment or even medial to the joint. With axial loading, varus malalignment causes increased pressure in the medial compartment cartilage(Loening, James et al. 2000). Increased stress may negatively impact cartilage repair and restoration procedures. Without correction of the alignment to at neutral, the outcomes of cartilage procedures have been less successful in the presence of varus malalignment. This has led to increased performance of valgus-producing high tibial osteotomy (HTO) either via an opening- (OW-HTO) or closing-wedge (CW-HTO) technique. Mechanical axis correction to neutral or slight valgus is adequate in conjunction with cartilage repair or restoration procedures(Mina, Garrett et al. 2008). For medial compartment osteoarthritis, overcorrection to up to 62% of the width of the tibial plateau from the medial tibial border is warranted(Miller, Cole et al. 2008). A similar technique is used for lateral compartment chondral pathology in the setting of valgus malalignment via a laterally-based opening wedge technique.

6.1.1 Outcomes

Outcomes after combined HTO and cartilage surgery for medial compartment cartilage pathology and varus malalignment have demonstrated significant improvements in subjective and objective clinical measures. Both CW-HTO and OW-HTO techniques have seen similar success concurrent with microfracture(Sterett and Steadman 2004; Sterett, Steadman et al. 2010; Pascale, Luraghi et al. 2011), abrasion arthroplasty(Matsunaga, Akizuki et al. 2007), and ACI(Franceschi, Longo et al. 2008; Gomoll, Kang et al. 2009; Minas, Gomoll et al. 2009).

6.2 Role of patellofemoral alignment

Similar to unloading osteotomy and cartilage surgery for tibiofemoral joint articular cartilage lesions with malalignment, patellofemoral joint chondral pathology in the setting of patellofemoral malalignment also warrants unloading via tibial tubercle osteotomy when combined with cartilage surgery. In the setting of lateral patellar or trochlear defects, unloading via osteotomy should include either medialization (Elmslie-Trillat) or anteromedialization (Fulkerson). The degree of medialization needed may be estimated with pre-operative measurement of the TT-TG (tibial tubercle-trochlear groove) distance. Nevertheless, the surgeon must be cognizant during the pre-operative workup and the operation itself to assure that no medial patellar or trochlear pathology exists if planning to unload the lateral patellofemoral compartments, as this will increase stress on degenerative cartilage(Kuroda, Kambic et al. 2001). Distal patellar cartilage pathology may warrant anteromedialization to allow the patella to enter the trochlea in earlier degrees of flexion and unload the distal cartilage pathology(Colvin and West 2008). In the presence of lateral patellar tilt, a lateral retinacular release may be indicated(Arendt 2009). Medial patellofemoral ligament (MPFL) insufficiency may warrant reconstruction(Arendt 2009).

6.2.1 Outcomes

The clinical outcomes following patellofemoral realignment osteotomy have demonstrated success with the proper indications. In patients with lateral and distal patellar defects, anteromedialization led to 100% patient satisfaction with 87% good to excellent results, while patients with medial, proximal, or diffuse defects had only 43% good to excellent results(Pidoriano, Weinstein et al. 1997). Excellent short- and mid-term outcomes have been demonstrated when distal patellofemoral realignment has been combined with ACI(Bentley, Biant et al. 2003; Minas and Bryant 2005; Henderson and Lavigne 2006; Farr 2007; Gigante, Enea et al. 2009; Gobbi, Kon et al. 2009).

7. Role of meniscus in cartilage surgery

7.1 Post-meniscectomy knee and meniscus allograft transplantation (MAT)

Primary functions of the meniscus include load transmission, shock absorption, and secondary joint stability. When the meniscus is anatomically (post-meniscectomy) or functionally (complete radial tears, root tears) lost, the ipsilateral articular cartilage now wholly bears the compartmental load. Thus, meniscal preservation is key to articular chondroprotection. In the young patient with meniscal deficiency, MAT is a viable treatment option. Key surgical tenets include proper sizing, graft bank source, bony rather than suture fixation, and recognition of associated chondral disease. Historically, ipsilateral full-thickness cartilage pathology was considered a contraindication to MAT due to the poor clinical outcomes seen after MAT in this patient group(Noyes and Barber-Westin 1995; van Arkel and de Boer 1995). Given the recent improvements in outcomes following cartilage surgery and MAT when considered in isolation, the combined procedure (either simultaneous or staged) has received much attention. In the presence of combined meniscal deficiency and advanced chondral pathology, cartilage surgery may be a necessary adjunct to MAT for optimal biological joint preservation.

7.1.1 Outcomes

Outcomes following combined MAT and cartilage surgery (ACI, OAT, osteochondral allograft) have demonstrated equivalent subjective and objective clinical outcomes as either procedure performed in isolation(Harris, Cavo et al. 2011). In these studies, failure rate is low (12%), but the rate of re-operation is high (~50%). Most of the failures (86%) that occur following combined MAT and cartilage surgery were due to failure of the MAT. In addition to consideration of meniscal status, coronal plane alignment must also be accounted for so as to not overload the ipsilateral compartment that receives cartilage surgery and MAT.

8. Articular cartilage defect management algorithm

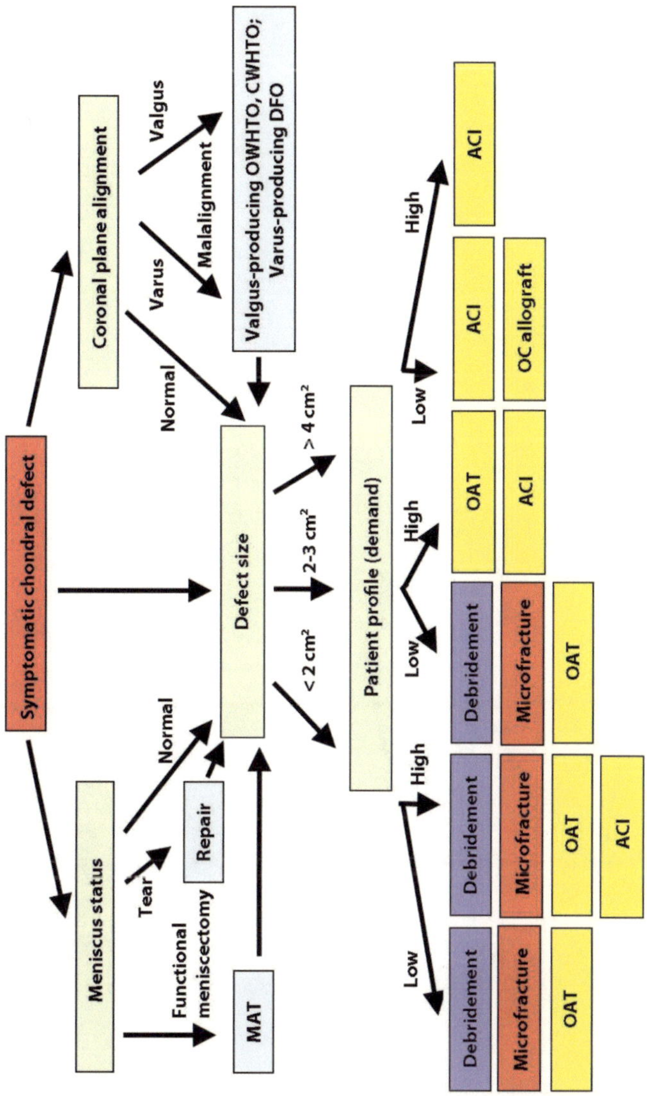

Fig. 12. Management of symptomatic chondral defect of medial or lateral femoral condyle. Concurrent issues, such as meniscal deficiency and coronal plane malalignment, need to be addressed, either simultaneously or sequentially in a staged manner. The most important defect-specific parameter is size (area in cm²), dictating treatment choice. MAT (meniscus allograft transplantation), HTO (high tibial osteotomy), OWHTO (opening wedge HTO), CWHTO (closing wedge HTO), DFO (distal femoral osteotomy), OAT (osteochondral autograft), ACI (autologous chondrocyte implantation), OC (osteochondral) allograft. Yellow (cartilage restorative technique); Red (cartilage reparative technique); Purple (cartilage palliative technique).

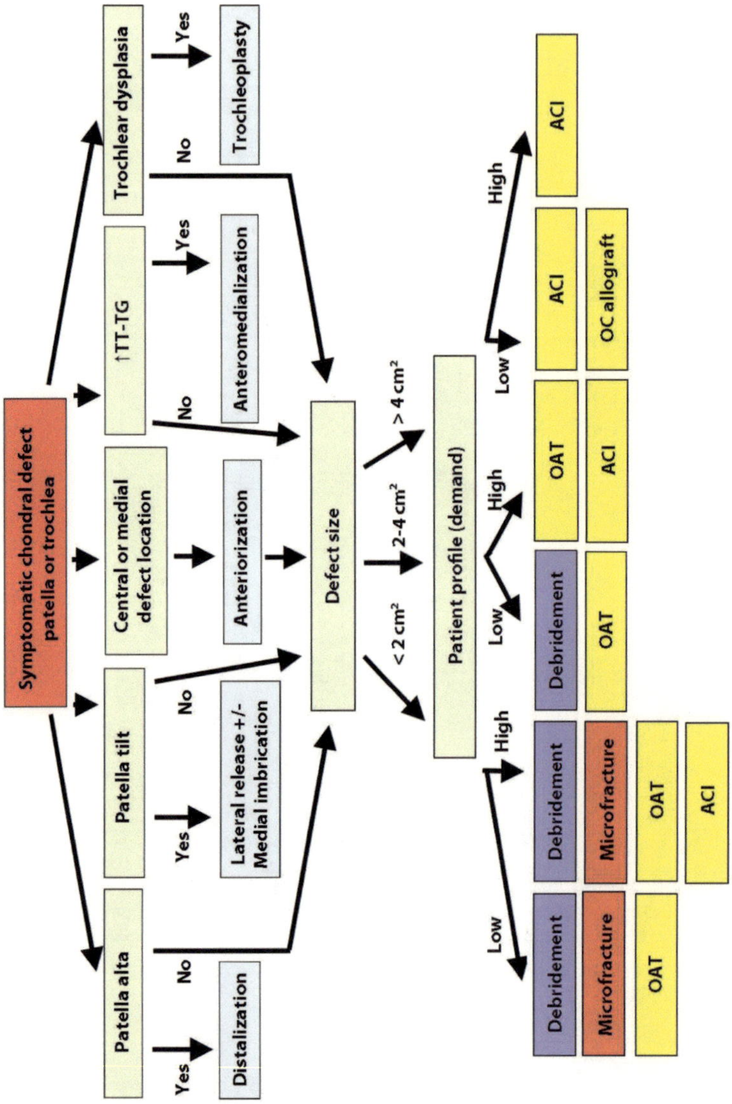

Fig. 13. Management of symptomatic chondral defect of femoral trochlea or patella. Concurrent issues, such as patella alta, patella tilt, increased extensor mechanism lateral vector (tibial tubercle - trochlear groove [TT-TG] distance), and trochlear dysplasia, need to be addressed, either simultaneously or sequentially in a staged manner. Centrally or medially located defects warrant different unloading osteotomy techniques, pending normal alignment. Medial patellofemoral compartment articular cartilage pathology is a contraindication to medializing osteotomy. The most important defect-specific parameter is size (area in cm^2), dictating treatment choice. OAT (osteochondral autograft), ACI (autologous chondrocyte implantation), OC (osteochondral) allograft. Yellow (cartilage restorative technique); Red (cartilage reparative technique); Purple (cartilage palliative technique).

9. Conclusions

Articular cartilage defects of the knee are a common source of pain and disability. Their natural history progression to osteoarthrosis of the knee is not completely understood. The management of these lesions is clearly multifactorial, involving factors specifically related to the patient, the lower extremity, the knee and the defect. Several surgical procedures exist to treat these injuries when non-operative management has failed. These include palliative, reparative, and restorative techniques. Both subjective and objective outcomes demonstrate significant improvement following these procedures. The future of cartilage surgery will need high-quality randomized clinical trials, using minimally-invasive techniques with the goal of obtaining normal hyaline articular cartilage, in the hopes of delay or prevention of defect progression to osteoarthrosis of the knee.

10. References

Aaron, R. K., A. H. Skolnick, et al. (2006). "Arthroscopic debridement for osteoarthritis of the knee." J Bone Joint Surg Am 88(5): 936-43.

Ahmad, C., Z. Cohen, et al. (2001). "Biomechanical and topographic considerations for autologous osteochondral grafting in the knee." American Journal of Sports Medicine 29(2): 201-206.

Ahmed, A. and D. Burke (1983). "In-vitro measurement of static pressure distribution in synovial joints. Part 1. Tibial surface of the knee." Journal of Biomechanical Engineering 105(3): 216-225.

Arendt, E. A. (2009). "MPFL reconstruction for PF instability. The soft (tissue) approach." Orthop Traumatol Surg Res 95(8 Suppl 1): S97-100.

Aroen, A., S. Loken, et al. (2004). "Articular cartilage lesions in 993 consecutive knee arthroscopies." American Journal of Sports Medicine 32: 211-215.

Baumgaertner, M. R., W. D. Cannon, Jr., et al. (1990). "Arthroscopic debridement of the arthritic knee." Clin Orthop Relat Res(253): 197-202.

Bentley, G., L. Biant, et al. (2003). "A prospective, randomized comparison of autologous chondrocyte implantation versus mosaicplasty for osteochondral defects in the knee." Journal of Bone and Joint Surgery, British 85B(2): 223-230.

Blankevoort, L., R. Huiskes, et al. (1988). "The envelope of passive knee joint motion." J Biomech 21(9): 705-20.

Brittberg, M. and C. Winalski (2003). "Evaluation of cartilage injuries and repair." Journal of Bone and Joint Surgery, American 85A(Supplement 2): 58-69.

Buckwalter, J. (1998). "Articular Cartilage: Injuries and potential for healing." Journal of Orthopaedic and Sports Physical Therapy 28: 192-202.

Burr, D. and E. Radin (2003). "Microfractures and microcracks in subchondral bone: Are they relevant to osteoarthrosis." Rheumatic Diseases in Clinics of North America 29: 675-685.

Cerynik, D., G. Lewullis, et al. (2009). "Outcomes of microfracture in professional basketball players." Knee Surgery, Sports Traumatology, Arthroscopy.

Clark, C. R. and J. A. Ogden (1983). "Development of the menisci of the human knee joint. Morphological changes and their potential role in childhood meniscal injury." J Bone Joint Surg Am 65(4): 538-47.

Colvin, A. C. and R. V. West (2008). "Patellar instability." J Bone Joint Surg Am 90(12): 2751-62.

Conlan, T., W. P. Garth, Jr., et al. (1993). "Evaluation of the medial soft-tissue restraints of the extensor mechanism of the knee." J Bone Joint Surg Am 75(5): 682-93.

Crema, M. D., F. W. Roemer, et al. (2011). "Articular cartilage in the knee: current MR imaging techniques and applications in clinical practice and research." Radiographics 31(1): 37-61.

Curl, W., J. Krome, et al. (1997). "Cartilage Injuries: A Review of 31,516 Knee Arthroscopies." Arthroscopy: The Journal of Arthroscopic and Related Surgery 13(4): 456-460.

Drawer, S. and C. Fuller (2001). "Propensity for osteoarthritis and lower limb joint pain in retired professional soccer players." British Journal of Sports Medicine 35(6): 402-408.

Dunn, T. C., Y. Lu, et al. (2004). "T2 relaxation time of cartilage at MR imaging: comparison with severity of knee osteoarthritis." Radiology 232(2): 592-8.

Emmerson, B. C., S. Gortz, et al. (2007). "Fresh osteochondral allografting in the treatment of osteochondritis dissecans of the femoral condyle." Am J Sports Med 35(6): 907-14.

Farr, J. (2007). "Autologous chondrocyte implantation improves patellofemoral cartilage treatment outcomes." Clinical Orthopaedics and Related Research 463: 187-194.

Flanigan, D. C., J. D. Harris, et al. (2010). "The effects of lesion size and location on subchondral bone contact in experimental knee articular cartilage defects in a bovine model." Arthroscopy 26(12): 1655-61.

Flanigan, D. C., J. D. Harris, et al. (2010). "Prevalence of chondral defects in athletes' knees: a systematic review." Med Sci Sports Exerc 42(10): 1795-801.

Fond, J., D. Rodin, et al. (2002). "Arthroscopic debridement for the treatment of osteoarthritis of the knee: 2- and 5-year results." Arthroscopy 18(8): 829-34.

Franceschi, F., U. Longo, et al. (2008). "Simultaneous arthroscopic implantation of autologous chondrocytes and high tibial osteotomy for tibial chondral defects in the varus knee." The Knee 15(4): 309-313.

Fraser, A., U. Fearon, et al. (2003). "Turnover of type II collagen and aggrecan in cartilage matrix at the onset of inflammatory arthritis in humans: relationship to mediators of systemic and local inflammation." Arthritis and Rheumatism 48(11): 3085-3095.

Frisbie, D., G. Trotter, et al. (1999). "Arthroscopic subchondral bone plate microfracture technique augments healing of large chondral defects in the radial carpal bone and medial femoral condyle of horses." Veterinary Surgery 28(4): 242-255.

Frisbie, D. D., S. Morisset, et al. (2006). "Effects of calcified cartilage on healing of chondral defects treated with microfracture in horses." Am J Sports Med 34(11): 1824-31.

Fukubayashi, T. and H. Kurosawa (1980). "The contact area and pressure distribution pattern of the knee - A study of normal and osteoarthritic knee joints." Acta Orthopaedica Scandinavica 51: 871-879.

Garrett, J. C. (1994). "Fresh osteochondral allografts for treatment of articular defects in osteochondritis dissecans of the lateral femoral condyle in adults." Clin Orthop Relat Res(303): 33-7.

Gigante, A., D. Enea, et al. (2009). "Distal realignment and patellar autologous chondrocyte implantation: Mid-term results in a selected population." Knee Surgery, Sports Traumatology, Arthroscopy 17(1): 2-10.

Gobbi, A., E. Kon, et al. (2009). "Patellofemoral full-thickness chondral defects treated with second-generation autologous chondrocyte implantation: results at 5 years' follow-up." Am J Sports Med 37(6): 1083-92.

Gomoll, A., R. Kang, et al. (2009). "Triad of cartilage restoration for unicompartmental arthritis treatment in young patients." Journal of Knee Surgery 22: 137-141.

Gross, A. E., N. Shasha, et al. (2005). "Long-term followup of the use of fresh osteochondral allografts for posttraumatic knee defects." Clin Orthop Relat Res(435): 79-87.

Guettler, J., C. Demetropoulos, et al. (2004). "Osteochondral defects in the Human Knee- Influence of defect size on cartilage rim stress and load redistribution to surrounding cartilage." American Journal of Sports Medicine 32(6): 1451-1458.

Hangody, L., J. Dobos, et al. (2010). "Clinical experiences with autologous osteochondral mosaicplasty in an athletic population: a 17-year prospective multicenter study." Am J Sports Med 38(6): 1125-33.

Hangody, L., G. Vasarhelyi, et al. (2008). "Autologous osteochondral grafting--technique and long-term results." Injury 39 Suppl 1: S32-9.

Harris, J., R. Brophy, et al. (2010). "Treatment of chondral defects in the athlete's knee." Arthroscopy: The Journal of Arthroscopic and Related Surgery 26(6): 841-852.

Harris, J. D., M. Cavo, et al. (2011). "Biological knee reconstruction: a systematic review of combined meniscal allograft transplantation and cartilage repair or restoration." Arthroscopy 27(3): 409-18.

Harris, J. D., R. A. Siston, et al. (2011). "Failures, re-operations, and complications after autologous chondrocyte implantation - a systematic review." Osteoarthritis Cartilage.

Harris, J. D., R. A. Siston, et al. (2010). "Autologous chondrocyte implantation: a systematic review." J Bone Joint Surg Am 92(12): 2220-33.

Harris, J. D., K. K. Solak, et al. (2011). "Contact pressure comparison of proud osteochondral autograft plugs versus proud synthetic plugs." Orthopedics 34(2): 97.

Heir, S., T. Nerhus, et al. (2010). "Focal cartilage defects in the knee impair quality of life as much as severe osteoarthritis." American Journal of Sports Medicine 38(2): 231-237.

Henderson, I. and D. LaValette (2005). "Subchondral bone overgrowth in the presence of full-thickness cartilage defects in the knee." The Knee 12: 435-440.

Henderson, I. and P. Lavigne (2006). "Periosteal autologous chondrocyte implantation for patellar chondral defect in patients with normal and abnormal patellar tracking." The Knee 13: 274-279.

Hjelle, K., E. Solheim, et al. (2002). "Articular cartilage defects in 1,000 knee arthroscopies." Arthroscopy: The Journal of Arthroscopic and Related Surgery 18(7): 730-734.

Huberti, H. H. and W. C. Hayes (1984). "Patellofemoral contact pressures. The influence of q-angle and tendofemoral contact." J Bone Joint Surg Am 66(5): 715-24.

Hughston, J., P. Hergenroeder, et al. (1984). "Osteochondritis dissecans of the femoral condyles." Journal of Bone and Joint Surgery, American 66(9): 1340-1348.

Iwaki, H., V. Pinskerova, et al. (2000). "Tibiofemoral movement 1: the shapes and relative movements of the femur and tibia in the unloaded cadaver knee." Journal of Bone and Joint Surgery, British 82B(8): 1189-1195.

Jackson, R. W. and C. Dieterichs (2003). "The results of arthroscopic lavage and debridement of osteoarthritic knees based on the severity of degeneration: a 4- to 6-year symptomatic follow-up." Arthroscopy 19(1): 13-20.

Jakobsen, R., L. Engebretsen, et al. (2005). "An analysis of the quality of cartilage repair studies." Journal of Bone and Joint Surgery, American 87A(10): 2232-2239.

Kettelkamp, D. B. and A. W. Jacobs (1972). "Tibiofemoral contact area--determination and implications." J Bone Joint Surg Am 54(2): 349-56.

Koff, M. F., K. K. Amrami, et al. (2007). "Clinical evaluation of T2 values of patellar cartilage in patients with osteoarthritis." Osteoarthritis Cartilage 15(2): 198-204.

Koh, J., K. Wirsing, et al. (2004). "The effect of graft height mismatch on contact pressure following osteochondral grafting: a biomechanical study." American Journal of Sports Medicine 32(2): 317-320.

Kuroda, R., H. Kambic, et al. (2001). "Articular cartilage contact pressure after tibial tuberosity transfer. A cadaveric study." Am J Sports Med 29(4): 403-9.

Lieberman, J. (2009). AAOS Comprehensive Orthopaedic Review. Rosemont, Illinois, American Academy of Orthopaedic Surgeons.

Linden, B. (1977). "Osteochondritis dissecans of the femoral condyles: a long-term follow-up study." Journal of Bone and Joint Surgery, American 59: 769-776.

Loening, A. M., I. E. James, et al. (2000). "Injurious mechanical compression of bovine articular cartilage induces chondrocyte apoptosis." Arch Biochem Biophys 381(2): 205-12.

Mach, D. B., S. D. Rogers, et al. (2002). "Origins of skeletal pain: sensory and sympathetic innervation of the mouse femur." Neuroscience 113(1): 155-66.

Madry, H., C. N. van Dijk, et al. (2010). "The basic science of the subchondral bone." Knee Surg Sports Traumatol Arthrosc 18(4): 419-33.

Mandelbaum, B., J. Browne, et al. (2007). "Treatment outcomes of autologous chondrocyte implantation for full-thickness articular cartilage defects of the trochlea." American Journal of Sports Medicine 35(6): 915-921.

Marlovits, S., P. Singer, et al. (2006). "Magnetic resonance observation of cartilage repair tissue (MOCART) for the evaluation of autologous chondrocyte transplantation: determination of interobserver variability and correlation to clinical outcome after 2 years." Eur J Radiol 57(1): 16-23.

Matsunaga, D., S. Akizuki, et al. (2007). "Repair of articular cartilage and clinical outcome after osteotomy with microfracture or abrasion arthroplasty for medial gonarthrosis." The Knee 14(6): 465-471.

Messner, K. and W. Maletius (1996). "The long-term prognosis of severe damage to weight-bearing cartilage in the knee." Acta Orthopaedica Scandinavica 67: 165-168.

Miller, B., J. Steadman, et al. (2004). "Patient satisfaction and outcome after microfracture of the degenerative knee." Journal of Knee Surgery 17: 13-17.

Miller, M., B. Cole, et al. (2008). Operative Techniques: Sports Knee Surgery. Philadelphia, PA, Saunders Elsevier.

Mina, C., W. Garrett, et al. (2008). "High tibial osteotomy for unloading osteochondral defects in the medial compartment of the knee." American Journal of Sports Medicine AJSM PreView(Published April 15, 2008 as doi: 10.1177/0363546508315471): 949-955.

Minas, T. (1999). "The role of cartilage repair techniques, including chondrocyte transplantation, in focal chondral knee damage." Instructional Course Lectures 48: 629-643.

Minas, T. and T. Bryant (2005). "The role of autologous chondrocyte implantation in the patellofemoral joint." Clinical Orthopaedics and Related Research 436: 30-39.

Minas, T., A. Gomoll, et al. (2009). "Increased failure rate of autologous chondrocyte implantation after previous treatment with marrow stimulation techniques." American Journal of Sports Medicine 37: 902-908.

Minas, T., A. Gomoll, et al. (2009). "Autologous chondrocyte implantation for joint preservation in patients with early osteoarthritis." Clinical Orthopaedics and Related Research Epub Aug 4, 2009.

Minas, T. and S. Nehrer (1997). "Current concepts in the treatment of articular cartilage defects." Orthopedics 20(6): 525-538.

Mithoefer, K., T. McAdams, et al. (2009). "Clinical efficacy of the microfracture technique for articular cartilage repair in the knee: an evidence-based systematic analysis." Am J Sports Med 37(10): 2053-63.

Mlynarik, V., S. Trattnig, et al. (1999). "The role of relaxation times in monitoring proteoglycan depletion in articular cartilage." J Magn Reson Imaging 10(4): 497-502.

Namdari, S., K. Baldwin, et al. (2009). "Results and performance after microfracture in National Basketball Association Athletes." American Journal of Sports Medicine 37: 943-949.

Noyes, F. and S. Barber-Westin (1995). "Irradiated meniscus allografts in the human knee. A two to five year follow-up study. ." Orthop Trans 19: 417.

Ogilvie-Harris, D. J. and D. P. Fitsialos (1991). "Arthroscopic management of the degenerative knee." Arthroscopy 7(2): 151-7.

Outerbridge, R. (1961). "The etiology of chondromalacia patellae." Journal of Bone and Joint Surgery, British 43: 752-757.

Pascale, W., S. Luraghi, et al. (2011). "Do microfractures improve high tibial osteotomy outcome?" Orthopedics 34(7): e251-5.

Peterfy, C. G., A. Guermazi, et al. (2004). "Whole-Organ Magnetic Resonance Imaging Score (WORMS) of the knee in osteoarthritis." Osteoarthritis Cartilage 12(3): 177-90.

Peterson, L., T. Minas, et al. (2000). "Two- to 9-Year Outcome After Autologous Chondrocyte Transplantation of the Knee." Clinical Orthopaedics and Related Research 374: 212-234.

Peterson, L., H. Vasiliadis, et al. (2010). "Autologous chondrocyte implantation - A long-term follow-up." American Journal of Sports Medicine 38(6): 1117-1124.

Pidoriano, A. J., R. N. Weinstein, et al. (1997). "Correlation of patellar articular lesions with results from anteromedial tibial tubercle transfer." Am J Sports Med 25(4): 533-7.

Radin, E. and R. Rose (1986). "Role of subchondral bone in the initiation and progression of cartilage damage." Clinical Orthopaedics and Related Research 213: 34-40.

Reilly, D. T. and M. Martens (1972). "Experimental analysis of the quadriceps muscle force and patello-femoral joint reaction force for various activities." Acta Orthop Scand 43(2): 126-37.

Richmond, J., D. Hunter, et al. (2009). "Treatment of osteoarthritis of the knee (nonarthroplasty)." J Am Acad Orthop Surg 17(9): 591-600.

Roos, H. (1998). "Are there long-term sequelae from soccer?" Clinics in Sports Medicine 17: 819-883.

Rosenberg, T. D., L. E. Paulos, et al. (1988). "The forty-five-degree posteroanterior flexion weight-bearing radiograph of the knee." J Bone Joint Surg Am 70(10): 1479-83.

Scott, W. (2005). Insall & Scott Surgery of the Knee, Churchill Livingstone.
Sharma, L., J. Song, et al. (2001). "The role of knee alignment in disease progression and functional decline in knee osteoarthritis." JAMA 286(2): 188-95.
Shasha, N., S. Krywulak, et al. (2003). "Long-term follow-up of fresh tibial osteochondral allografts for failed tibial plateau fractures." J Bone Joint Surg Am 85-A Suppl 2: 33-9.
Simonian, P. T., P. S. Sussmann, et al. (1998). "Contact pressures at osteochondral donor sites in the knee." Am J Sports Med 26(4): 491-4.
Sprague, N. F., 3rd (1981). "Arthroscopic debridement for degenerative knee joint disease." Clin Orthop Relat Res(160): 118-23.
Stahl, R., A. Luke, et al. (2009). "T1rho, T2 and focal knee cartilage abnormalities in physically active and sedentary healthy subjects versus early OA patients--a 3.0-Tesla MRI study." Eur Radiol 19(1): 132-43.
Steadman, J., K. Briggs, et al. (2003). "Outcomes of microfracture for traumatic chondral defects of the knee: Average 11-year follow-up." Arthroscopy: The Journal of Arthroscopic and Related Surgery 19(5): 477-484.
Steadman, J., B. Miller, et al. (2003). "The microfracture technique in the treatment of full-thickness chondral lesions of the knee in NFL players." Journal of Knee Surgery 16: 83-86.
Sterett, W. and J. Steadman (2004). "Chondral Resurfacing and High Tibial Osteotomy in the Varus Knee." American Journal of Sports Medicine 32(5): 1243-1249.
Sterett, W., J. Steadman, et al. (2010). "Chondral Resurfacing and High Tibial Osteotomy in the Varus Knee." American Journal of Sports Medicine e-published on April 7, 2010.
Ulrich-Vinther, M., M. D. Maloney, et al. (2003). "Articular cartilage biology." J Am Acad Orthop Surg 11(6): 421-30.
van Arkel, E. and H. de Boer (1995). "Human meniscal transplantation. Preliminary results at 2 to 5-year follow-up." Journal of Bone and Joint Surgery, British 77B: 589-595.
Vavken, P. and D. Samartzis (2010). "Effectiveness of autologous chondrocyte implantation in cartilage repair of the knee: a systematic review of controlled trials." Osteoarthritis Cartilage 18(6): 857-63.
Welsch, G. H., T. C. Mamisch, et al. (2008). "Cartilage T2 assessment at 3-T MR imaging: in vivo differentiation of normal hyaline cartilage from reparative tissue after two cartilage repair procedures--initial experience." Radiology 247(1): 154-61.
Widuchowski, W., J. Widuchowski, et al. (2007). "Articular cartilage defects: Study of 25,124 knee arthroscopies." The Knee 14: 177-182.
Yang, S. S. and B. Nisonson (1995). "Arthroscopic surgery of the knee in the geriatric patient." Clin Orthop Relat Res(316): 50-8.

7

Articular Cartilage Regeneration with Stem Cells

Khay-Yong Saw[1], Adam Anz[2], Kathryne Stabile[2], Caroline SY Jee[3], Shahrin Merican[1], Yong-Guan Tay[1] and Kunaseegaran Ragavanaidu[4]

[1]*Kuala Lumpur Sports Medicine Centre,*
[2]*Wake Forest University Baptist Medical Center,*
[3]*The University of Nottingham Malaysia Campus;*
[4]*Clinipath, Klang*
[1,3,4]*Malaysia*
[2]*USA*

1. Introduction

Cartilage defects continue to be a clinical challenge as regards to articular cartilage regeneration. The structure and function of articular cartilage leads to non-healing lesions after injury occurs. Well-established arthroscopic methods utilize controlled healing with marrow stimulation or transferring of non-injured cartilage to areas of injury. These include: microfracture, chondral drilling, osteochondral autograft transfer system, ostechondral allograft transplant, and autologous chondrocyte implantation. However, more often than not the treatments result in the formation of fibrocartilage and similar results within all methods with no clear superior modality (Jakobsen et al, 2005; Lubowitz et al, 2007; Magnussen et al, 2008; Nakamura et al, 2009). Recent study has investigated synthetic and biologic adjuncts to current methodology, including the use of: hyaluronic acid (HA), platelet rich plasma, mesenchymal stem cells (MSC) and peripheral blood progenitor cells (PBPC). Cell therapy has produced exciting results in animal models and has been shown to regenerate hyaline cartilage clinically in the knee joint. Our current method utilizes arthroscopic subchondral drilling of cartilage lesions in combination with a postoperative adjunct treatment involving: stimulation of the release of PBPC with filgrastim, harvest of PBPC with apheresis, and postoperative intraarticular injection of PBPC in combination with HA. Our early results lead us to the conclusion that cell therapy will have an integral part in the future treatment of cartilage damage as well as other potential orthopedic, surgical, and medical applications.

2. Anatomy of articular cartilage

Understanding the form and function of articular cartilage is the cornerstone to developing successful treatments for articular cartilage damage. Articular cartilage is a tissue that bears load and forms the articulating surfaces of diarthrodial joints. Articular cartilage dissipates loads, has low friction, provides lubrication, and can last up to 8 decades.

Articular cartilage is predominately composed of extracellular matrix (ECM) with a sparse population of chondrocytes that help to maintain the ECM. The major components of the

ECM are water, collagen, and proteoglycans. These combine with the chondrocytes to form the complex structure of articular cartilage which varies throughout its depth. The structure of articular cartilage is typically divided into 4 zones (superficial, middle, deep, and zone of calcified cartilage). The superficial zone or tangential zone is adjacent to the joint cavity and forms a gliding surface. The superficial zone is characterized by thin collagen fibrils that are aligned parallel with the articular surface. This zone also has disk shaped chondrocytes, low proteoglycan content, with high collagen and water contents. The middle (transitional) zone is characterized by large diameter collagen fibers which are oriented obliquely, round chondrocytes, and an increased proteoglycan content. The deep (radial) zone has the highest proteoglycan content with collagen fibers oriented perpendicular to the joint surface. The chondrocytes in the deep zone are round and organized into columns. The deepest layer is the zone of calcified cartilage and separates the hyaline cartilage from the subchondral bone. This zone is characterized by collagen fibrils that are radially aligned with round chondrocytes that are buried in calcified matrix. This zone has a low concentration of proteoglycans and a high concentration of calcium salts (Fig 1).

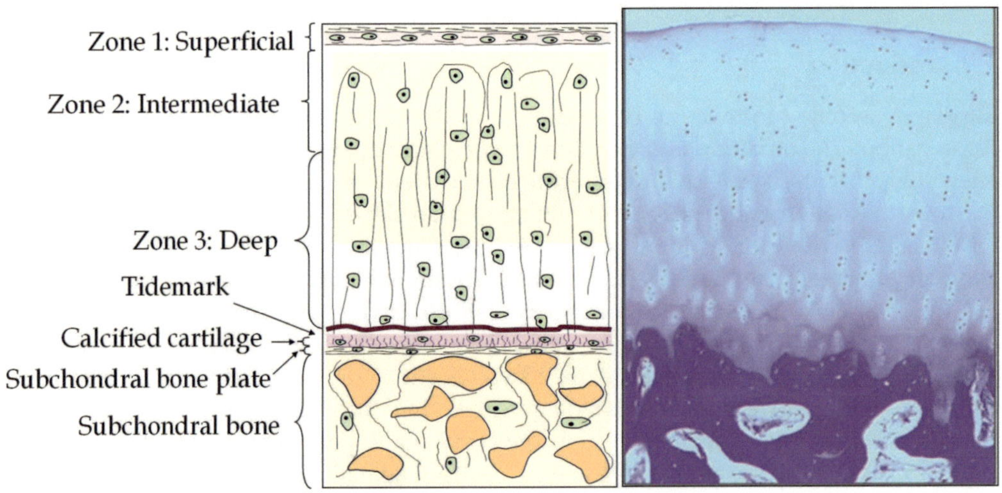

Fig. 1. This figure illustrates the zones of hyaline cartilage: superficial, middle, deep, and zone of calcified cartilage. Lacunae are present in hyaline cartilage and typically contains 1-2 chondrocytes. There is a periphery of increased proteoglycan content around each chondrocyte and lacuna.

Articular cartilage is avascular and obtains its nutrition from the diffusion of synovial fluid through the ECM and from underlying bone. Chondrocytes produce ECM components in response to chemical (growth factor and cytokines) and physical (mechanical load, hydrostatic pressure) stimuli. The ECM is composed primarily of water 65-80%, collagen (type II) 10-20%, and aggrecan 4-7%. Other components of the ECM make up less than 5% of articular cartilage. These include proteoglycans, biglycan, decorin, fibromodulin, various collagen types (V, VI, IX, X, XI), link protein, hyaluronate, fibronectin, and lipids. The role of each of these molecules is not fully understood. Collagen functions to provide shear and tensile strength to the cartilage. Proteoglycans are produced and secreted by the chondrocytes. Proteoglycans are tangled in between collagen fibers creating an ECM that inhibits the movement of water and provides compression strength of cartilage. Aggrecan molecules for example bind with hyaluronic acid to create macromolecules (proteoglycan aggregate). These macromolecules are effectively immobilized in the collagen ECM. There tends to be a higher concentration of proteoglycans in the ECM closest to the chondrocytes. Proteoglycans are made up of repeating dissacharaide subunits called glycosaminoglycans (GAG). There are 3 types of GAGs found in cartilage 1. chondroitin sulfate, 2. keratin sulfate, and 3. dermatan sulfate. Chondroitin sulfate is most abundant and with age chondroitin-4 sulfate is found to decrease while keratin sulfate increases. These changes with age or arthritis can directly affect the properties of the cartilage. For example, with age, articular cartilage has decreased water content but with osteoarthritis it has increased water content (Mankin et al, 2000).

2.1 Histology of cartilage

To image articular cartilage, standard hematoxylin and eosin (H&E) is sufficient to visualize cartilage damage and clinical use (Fig 2). However, additional stains can provide more specific information about the ECM, proteoglycans, and chondrocytes. For proteoglycans cationic dyes such as Safranin-O and Alcian blue are typically used. Safranin-O stains polysaccharides (both carboxylated and sulfated) orange. Alcian blue can stain for both types of polysaccharides (pH 2.5) or be more specific for sulfated polysaccharides (pH 1.0) such as chondroitin sulfate, turning them turquoise (Horvai 2011). A Trichrome (Gomori or Masson's) stain highlights the orientation of collagen fibrils with a bright blue stain, while staining cytoplasm and other proteins red. Additionally, elastin fibers which are abundant in elastic cartilage are typically visualized with a silver stain such as a Verhoff stain where the fibers stain black. Cartilage staining can provide clear visualization of the cartilage profile in a specific location, however it is more qualitative than quantitative. To obtain more quantitative measurements of protein content Polymerase Chain Reaction (PCR) and other molecular techniques are needed.

3. Cartilage injury

Partial and full thickness cartilage defects have a limited ability for healing. This is in part attributed to the avascular properties of cartilage, limited stem cell population, as well as the hypoxic environment of diarthrodial joints. Additionally the mechanical loads in the joint can make articular cartilage healing a challenge. The full natural history of full thickness chondral defects is not well documented in the literature. However it is thought that full thickness defects left untreated lead to joint space narrowing and degenerative arthritis (Messner & Maletius, 1996).

Cartilage injuries can occur with a twisting, shearing type injury in combination with axial loading. These defects are commonly associated with concomitant knee pathology such as meniscus tears, anterior cruciate ligament tears, medial collateral or lateral collateral ligament tears. There is a 5-10% incidence of full thickness chondral lesions following acute hemarthrosis (Noyes et al, 1980). In athletes, there is approximately a 36% prevalence of full thickness focal chondral defects, with 14% being asymptomatic (Flanigan et al, 2010).

Patients who have symptomatic chondral lesions typically present with pain localized to the compartment of injury, increased with weight-bearing of that compartment. They may also have recurrent effusions, catching, locking, or other mechanical symptoms. The physical examination typically will demonstrate crepitance, joint effusion, tenderness along ipsilateral joint line, signs of concomitant injury (meniscus or ligamentous), or malalignment. Coexisting malalignment can contribute to chondral injuries, i.e. patella maltracking, high Q angle, tight lateral patellar retinaculum, or varus/valgus alignment (Fig 3) (Freedman et al, 2004).

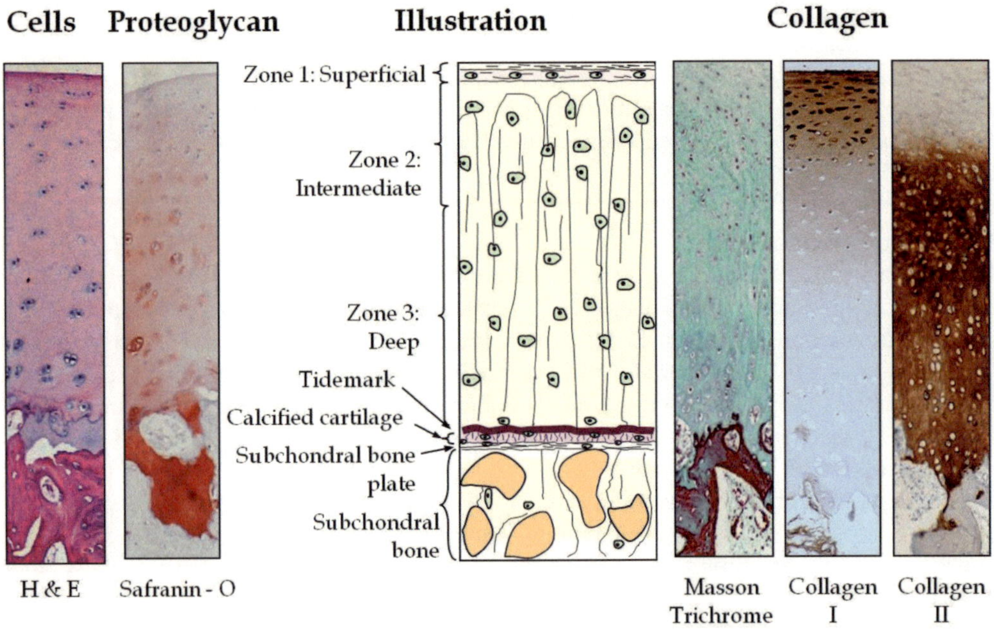

Fig. 2. This figure demonstrates how cartilage can be visualized differently with varying histological stains. From left to right: hemotoxylin & eosin (H&E) shows cellular content, Safranin-O highlights proteoglycan content, Masson's Trichrome shows collagen fibers and orientation of fibers, and immunohistochemistry can illustrate the different collagen types. Histological stains provide visualization and qualitative analysis of cartilage.

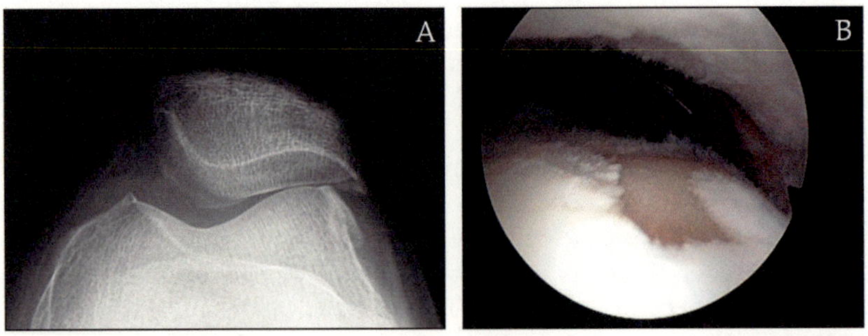

Fig. 3. Illustration of lateral patellar maltracking and its effects on chondral wear in the patellofemoral joint. (A) Radiograph with lateral patella maltracking, and (B) arthroscopic view showing chondral injury in a patient with lateral patella maltracking and the "kissing lesion" associated.

4. Cartilage regeneration methods

In 1959, abrasion arthroplasty was developed by Pridie to address chondral defects (Pridie, 1959). Originally developed as an open procedure, it was later adapted for arthroscopy by Johnson (Johnson, 1986). Today, abrasion arthroplasty is used primarily for osteoarthritic knees. However, for small focal chondral defects, microfracture is most commonly used.
Microfracture is a marrow stimulating technique that penetrates the subchondral bone in the cartilage defect (Fig 4). This allows marrow to communicate with the cartilage defect populating it with MSC, inflammatory mediators, and blood. This technique is simple to perform and has good to excellent clinical results (Gill, 2000; Steadman et al, 2003; Asik et al, 2008). Postoperative management requires prolonged non-weight-bearing (4 to 6 weeks) followed by the use of continuous passive motion. However, microfracture generates fibrocartilage in the defect and has a shorter functional lifespan compared with hyaline cartilage (Menche et al, 1996; McGuire et al, 2002; Steinwachs et al, 2008).

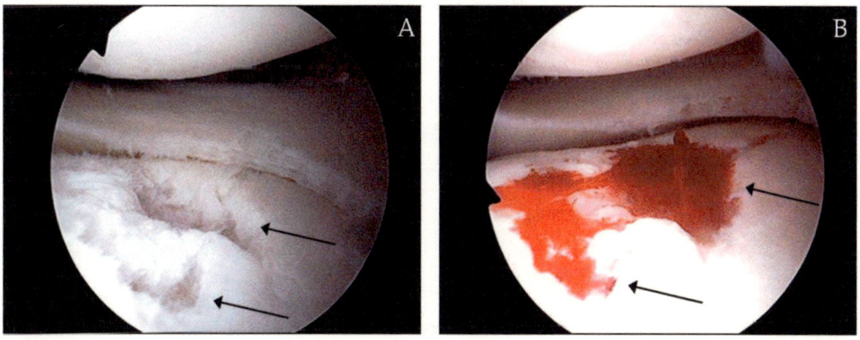

Fig. 4. Marrow stimulation with: (A) microfracture provides a source of (B) blood cells and bone marrow mesenchymal stem cells for cartilage regeneration. Healing response typically results in fibrocartilage formation.

Other techniques to address focal cartilage defects are osteoarticular transfer system with auto/allograft transplantation (OATS). This technique involves transplanting the defect with an intact cartilage and subchondral bone plug. This technique is typically used for small to medium sized lesions (0.5-3cm^2) (Fig 5). If a larger area is to be addressed a mosaicplasty is performed with multiple plugs. The main disadvantages are donor site morbidity, breakdown between the implanted cartilage and subchondral bone, gaps that remain between plugs, as well as technical difficulty.
More recently autologous chondrocyte implantation (ACI) was developed to regenerate cartilage closer to hyaline cartilage. This technique can be used for larger defects (2-10 cm^2), in patients who are symptomatic, and primarily located on the femoral condyles. To perform ACI requires 2 stages. The first stage involves harvesting cartilage from a biopsy to acquire cartilage cells. These cells are cultured to produce expanded autologous chondrocytes, which are subsequently implanted in the defect and held in place with a periosteal patch or collagen sheet sewn in place and sealed with a fibrin glue (Gooding et al, 2006). The postoperative course is challenging with a prolonged course of protected weight-bearing and continuous passive motion for 4 to 6 weeks. It can take up to 1-1.5 years for larger lesions to fill in. Second generation ACI is currently undergoing development to overcome the technical disadvantages of the first generation. Second generation ACI uses

tissue engineered 3- dimensional scaffolds that are seeded with autologous chondrocytes to promote cartilage regeneration. Despite continued technological improvements, clinical outcomes have yielded primarily symptomatic relief with fibrocartilage generation. The regeneration of long lasting hyaline cartilage continues to be a challenge (Ossendorf et al, 2007; Tuan, 2007).

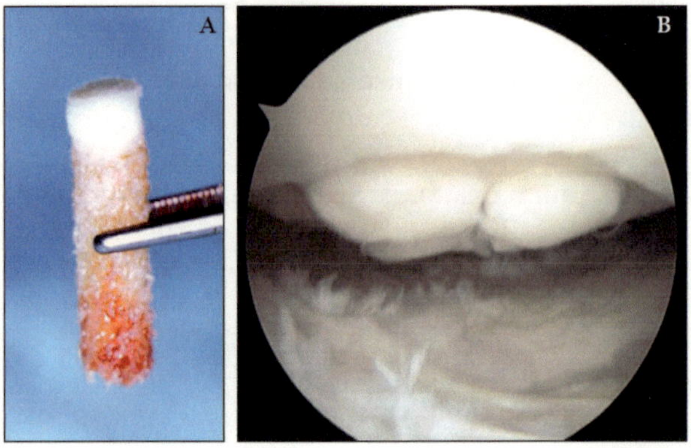

Fig. 5. Transfer system with auto/allograft transplantation (OATS) is illustrated in this figure with (A) harvesting and (B) second-look at one year showing chondral defects between the osteochondral plugs.

5. Adjuncts to current methods

Recent literature has illustrated that postoperative additions of HA to arthroscopic cartilage procedures yield better results (Johnson 1986; Kujawa & Caplan 1986; Gill, 2000; Freedman et al, 2004; Jakobsen et al, 2005; Gooding et al, 2006; Lee et al, 2007; Kang et al, 2008; Horvai et al, 2011; Fortier et al, 2011). High molecular weight hyaluronic acid is a component found in synovial fluid that has been investigated as adjunct for full thickness cartilage injury, microfracture, mesenchymal stem cells, and osteochondral allografting. Studies indicated that hyaluronic acid may play a role with differentiation of stem cells to chondrocytes, decreased joint inflammation, increased proteoglycan content, improved histologic scores, defect filling and incorporation, as well as decreased friction in the joint.

Another approach in attempts to regenerate hyaline cartilage are to use cells delivered either seeded on a matrix or transplanted to the defect similar to ACI. There are many cells that have been investigated, these include: mesenchymal stem cells (adipose versus bone marrow derived), chondrocytes, periostium, perichondrium. Short term results for these cellular based treatment modalities have been positive. However, long term clinical results are uncertain and have had limitations. Chondrocytes for example, lose chondrocyte phenotype with monolayer cell culture expansion and change to a fibroblastic appearance.

When chondrocytes are combined with matrix/scaffold materials the result is predominately fibrocartilage. Perichondral/periosteal cells also have chondrogenic potential in vitro and in vivo when seeding matrices. However limitations have included, variable results, the need for 2 surgeries for harvest and implantation, and instability of repair tissue. Mesenchymal stem cells either adipose derived or bone marrow derived have multilineage potential and in the appropriate microenvironment will differentiate to chondrocytes. In vivo studies have yielded short term success in generating hyaline cartilage. However, long term results and stability of the repair tissue remain to be demonstrated (Steinert et al, 2007). Stem cell transplantations are widely used in treatments where they are induced to differentiate into specific cell types required in repairing damaged or destroyed cell tissues (Chung et al., 2006). Stem cells are capable of differentiating in vitro and in vivo along multiple pathways that include bone, cartilage, cardiac and skeletal muscle, neural cells, tendon, adipose, and connective tissue (Panagiota et al., 2005). There has been a vast and increasing interest in the research and application of human mesenchymal stem cells (hMSC) in the area of regenerative medicine over the last decade. The reasons are due to the multipotency and stability of the cellular characteristics of hMSC. However, stem cell growth and differentiation, particularly for hMSC, requires a complex and tightly regulated system consisting of medium, growth factors and serum components.

hMSC has been studied for many years and there are a set of tests that can be performed as the minimal criteria for defining multipotency of mesenchymal stromal cells (Dominici et al, 2006). These are:

1. Plastic adherent assessment: hMSC is known to be able to adhere to plastic and hence the first observation is whether the cultured hMSCs exhibit the "plastic-adherent" behaviour using standard tissue culture flasks at standard culture conditions.
2. Surface antigen expression: more than 95% of the hMSC population is to express positive for CD105, CD73 and CD90. These can be easily measured using flow cytometry. In addition, the cells have to show negative expression (less or equal to 2%) of CD45, CD34, CD14 or CD11b, CD79a or CD19 and HLA class II.
3. Multipotent differentiation potential assessment: One of the criteria that defines hMSC is that the cells must differentiate under in vitro culture conditions to osteoblasts, adipocytes and chondroblasts. The identification of these differentiated cells can be done via Alizarin Red or von Kossa staining (for osteoblast), Oil Red O (for adipocytes) and Alcian blue or immunohistochemical staining for collagen type II (for chondroblasts).

There are numerous reports in the literature using MSC to regenerate bone and cartilage. A few of the examples are outlined in Table 1 below. Generally, the use of MSC will involve either direct injection or incorporation with a scaffold or matrix to aid delivery of the cells to the intended site (Nöth et al, 2008). Nevertheless, not all cases use MSC directly, most often the MSC are differentiated in vitro for various purposes. This involves some form of benchtop work either with isolation of cells or culture expansion thus leading to increased costs.

The literature has not shown any strong evidence that any of the above methods actually generated fully function cartilage matching the original cartilage although evidence has suggested an improvement of the condition with these treatments. It is theorized that MSC have an unknown number of bioactive molecules that are immunoregulatory and able to promote regenerative activities (Chen et al 2006 & Uccelli et al, 2007). There are cases whereby MSC are used with or without a matrix as a vehicle to deliver gene therapy site specific. However, these are still experimental and will not be covered in this chapter.

Additional approaches to regenerate hyaline cartilage are to adjunct bone marrow stimulation with growth factors and hyaluronic acid which is rich in glycosaminoglycans and provide the building blocks necessary for cartilage regeneration. Investigators are beginning to evaluate platelet rich plasma (PRP). There are numerous proteins found in platelets including growth factors involved in the healing response such as platelet derived growth factor (PDGF), vascular endothelial growth factor (VEGF), transforming growth factor (TGF-M1), fibroblast growth factor (FGF). Early research has shown that mesenchymal stem cells and chondrocytes exposed to PRP have increased cell proliferation and production of proteoglycans and collagen type II (Fortier et al, 2011). In a clinical cohort comparing hyaluronic acid with PRP injections, PRP had improved pain scores (Sanchez et al, 2008). However, the quality and longevity of the repair tissue generated by the adjunct of PRP is still unproven.

Applications	**Techniques**	**Scaffolds used**	**Status**
Growth plate cartilage injury	Autologous mesenchymal stem cells seeded onto Gelform scaffold containing TGF-β1 growth factor, then transplanted to injury site (McCarty et al, 2010)	Gelform	Animal (ovine) study
Large cartilage defects	Direct intra-articular injection of autologous mesenchymal stem cells suspended in hyaluronic acid (Lee et al, 2007)	None	Animal (porcine model)
Osteoarthritis	Direct intra-articular injection of autologous mesenchymal stem cells in a dilute solution of hyaluronic acid (Murphy et al, 2003)	None	Animal (Caprine model)
Full-thickness cartilage defects	Autologous mesenchymal stem cells seeded with collagen type I hydrogels (Wakitani et al , 2004)	Collagen type I hydrogels	Human

Table 1. Examples of clinical applications of hMSC

6. Arthroscopic subchondral drilling augmented with peripheral blood progenitor cells (PBPC)

Our laboratory has had increased interest in the used of peripheral blood progenitor cells (PBPC) over the use of bone marrow derived progenitor cells (BMPC). A study report published in April 2011 by the first author's group (Saw et al, 2011) confirmed that articular hyaline cartilage regeneration was possible with arthroscopic subchondral drilling followed by postoperative intraarticular injections of autologous PBPC in combination with HA.

Treatment involving progenitor cells stems from the hematology/oncology profession: Given the potential morbidity associated with iliac crest harvest, cell collection for bone marrow repopulation now involves mobilization of multipotential progenitor cells through hormonal stimulation and collection via a peripheral automated cell separator machine. This process, commonly referred to as apheresis, has potential for increased magnitude of harvest. Studies involving review of healthy donors have shown this to be a safe and effective procedure for the production and harvest of cells (Ceselli et al, 2009 & Holig et al, 2009). Recent study into the properties of these PBPC has shown that they are similar to embryonal stem cells in that they express transcription factors specific to pluripotential cells, have proliferative potential, have the ability to differentiate into a multitude of cell types, and are more immature than

BMPC (Ceselli et al, 2009). In addition, when injected subcutaneously into mice, these cells were found to migrate to multiple organs and integrate and function as the surrounding cells (Ceselli et al, 2009). In addition to implementing evidence from recent animal studies, we have sought to make use of clinical evidence regarding the potential and safety of PBPC, preferring to use PBPC as opposed to BMPC because of the ease of harvest, decreased harvest-site morbidity, and increased potential with these cells (Ceselli et al, 2009; Holig et al, 2009 & Ordemann et al, 1998). In the clinical setting, we prefer to use PBPC as opposed to BMPC due to the ease of harvest and the increased potential with these cells. Subsequently, we have developed a method involving standard marrow stimulation in the form of subchondral drilling and novel postoperative intraarticular injections of autologous PBPC in combination with HA to regenerate articular cartilage.

7. Authors preferred method

7.1 Evolution of technique

Arthroscopic surgeons are regularly faced with the challenges of providing a satisfactory end result for the treatment of chondral lesions. Prior to the development of the current method, the first author was treating chondral lesions with standard subchondral drilling followed by postoperative intraarticular injections of hyaluronic acid (HA). This being a variant of marrow stimulation technique, produces fibrocartilage which is not as resilient as the original hyaline cartilage. The newly regenerated fibrocartilage gradually deteriorated with time. Since Year 2005, the first author has been dissatisfied with the inconsistent end results following this method of cartilage repair as shown in Fig 6.

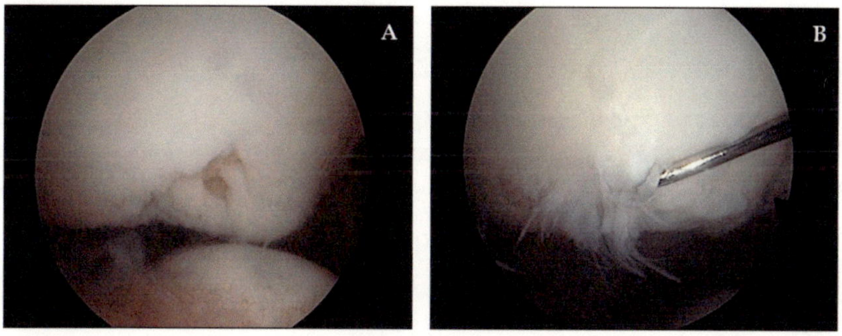

Fig. 6. Intraoperative view after subchondral drilling of the lateral patella facet - right knee (A). Second-look at 18 months (B) showing partial coverage of the defect with fibrocartilage.

At the same time, veterinary surgeons have shown that injections of bone marrow aspirate into race horse's flexor tendon injuries resulted in satisfactory healing (Pacini et al, 2007; Taylor et al, 2007; Thomas et al, 2008 & Violini et al, 2009). This gave rise to the idea of utilizing stem cells in the knee joint to initiate articular cartilage repair after subchondral drilling.

A literature search suggests that the mesenchymal stem cell (MSC) is a better alternative to the chondrocyte as it is a less differentiated cell and is capable of differentiating into both bone and articular cartilage. As most chondral lesions involve both these components, cells that are capable of forming both bone and cartilage should theoretically be able to regenerate into tissue that will integrate better with the surrounding native structures. This may minimize of delamination which is occasionally seen by the autologous chondrocyte implantation (ACI) technique. Fig 7 shows the potential differentiation process of MSC.

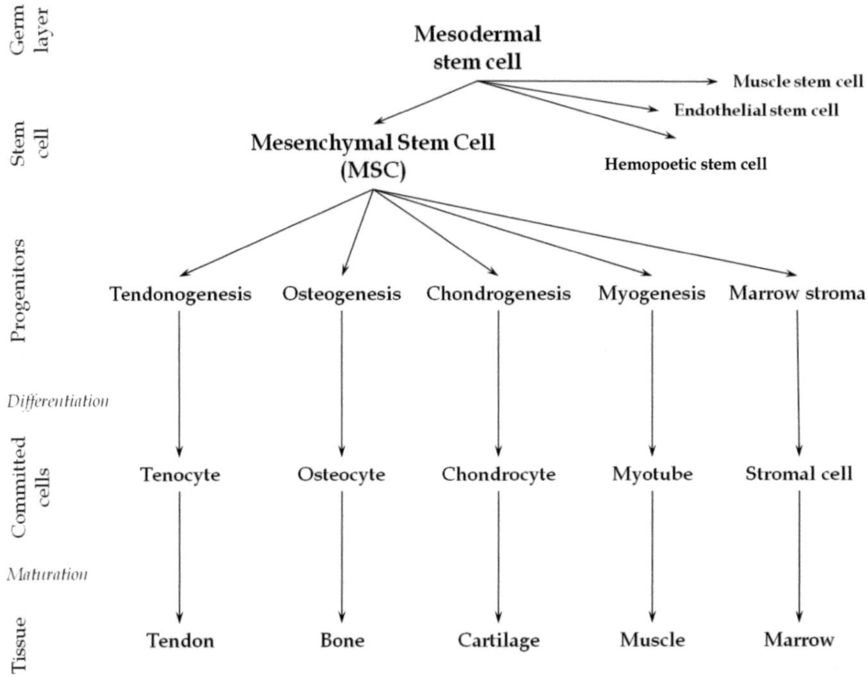

Fig. 7. Potential differentiation process of MSC.

Open surgery does not appeal to arthroscopic surgeons. The ideal method of articular cartilage repair would be a single arthroscopic procedure followed by an adjunct cell therapy which could be performed in the out-patient setting. Obviously the desired end result should be the regeneration of the original hyaline cartilage with clinical improvement. The arthroscopic surgeon's wish list for chondrogenesis is listed below:

- Single arthroscopic procedure
- Able to treat multiple/kissing lesions
- Applicable in large osteochondral defects
- Simple delivery - intraarticular injections
- Scaffold free
- Treat associated injuries
- Regeneration of soft tissues
- Cost effective
- Hyaline cartilage regeneration

7.2 Animal model

The following work has been published in *Arthroscopy: The Journal of Arthroscopic and Related Surgery, Vol 25, No 12 (December), 2009: pp 1391-1400* (Saw et al, 2009). An excerpt of the published work is described.

In the animal model, we wished to find out whether postoperative intraarticular injections of autologous marrow aspirate (MA) and HA after subchondral drilling could result in a better cartilage repair.
A 4 mm full thickness articular cartilage defect was created in the stifle joint, followed by subchondral drilling as shown in Fig 8. The animals were divided into three groups: group A (control), no injections; group B (HA), weekly injection of 1 mL of sodium hyaluronate for 3 weeks; and group C (HA + MA), similar to group B but with 2 mL of autologous MA in addition to HA. MA was obtained by bone marrow aspiration, centrifuged, and divided into aliquots for cryopreservation. 15 animals were equally divided between the groups and sacrificed 24 weeks after surgery, when the joint was harvested, examined macroscopically and histologically (Fig 9).

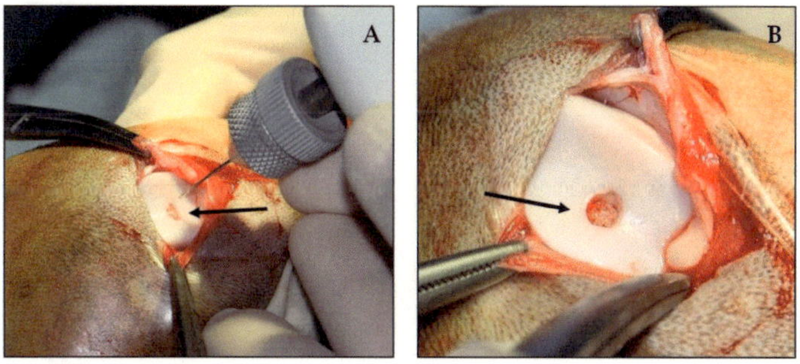

Fig. 8. (A&B) A 4mm full thickness articular cartilage defect was created in the stifle joint, followed by subchondral drilling.

7.2.1 Macroscopic findings

The chondral defects were covered with repair tissue in all groups, without evidence of synovitis or synovial thickening (Fig 9). In group A the defects were covered with semitransparent tissue having recognizable margins but with an irregular surface. A similar appearance was seen in group B goats. In group C the defect coverage was almost complete, and the color of the repair tissue was indistinct from surrounding cartilage. The surfaces were smooth and appeared level with adjacent normal cartilage.

7.2.2 Histologic findings

Under H&E staining, scar tissue was present in group A, which was characterized by a disordered arrangement of fibroblasts in an edematous stroma (Fig 9). The interface of scar tissue with subchondral bone was marked by the presence of dilated capillaries and venules. In group B scar tissue was less pronounced, and islands of hyaline-like cartilage were seen at the interface with subchondral bone and also adjacent to normal cartilage at the defect margins. Edema was also less marked than in the control group. In group C there was chondrogenesis with evidence of hyaline cartilage formation. The hyaline cartilage also showed features of maturation as evidenced by a linear arrangement of chondrocytes extending from the subchondral bone toward the surface. No edema was seen in this group.
With Safranin-O staining, proteoglycans were notably absent from the repair tissue in group A. In group B proteoglycans were seen only at the base and sides of the defect in the same distribution as the hyaline-like cartilage. In group C there was marked proteoglycan accumulation in the deeper layers, excluding the perichondrium, which normally does not contain proteoglycans.

Under collagen staining, the scar tissue in group A was found to contain only type I collagen, with an absence of staining for type II collagen. In group B type I collagen staining in the repair tissue was less pronounced, with light staining for type II collagen around the areas of hyaline-like cartilage. In group C type I collagen staining was found only in the perichondrium, whereas the deeper cartilage stained strongly for type II collagen.

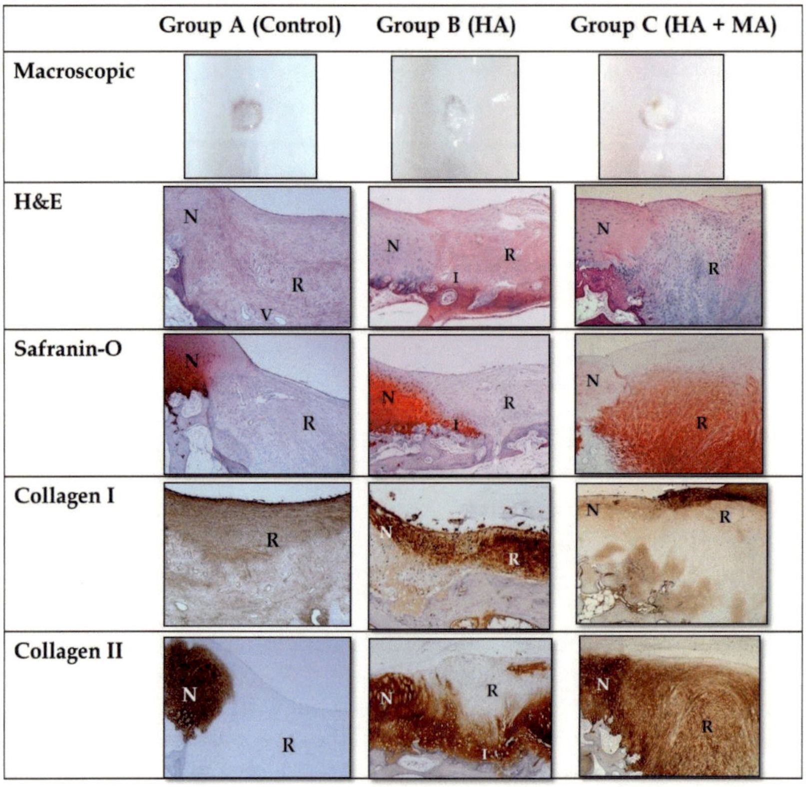

Fig. 9. Macroscopic and histologic findings for representative subjects from all 3 groups. (N, normal cartilage; R, repair cartilage; V, dilated capillaries and venules; I, islands of hyaline-like cartilage).

7.2.3 Discussion on the animal model

Penetration of the subchondral bone was shown to release the underlying marrow, which initiated repair of the chondral defect with fibrocartilage in a pattern that was observed in group A animals. The reason why fibrous tissue forms instead of hyaline cartilage is not known, but it is likely that the local microenvironment contains paracrine factors that either promote fibrous tissue formation, inhibit cartilage growth, or both.

The addition of HA in group B animals improved the quality of repair tissue by allowing hyaline-like cartilage to form. This suggests that HA modifies the microenvironment in such a way that neutralizes these paracrine factors. The incomplete regeneration could be because of HA being only partially effective or the duration of administration being too short. It appeared that the region adjacent to subchondral bone and the interface with normal cartilage seemed to be most favorable to cartilage formation.

The combination of HA and MA in group C yielded the best results in that the repair tissue was composed of true hyaline cartilage, showing vertical orientation of chondrocyte nests and the presence of type II collagen and proteoglycans in the intermediate and deep cartilage layers, with type I collagen confined to the superficial layer and perichondrium (Fig 9). This suggests that the combination of HA and MA is most effective in neutralizing the paracrine factors, and its effects persist for the duration of the repair process. One of the essential active components in MA is likely the MSC content, given that a previous study in a porcine model showed that cultured autologous MSCs injected intraarticularly together with HA could produce the same results as in the group C animals (Lee et al, 2007).
The presence of edema in the repair tissue appears to be proportional to the degree of fibrous scarring and was most marked in group A animals. The dilated capillaries and venules at the base of the defect suggest an inflammatory process that originates in the subchondral bone. These observations indicate that the paracrine factors, which promote fibrous tissue formation, are closely related to the inflammatory process that occurs after mechanical disruption of the chondral plate and that both HA and MA may be able to suppress inflammation locally.

7.2.4 Conclusion on the animal model

This preclinical experimental study in the goat model concluded that postoperative intraarticular injections of autologous MA in combination with HA after subchondral drilling resulted in a better cartilage repair.

7.2.5 Clinical relevance from the animal model

After arthroscopic subchondral drilling, postoperative intraarticular injections of autologous progenitor cells in combination with HA may result in better articular cartilage regeneration.

7.3 Clinical trial

A human clinical trial followed the preclinical animal studies. The surgical technique applied in the clinical trial involved standard marrow stimulation in the form of arthroscopic subchondral drilling and postoperative intraarticular injections of autologous peripheral blood progenitor cells (PBPC) in combination with HA. The objective of the trial was to assess whether the results of the preclinical animal model could be replicated in the human knee joint. The purpose of the clinical trial was to evaluate the quality of resultant articular cartilage regeneration. A hypothesis was made that articular hyaline cartilage regeneration was possible with this novel approach.
The early results with histology were published in *Arthroscopy: The Journal of Arthroscopic and Related Surgery, Vol 27, No 4 (April), 2011: pp 493-506* . An excerpt of the paper is presented in the following sections (Saw et al, 2011).

7.3.1 Patient selection – indication for surgery

The diagnosis of chondral injury was made after clinical and radiologic evaluation. Chondral lesions were graded according to the International Cartilage Repair Society (ICRS) Cartilage Injury Evaluation Package (Brittberg & Peterson, 1998) The inclusion criteria were patients with ICRS grade III and IV lesions, defects of any size and number, age 18 to 60 years, deformity (lateral patella maltracking or axis correction) correctable at the time of surgery, and ligamentous instability deemed reconstructable at the same time. The exclusion criteria were patients with disease progression such that total knee arthroplasty was indicated; a history of infected knees, gross bone defects, rheumatoid arthritis, or intraarticular corticosteroids within the previous 6 weeks; and gross valgus or varus deformity not correctable during surgery.

7.3.2 Surgical procedure

All surgical procedures were performed by a single surgeon (by the first author) involving standard arthroscopic techniques in the supine position without a tourniquet. Saline solution irrigation bags were chilled in an ice-water bath before use to minimize bleeding during the arthroscopic procedure. In our experience, we have had difficulty performing microfracture to the patella and areas of the plateau. For this reason, our preferred method is arthroscopic subchondral drilling modified from the principles established by Steadman et al (Steadman et al, 1999), for microfracture and Pridie (Pridie, 1959) for drilling. We begin by defining the extent of cartilage injury with a probe. A 3.5 mm full-radius shaver is used to debride loose cartilage to a stable margin; often a straight or curved arthroscopic biter is required as well. A 2 mm burr, with its guard removed, "drills" from the surface of the defect to the bone marrow, creating a conduit. The remaining area within the margin is also drilled to a depth of 5 to 10 mm. Initially, we spaced drill holes 3 to 4 mm apart. The methods have subsequently been refined such that a goal of 1 to 2 mm between drill holes is now preferred based on the results of second-look arthroscopy. It is not crucial that the subchondral drilling be performed perpendicular to the bone surface because a lesser angle of drilling capable of penetrating into the subchondral bone is sufficient. Abrasion chondroplasty up to a depth of 1 mm is performed with burring of the bony area between drill holes. The result is an extended area of bleeding bone, hence a larger surface area for the initiation of articular cartilage repair with PBPC and HA (Fig 10). The arthroscopic portals are closed with No. 3-0 nylon suture. A mixture of 20 mL of 0.5% bupivacaine hydrochloride and epinephrine, 3 mL of 1 mg/mL morphine, and 2 mL of HA (Hyalgan; Fidia Farmaceutici, Abano Terme, Italy) is injected into the operated knee at the end of the surgical procedure.

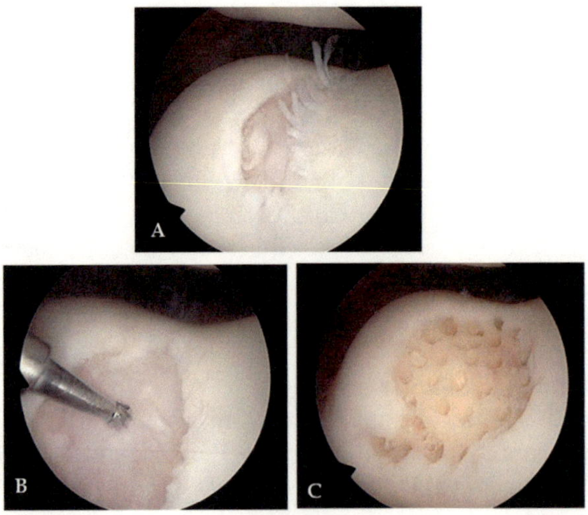

Fig. 10. Subchondral drilling. (A) A delaminated flap tear on the medial & central trochlear of a left knee. (B) A 2 mm burr with guard removed allows for drilling with light suction. (C) View after debridement, subchondral drilling and abrasion chondroplasty.

7.3.3 Postoperative rehabilitation

Cold therapy is initiated for one hour 2 to 3 times a day immediately in the postanesthesia period and continued throughout the first month after surgery. On the first postoperative day, continuous passive motion is used on the operated knee for a duration of 2 hours (Fig 11). This is continued daily for a period of 4 weeks. The range of motion is initially set from 0° to 30° and progresses as the clinical situation improves. Patients with subchondral drilling to the weight-bearing femorotibial joint are instructed on crutch-assisted partial weight-bearing (15 to 20 kg) for the first 4 weeks. This progresses to full weight-bearing in 6 to 8 weeks. Patients with drilling to the patellofemoral joint are allowed full weight-bearing as tolerated with restrictions from weight-bearing on stairs for the first 3 months after surgery. This is to avoid overloading the patellofemoral joint.

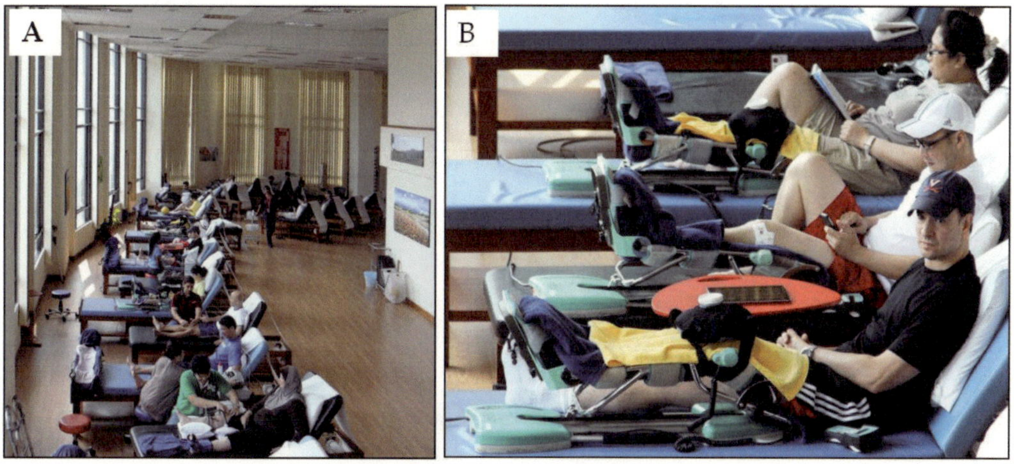

Fig. 11. Patients undergoing postoperative rehabilitation (A). A closer view of patients showing continuous passive motion applied on the operated knee (B).

7.3.4 Neupogen administration, apheresis, and cryopreservation

Human granulocyte colony-stimulating factor is a glycoprotein that regulates the production and release of functional neutrophils from the bone marrow. Neupogen contains recombinant granulocyte colony-stimulating factor and causes marked increases in peripheral blood neutrophil counts with a minor increase in monocytes within 24 hours. On postoperative days 4, 5, and 6, patients were given a morning dose of 300 micro-grams of Neupogen (Filgrastim, Amgen, Thousand Oaks, CA) subcutaneously. On postoperative day 7, autologous PBPC were collected by an automated cell separator (apheresis) via central venous access. Venous access was achieved through a femoral double-lumen catheter placed into the contralateral leg, under ultrasound guidance, performed by a trained specialist. Apheresis was performed by use of the Spectra Optia Apheresis Machine (Caridian BCT, Denver, CO). A fresh aliquot of 8 mL of PBPC was separated for fresh intraarticular injection into the operated knee. The remaining PBPC were cryopreserved in 10% dimethyl sulfoxide and divided into 4 mL cryovials for storage in liquid nitrogen at -196°C. Flow cytometry with CD34+ (hematopoietic stem cells) and CD105+ (markers for mesenchymal stem cells) was quantified. Flow cytometry was performed with a Beckman Coulter FC500 device (Beckman Coulter, Fullerton, CA). Fig 12 showing the apheresis process. The cryopreservation of the harvested PBPC in cryovials can be seen in Fig 13.

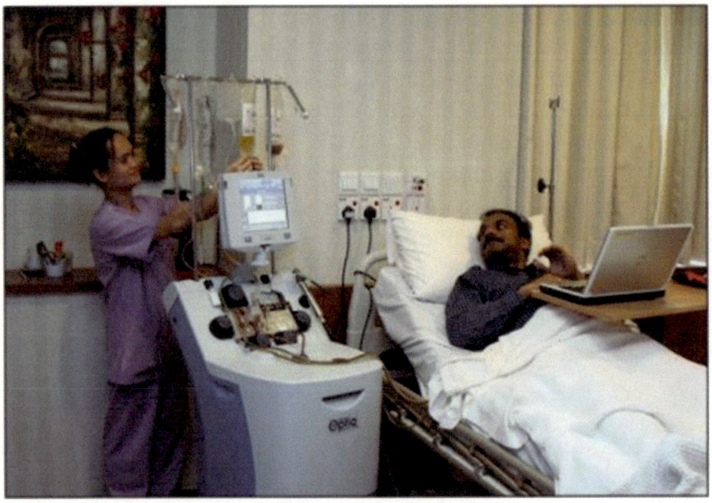

Fig. 12. A typical apheresis process.

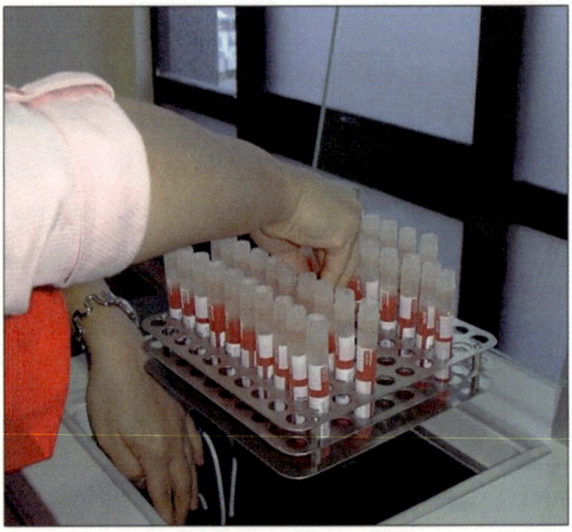

Fig. 13. Cryopreservation of the harvested PBPC in cryovials.

7.3.5 Intraarticular injection

On postoperative day 7, 8 mL of the fresh PBPCs is mixed with 2 mL of HA and injected into the operated knee joint under aseptic conditions in the out-patient clinic. Prior to this, the knee is first aspirated for hemarthrosis. At weekly intervals, 8 mL (from two 4 mL cryovials) of the frozen PBPC were obtained from the laboratory, allowed to thaw to room temperature, mixed with 2 mL of HA, and injected into the operated knee joint for 4 subsequent weeks. A flow chart of the protocol for patients undergoing articular cartilage regeneration is shown in Fig 14. Table 2 shows the PBPC count of 20 recent consecutive patients after refinement of our processing methods, showing data of fresh and frozen samples with white blood cell count, CD34+ and CD105+ counts, and cell viability.

	White Cell Count 10^3 / uL	CD 34+ (10^6) Cells per 4ml Vial		CD 105+ (10^6) Cells per 4ml Vial		Viability %	
		Fresh	Frozen	Fresh	Frozen	Fresh	Frozen
	32.00	6.86	4.58	7.42	8.14	99.30	79.90
	24.40	1.04	0.66	9.98	14.41	99.30	89.65
	30.00	0.33	0.23	3.32	5.08	99.10	89.99
	35.60	1.03	0.74	15.44	20.33	99.01	91.97
	14.80	3.88	2.86	2.69	8.87	99.40	87.90
	33.50	0.44	0.37	8.95	7.04	99.60	95.30
	33.50	3.28	2.33	5.41	7.75	99.00	82.90
	34.80	2.02	1.34	13.60	14.01	99.50	94.04
	23.00	2.53	1.69	7.01	13.77	99.50	88.10
	37.10	2.42	1.32	3.37	5.72	98.90	88.10
	26.50	1.55	1.07	4.54	6.98	99.00	84.80
	52.10	2.76	2.17	8.89	4.56	99.40	90.30
	38.80	3.15	1.82	15.50	11.62	99.30	79.30
	32.10	0.86	0.75	12.79	6.35	98.90	91.30
	33.00	5.71	3.14	6.30	8.53	99.10	78.40
	20.00	1.02	0.62	14.80	15.40	97.80	88.40
	37.50	3.19	2.08	4.15	1.66	99.30	82.20
	26.90	2.78	1.90	1.43	4.44	99.30	82.30
	31.00	1.55	1.01	23.45	31.15	99.10	89.10
	44.60	1.16	0.67	16.62	19.40	98.50	91.80
AVERAGE	32.06	2.38	1.57	9.28	10.76	99.12	87.29

Table 2. Example of 20 consecutive PBPC counts from patients following 3 neupogen injections. Data of fresh and frozen samples with white cell count, CD34+ and CD105+ counts, and cell viability.

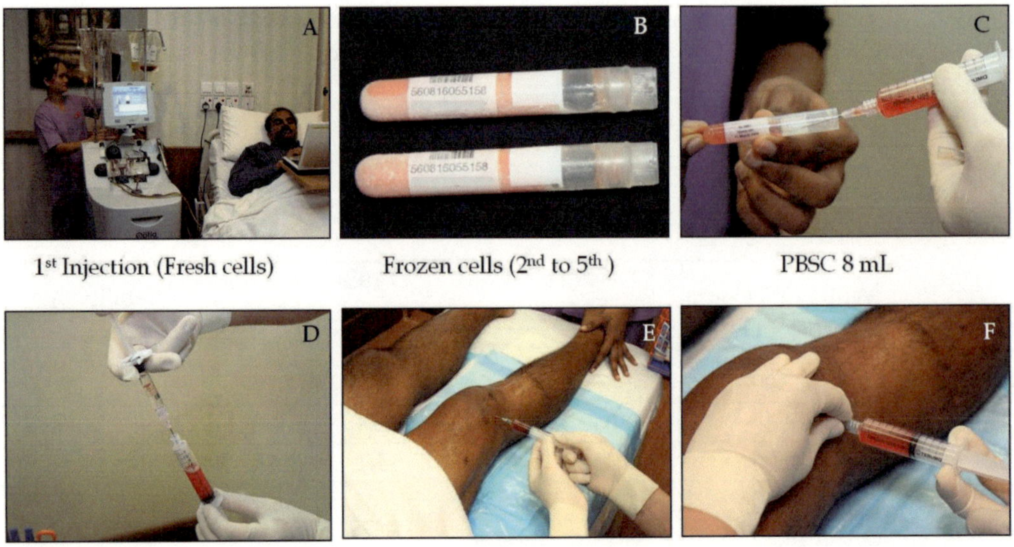

1st Injection (Fresh cells) | Frozen cells (2nd to 5th) | PBSC 8 mL

PBSC + 2 mL HA | Aspiration of hemarthrosis | PBSC + HA injection

Fig. 14. Flow chart showing the standard protocol for articular cartilage regeneration with PBPC and HA.

Fresh cells are used preferably for the first injection because of a mean viability of 99% compared with frozen cells, which have a mean viability of 87%. It should be noted that 8 mL of PBPC injected into the operated knee has a mean of 20 million CD105+ cells. Historically, the cell marker CD34+ (hematopoietic stem cells) has been used to identify functional cells for bone marrow transplant. We have begun to draw interest in CD105+ cells, because this is the marker for mesenchymal stem cells.

Five weekly injections are based on the HA protocol for osteoarthritis, as well as the suggestion from preclinical animal studies involving Bone Marrow Progenitor Cells (BMPC) that an increased number of intraarticular injections is more efficacious (Saw et al, 2009). Table 3 shows the viability of 5 consecutive frozen PBPC samples after mixing with HA. As can be seen, there is no effects of HA on the viability of the PBPC.

Frozen PBPC from -196°c Storage Tank						
Patient	Before addition of HA			After addition of HA		
	CD34+ (10^6) Based-4ml per vial	CD105+ (10^6) Based-4ml per vial	Viability	CD34+ (10^6) Based-4ml per vial	CD105+ (10^6) Based-4ml per vial	Viability
A	3.000	2.010	75.10%	3.380	6.050	77.50%
B	1.060	10.800	78.90%	0.980	3.750	83.00%
C	3.220	16.800	68.20%	2.660	8.230	68.90%
D	1.020	5.150	85.10%	0.550	2.370	86.60%
E	0.720	7.710	82.20%	0.750	2.780	84.80%
AVERAGE	**1.804**	**8.494**	**77.90%**	**1.664**	**4.636**	**80.16%**

Table 3. Cell count viability.

7.4 Introduction to clinical cases

Five cases are presented here with their respective chondral biopsies and histology. These cases provided explanation to the principles of chondrogenesis in our novel approach.
The patients are part of a larger pilot study in which 180 patients who presented with chondral defects of the knee joint were recruited. Postoperatively, the clinical course of these 5 patients presented an opportunity for a second-look arthroscopy. Two patients underwent contralateral knee surgery, and one patient had removal of a Tomofix plate and screw construct (Synthes, West Chester, PA), providing an opportune setting of anesthesia for second-look arthroscopy. One patient had recurrence of discomfort attributed to a prominent osteophyte and elected for a further arthroscopic procedure. The last patient had returned to football 18 months after articular cartilage repair and sustained a torn anterior cruciate ligament of the previously treated knee. He elected for arthroscopic reconstruction, which provided an opportunity for second-look arthroscopy. Informed consent after discussion of risks and benefits, as well as local ethics committee approval, was obtained before biopsy.

7.4.1 Second-look arthroscopy with chondral core biopsy

During the second-look procedures, a chondral core biopsy specimen was procured. This was performed arthroscopically with a 5.5 mm sterilized BioCorkscrew anchor driver (Arthrex, Naples, FL). Typically, a 2 mm diameter specimen of cartilage together with a core of bone up to 1 cm in length is obtained (Fig 15).
Arthroscopically, the regenerated articular cartilage appeared smooth and had excellent integration with the surrounding native cartilage without any delamination or hypertrophy. The exception was case 2, in which the drill holes over the lateral patellofemoral joint were too far apart with resultant tufts of cartilage seen between areas devoid of regenerated cartilage (Fig 16).

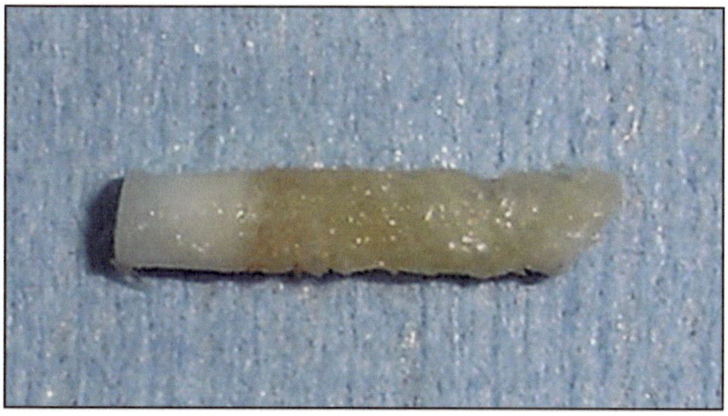

Fig. 15. Solid articular cartilage core biopsy with a 2 mm diameter including the underlying subchondral bone.

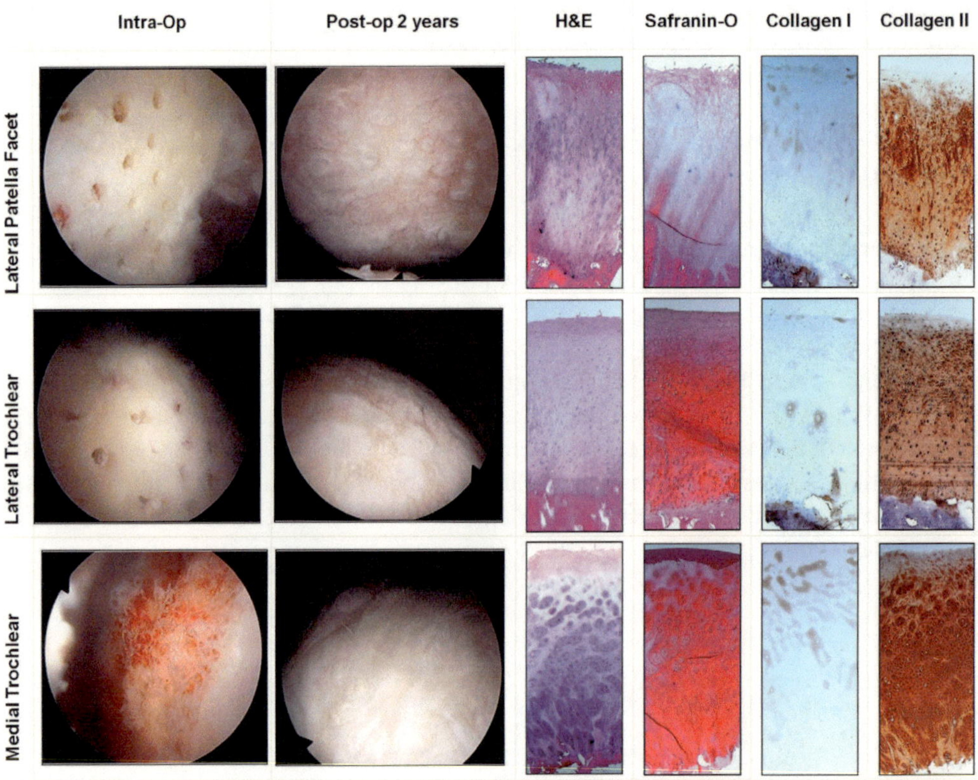

Fig. 16. 34-year-old female from Fig 22. Second-look arthroscopy from the lateral patella facet and lateral trochlear showed tufts of cartilage forming at each individual drill hole. Upon histological stains, notice the red staining with Safranin-O representing proteoglycans and the brown staining of collagen type II diffuse throughout the regenerated tissue. Collagen type I stain is minimal and localized near the superficial layers.

7.4.2 Histology

Histologic samples were stained as follows: hematoxylin-eosin (H&E) stain was used to visualize overall morphology, Safranin-O was used to highlight proteoglycans, immunohistochemistry staining with anti-collagen type I mouse Ab I-8H5 stain (catalog No. CP 17; Calbiochem Merck, Darmstadt, Germany) was used to highlight collagen type I, and immunohistochemistry staining with anti-collagen type II mouse monoclonal antibody Ab 3 (clone 6B3) (catalog No. MAB8887; Millipore, Billerica, MA) was used to highlight collagen type II. Optimal dilution and predigestion with pepsin were determined by the investigator with the protocol being saved by use of software of an automated immunohistochemical slide preparation system (Ventana Benchmark; Ventana Medical Systems, Tucson, AZ).

Cases 1 and 2 with gross grade IV kissing lesions are presented with multiple biopsy specimens and histologic analyses after second-look arthroscopy. Cases 3, 4, and 5 are patients with smaller isolated lesions.

Case 1: Biopsy was performed 22 months after the initial surgery in a 49-year-old woman with a varus deformity who underwent debridement, subchondral drilling, and an open wedge high tibial osteotomy with Tomofix fixation (Fig 17).

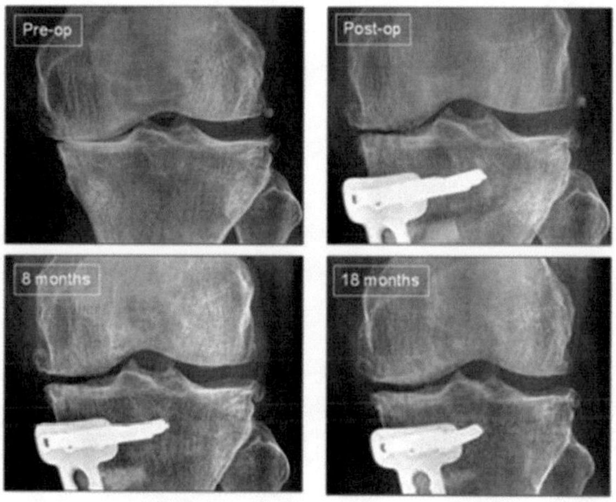

Fig. 17. Progressive serial weight-bearing radiographs of Case 1 with high tibial osteotomy. Notice re-appearance of the medial articulation.

Approximately 80% of the weight-bearing medial compartment had grade III and IV lesions. Weight-bearing radiographs at 8 and 18 months showed reappearance of the medial femorotibial joint space. Second-look arthroscopy of the regenerated cartilage showed a stable, smooth surface with no delamination. On probing, the regenerated cartilage had the same consistency as the surrounding normal cartilage. The second-look images and biopsy specimens are included in Fig 18.

Immunohistochemistry staining was performed to assess the collagen type I and type II content of the biopsy specimens. Specimens from the medial femoral condyle and medial tibial plateau showed the presence of collagen type I confined to the superficial layer. Collagen type II was present throughout the deeper layers. These are features of hyaline cartilage as opposed to fibrocartilage (Fig 18). Fig 19 shows a higher magnification of the histological sections from the medial tibial plateau.

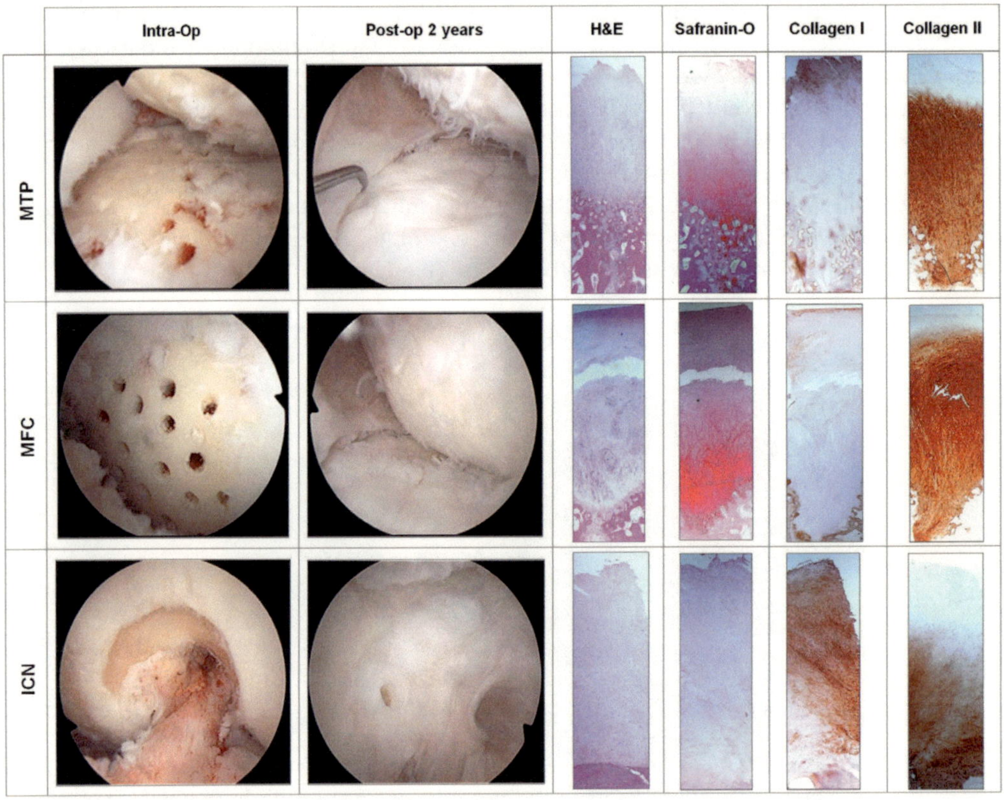

Fig. 18. Medial tibial plateau (MTP), medial femoral condyle (MFC) and intercondylar notch (ICN) biopsy results at 22 months after surgery. Biopsies from the MTP and MFC with H&E staining illustrate columnar morphology of cells with pale background. Safranin-O staining highlights abundance of proteoglycans throughout the regenerated cartilage layer. Collagen type I staining was limited to the superficial layer except in the non-weight-bearing ICN biopsy which showed a higher percentage of collagen type I and a disorganized pattern of healing. Collagen type II was concentrated in the deeper layers.

One full-thickness biopsy specimen from the medial tibial plateau captured a drill hole and adjacent bone (Fig 20). This sample shows full-thickness regenerated articular cartilage with a fairly smooth articular surface, subchondral bone, and marrow space. A streaming, linear pattern of chondrocytes is seen arising from the subchondral bone region from the area of previous subchondral drilling. Incidental findings of cartilage clusters with early ossification are also seen within the tract. The chondrocytes are involved in ongoing remodelling and are present beneath the calcified cartilage layer. A biopsy specimen from the medial femoral condyle of the patient also showed the presence of a previous drill hole lined with chondrocytes. This sample illustrated an area of regeneration undergoing ossification, showing re-establishment of the calcified cartilage layer and the tidemark (Fig 21). The tidemark is seen as an undulating basophilic line on routine H&E staining and is the point at which the articular cartilage becomes calcified. The subchondral drill defect area is replaced by the presence of chondrocytes with varying degrees of maturation surrounded by a ground substance matrix. In addition, ossification is evident with new trabecular bone formation. Ossification changes were not seen over the new hyaline cartilage formation zone.

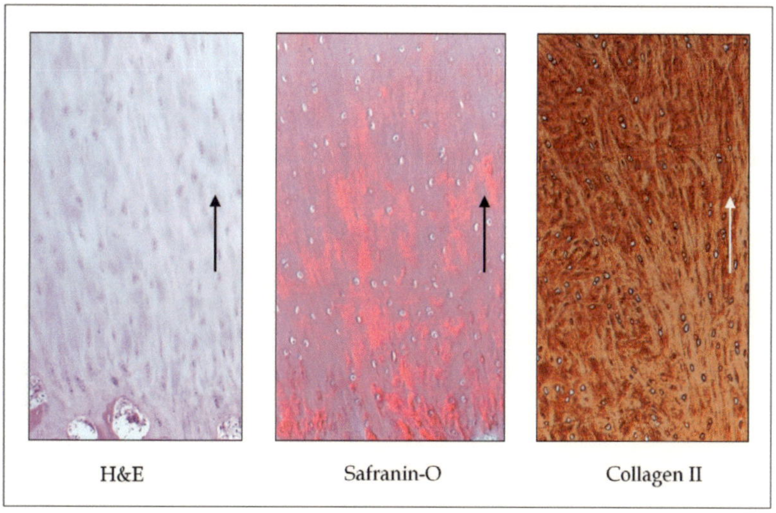

Fig. 19. Biopsy from the medial tibial plateau in case 1 showing the presence of chondrocytes and collagen fibres aligning to the axis of weight transmission with their specific stains (Original magnification X 100).

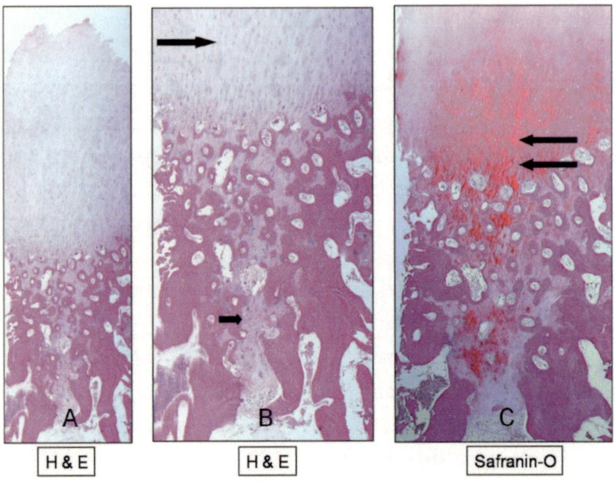

Fig. 20. (A) H&E sample as in Figure 18 from the medial tibial plateau managed to biopsy an area of previous drilling. (B) Upon higher magnification, chondrocytes appeared deep to the subchondral bone with areas of ossification. Notice the chondrocytes below the subchondral bone region beginning as immature cells (short arrow) and progressing toward the joint surface as mature chondrocytes in rows (long arrow). (C) Upon staining with Safranin-O, there was a high concentration of proteoglycans at the base of the regenerated tissue represented as red coloration (double arrow).

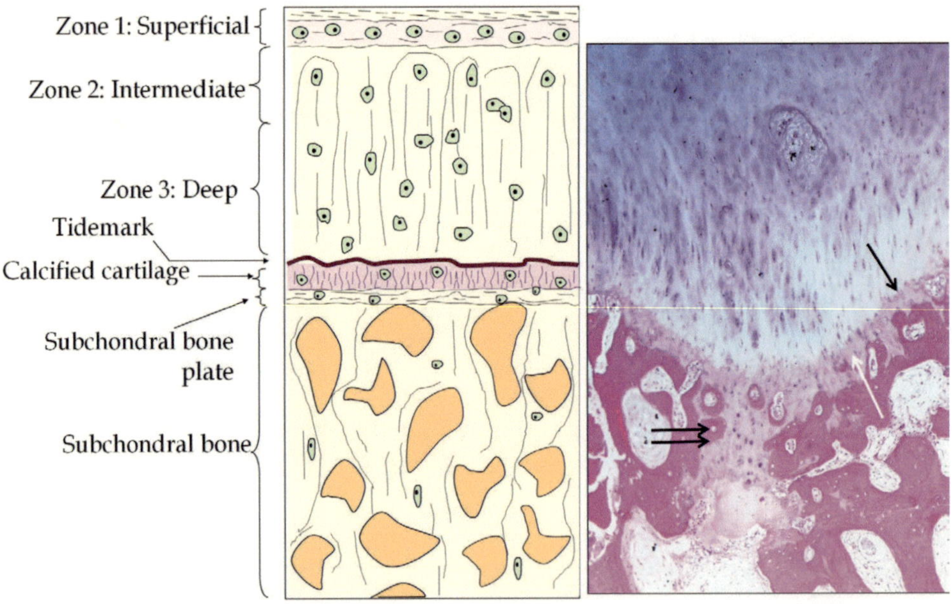

Fig. 21. A biopsy from the medial femoral condyle illustrating ossification of regenerated cartilage and the re-establishment of the calcified cartilage (white arrow) layer with tidemark (black arrow). Note the presence of chondrocytes below the calcified cartilage (double arrow) with areas of ossification.

The intercondylar notch sample was an area of previous roof-plasty and notchplasty with abrasion chondroplasty. This represents an area that is non–weight-bearing. Histologic biopsy examination here showed a mixed tissue with fibrocartilage and hyaline-like cartilage: the predominance of collagen type I, less collagen type II, and chondrocytes arranged in a more disorganized pattern. We believe that the failure of the chondrocytes to exhibit a linear streaming pattern, as seen from the medial tibial plateau and medial femoral condyle biopsy specimens, is due to the absence of stimulation from weight-bearing forces on the intercondylar notch (Fig 18).

Case 2: A chondral core biopsy specimen was taken 26 months after surgery in a 34-year-old woman with previous multiple open surgeries for recurrent dislocation of the patella as an adolescent. She underwent arthroscopic debridement, lateral patella release, and subchondral drilling. There were grade III and IV lesions over the entire patellofemoral joint. Preoperative merchant-view radiographs showed severe patellofemoral osteoarthritis, a large medial trochlear osteophyte, and absence of the lateral patellofemoral joint space (Fig 22). During arthroscopic surgery, the medial trochlear osteophyte was burred and subchondral drilling was performed on the entire patellofemoral joint. An immediate postoperative radiograph showed evidence of subchondral drilling. Radiographs at 6 months and 2 years showed progressive reappearance of the lateral patellofemoral joint space (Fig 22). Fig 16 contains results of the second-look arthroscopy with chondral core biopsy specimens. The lateral patella facet and lateral trochlear areas showed tufts of cartilage between areas devoid of cartilage. In contrast, the medial trochlear area that underwent the removal and burring of a large osteophyte followed by subchondral drilling showed complete coverage by newly formed articular cartilage.

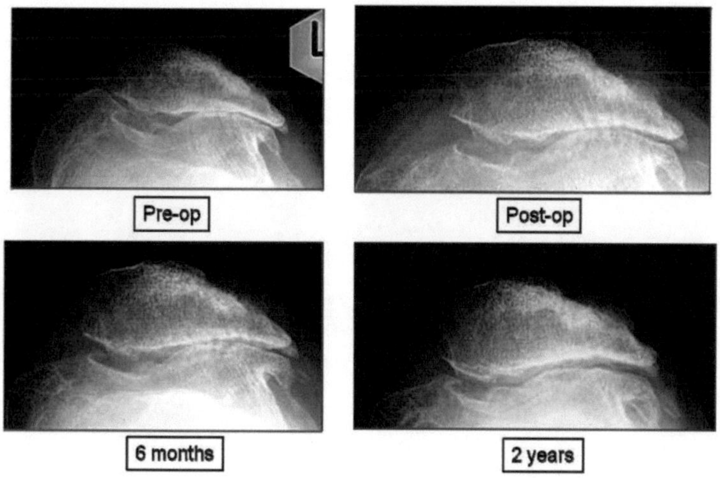

Fig. 22. 34-year-old female with recurrent dislocation of her patella as an adolescent. Immediate postoperative radiographs showed evidence of subchondral drilling while radiographs at 6 months and 2 years showed a progressive reappearance of the lateral patellofemoral articulation.

Case 3: A biopsy specimen was obtained 1 year after surgery from a 52-year-old woman with an isolated grade IV lesion of the lateral femoral condyle measuring 2 X 1 cm.

Case 4: A biopsy specimen was obtained 10 months after surgery in a 43-year-old woman with lateral patellar maltracking. There was a grade III/IV defect measuring 2.5 X 3.5 cm over the lateral patella facet. Lateral patella release was performed in addition to subchondral drilling.

Case 5: Biopsy was performed at 18 months after surgery in a 19-year-old man with lateral patellar maltracking and a lateral trochlear grade IV lesion measuring 0.8 cm in diameter. Subchondral drilling was performed followed by lateral patellar release (Fig 23).

Chondral core biopsy specimens in cases 2, 3, 4, and 5 with histologic staining with H&E showed columnar morphology of cells with a pale blue ground substance. Safranin-O showed intense orange / red staining of the newly regenerated cartilage zone throughout the regenerated cartilage layer with a propensity toward the deeper areas of cartilage above the subchondral bone. The matrix also showed a predominance of collagen type II deposits, whereas collagen type I was minimal and located mostly over the superficial regions of the articular surface. These compositional results are features of hyaline as opposed to fibrocartilage (Kang et al, 2008; Saw et al, 2009 & Lee et al, 2007).

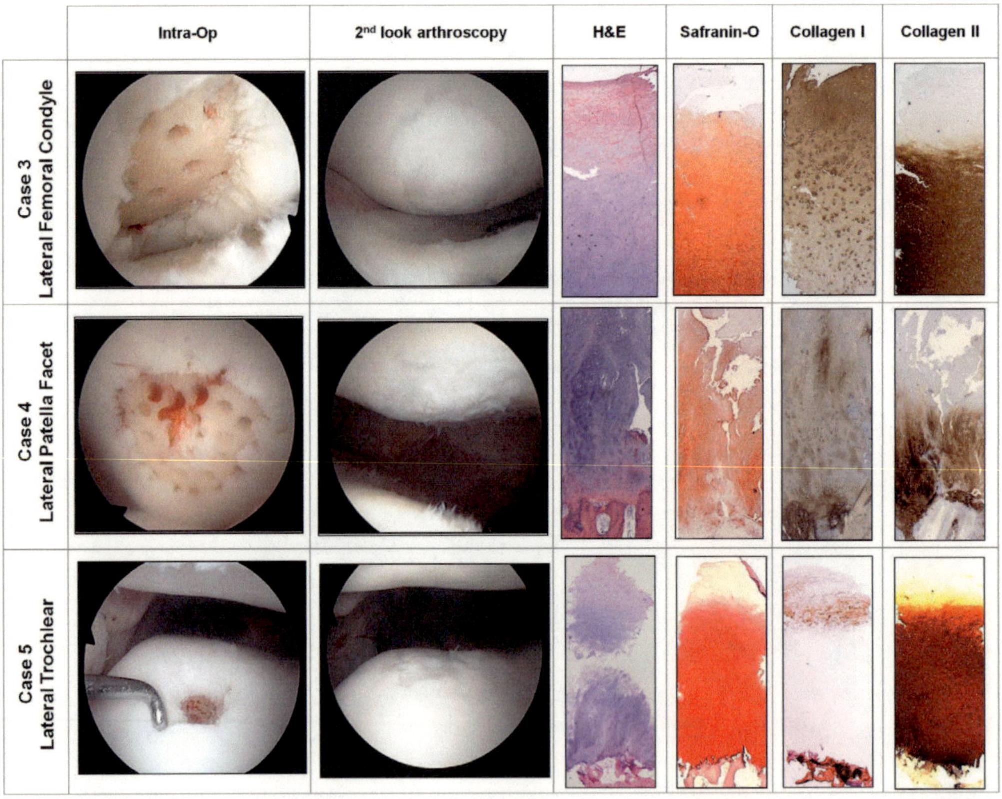

Fig. 23. Second-look arthroscopy and histological images of a lesion from the lateral femoral condyle (Case 3), a lesion from the lateral patella facet (Case 4) and a lesion from the lateral trochlear (Case 5).

7.4.3 Chondrogenesis with PBPC and HA

Findings from second-look arthroscopy presented in the above 5 case series confirmed that it was possible to replicate the results of our animal model (Saw et al, 2009) in the human knee joint using a combination of postoperative intraarticular injections of autologous PBPC with HA after arthroscopic subchondral drilling. This method uses marrow stimulation to create an autologous scaffold that is subsequently seeded with both intraarticular injections of autologous PBPC and in-situ progenitor cells from the underlying marrow (Fig 24).

7.4.4 Contained lesion

In a typical chondral lesion of the medial femoral condyle (Fig 24) measuring 2cm x 2cm, chondrogenesis progresses as described in Fig 24.

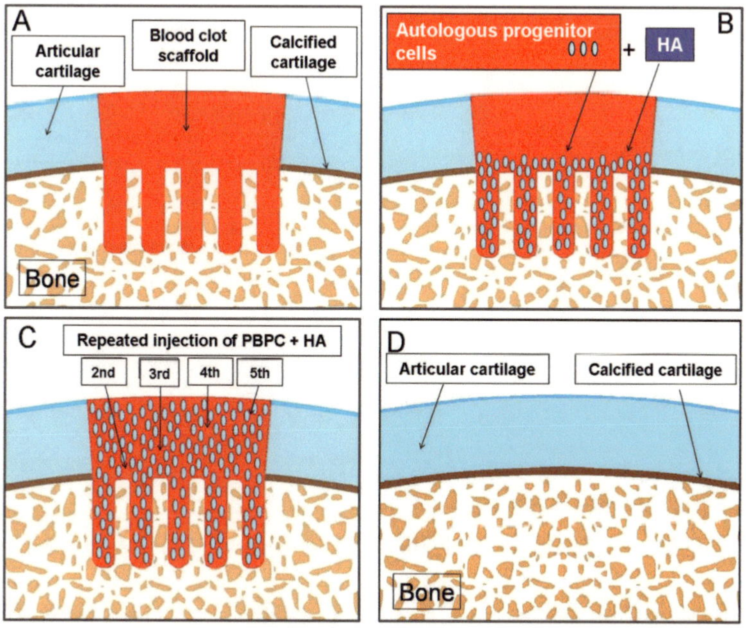

Fig. 24. Chondrogenesis: Contained lesion. (A) A blood clot scaffold is formed after subchondral drilling and abrasion chondroplasty between the drill holes. The surrounding articular cartilage is normal with the underlying calcified cartilage layer and subchondral bone. (B) Injection of fresh PBPC plus HA 1 week after surgery results in the homing of the PBPC into the blood clot scaffold. (C) The PBPC residing in the osteochondral junction and blood clot scaffold gradually transform to chondrocytes. HA helps to reduce inflammation and provide raw material for chondrogenesis. The injected PBPC exert paracrine effects and recruit in-situ progenitor cells to assist in chondrogenesis. Repeated injections of PBPC plus HA enable more cells to be recruited into the chondral defect and enhance chondrogenesis. (D) The final result is the formation of a new layer of articular cartilage with good integration to the surrounding tissues. The ossification of the chondrocytes below the articular cartilage results in repair of the subchondral bone with re-establishment of the calcified cartilage layer.

7.4.5 Uncontained Lesion – Sparse drilling

Second-look arthroscopy in case 2 revealed tufts of cartilage in between areas devoid of regenerated cartilage. The subchondral drilling over the lateral patellofemoral joint was spaced at 3 to 5 mm apart. Fig 25 provides an explanation. As a result, we have refined our techniques so that a goal of 1 to 2 mm between drill holes is now sought. Abrasion chondroplasty up to a depth of 1 mm is also performed.

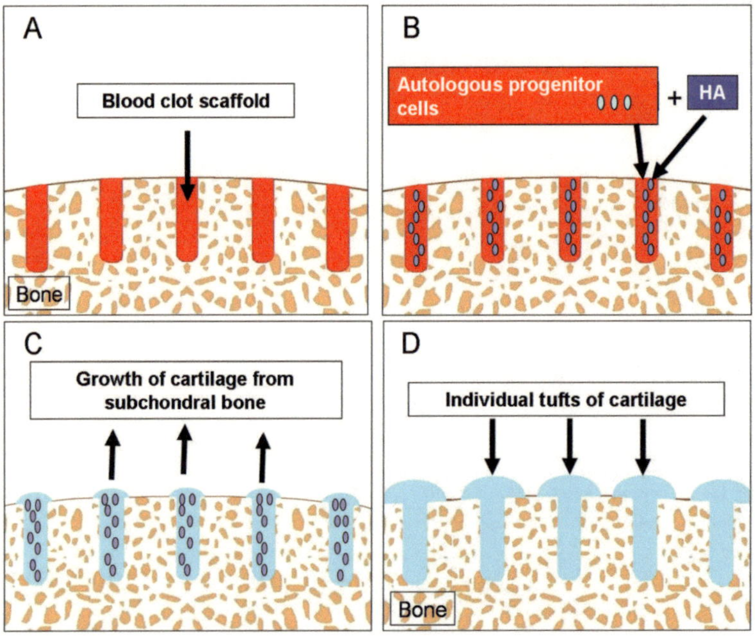

Fig. 25. Chondrogenesis: Uncontained lesion—sparse drilling. (A) In large chondral defects with areas of bare bone, the only available blood clot scaffold is from the areas after subchondral drilling. (B) Injection of fresh autologous PBPC plus HA 1 week after surgery will result in the homing of the PBPC into the subchondral blood clot scaffold, with the PBPC residing in the blood clot scaffold. (C) Because there is no blood clot scaffold superficial to the subchondral bone, chondrogenesis can only be achieved by the protruding tufts of cartilage from the subchondral bone drilling. (D) If the subchondral drill holes are placed too far apart, the end result is the incomplete coverage of the subchondral bone with individual tufts of cartilage seen between areas devoid of cartilage.

7.4.6 Uncontained Lesion – Ideal drilling

Ideally placed drill holes with abrasion chondroplasty allows for a larger surface area and volume of blood clot scaffold to form. When seeded with PBPC and HA, chondrogenesis progresses evenly and the individual tufts of growing cartilage coalesce to form a new layer of articular hyaline cartilage.

Our current method of subchondral drilling in large uncontained lesion is shown in Fig 26.

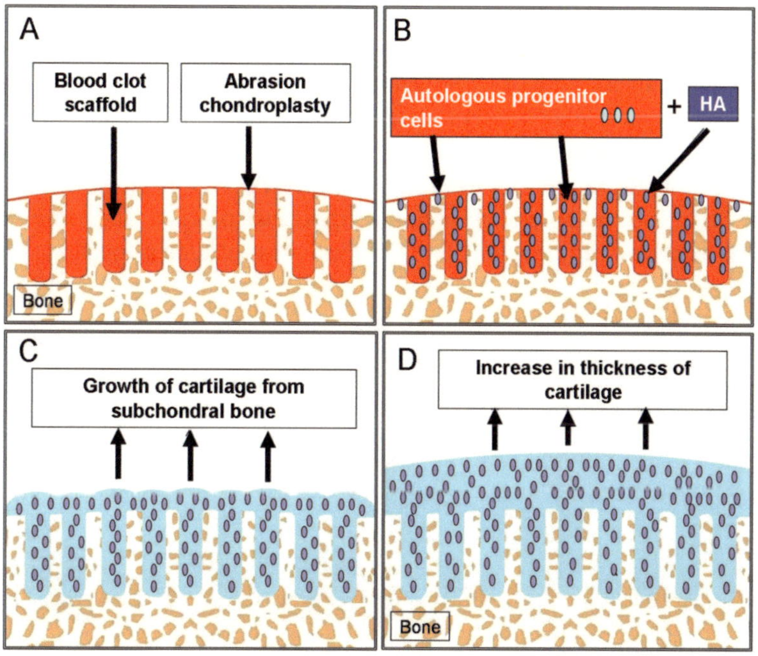

Fig. 26. Chondrogenesis: Uncontained lesion—ideal drilling. (A) Ideally placed subchondral drilling (1 to 2 mm apart) and abrasion chondroplasty between the drill holes increase the available bony areas for the homing of the PBPC. (B) Injected PBPC and HA have a larger surface area of raw bone providing homing signals for the recruitment of the PBPC. (C) Individual tufts of cartilage arise from the subchondral bone and coalesce to cover the bony defect. (D) Maturation will result in an increase in thickness of the regenerated cartilage covering the entire defect.

7.4.7 Further cases to support the theory of chondrogenesis with ideal drilling in uncontained lesion

The following cases illustrate the advances made in the light of the histological findings following second-look arthroscopy as regards to the importance of meticulous surgical technique, adjuvant PBPC & HA therapy and cell viability.

Chondral lesions in difficult to access region of the knee joint presented a special challenge to treatment. An example would be the posterior aspects of the medial and lateral tibial plateau. In the early phase of the clinical trial, the first author used a technique called the "Inkwell" (Fig 27) procedure in which a 4 mm burr was used to create multiple half moon-shaped pits into the bone surface.

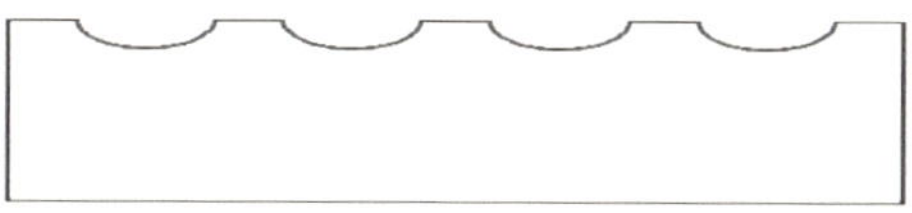

Fig. 27. Illustration of an "Inkwell" procedure.

Case 6: A 53-year-old man with a varus knee presented with the loss of the articular cartilage over the medial compartment. He underwent a high tibial osteotomy with the fixation of a Tomofix plate. Postoperative intraarticular injections of PBPC in combination with HA were given in accordance with the standard protocol.
The medial femoral condyle underwent ideal subchondral drilling of the uncontained lesion (Fig 28). In the medial tibial plateau, ideal subchondral drilling was performed over the anterior half of the tibial plateau. Due to poor access, it was not possible to perform subchondral drilling over the posterior half of the tibial plateau. Therefore the "Inkwell" procedure was applied over the posterior half of the tibial plateau (Fig 29).

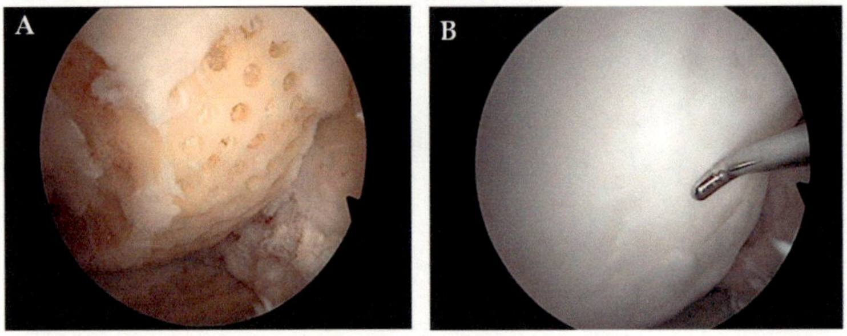

Fig. 28. The corresponding arthroscopic views over the medial femoral condyle. (A) Intraoperative view and (B) view at 18 months.

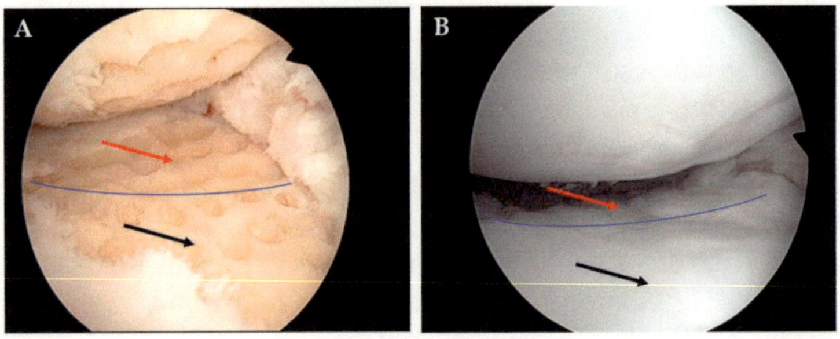

Fig. 29. (A) Arthroscopic view with black arrow showing ideal subchondral drilling over the anterior half of the medial tibial plateau. Red arrow showing the multiple "inkwells" created in the posterior half of the medial tibial plateau. The blue line indicates the border separating the two distinct procedures. (B) Second-look arthroscopy at 18 months showing ideal chondrogenesis in the anterior half of the tibial plateau as compared to the posterior half.

Fig 30 shows the radiological reappearance of the medial articulation at 7 months after surgery. MRI scan at 18 months confirmed the presence of repair cartilage over the anterior half of the medial compartment (Fig 31), confirmed on second-look arthroscopy (Fig 29). This is in contrast with the repair appearance of the posterior half of the tibial plateau (Figs 29 and 32).

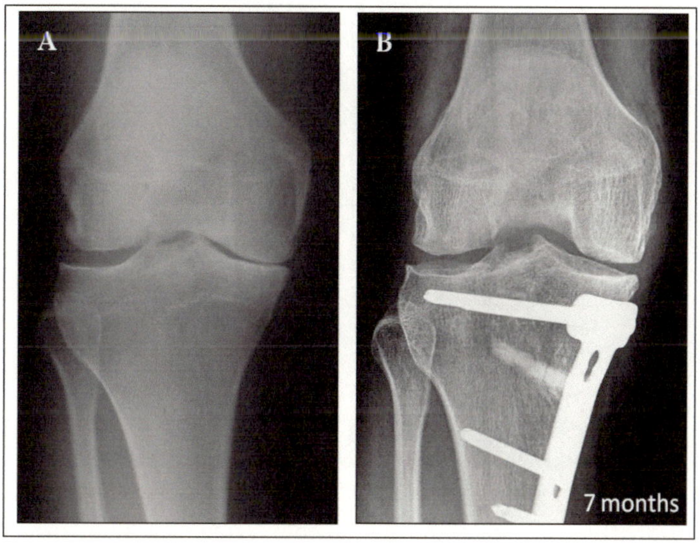

Fig 30. A 53-year-old male underwent high tibial osteotomy: (A) Preoperative XR showing narrowing of medial compartment; and (B) Postoperative view at 7 months showing re-appearance of the medial compartment.

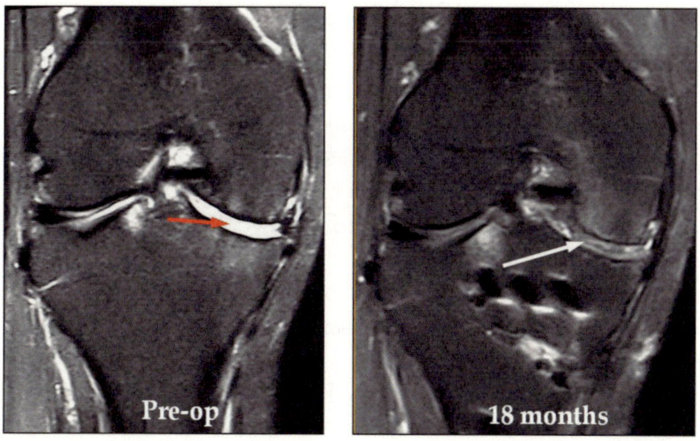

Fig. 31. Preoperative (Pre-op) MRI (STIR) showing 'bone on bone' over the medial compartment of the right knee (red arrow). White arrow showing regenerated articular cartilage at 18 months over the anterior half of both the medial femoral condyle and medial tibial plateau.

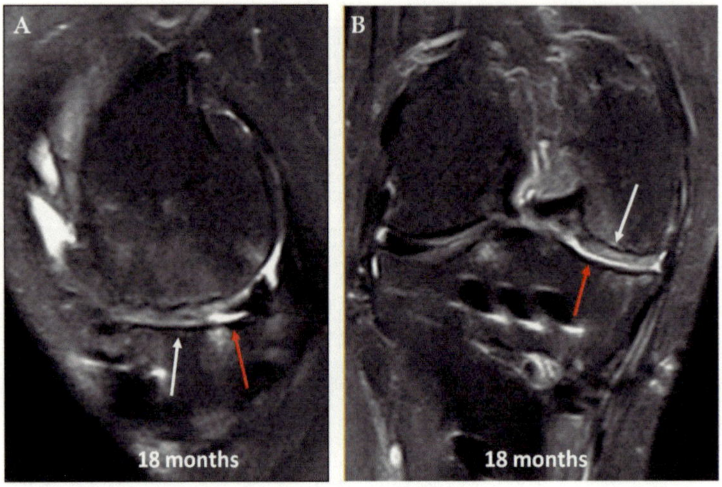

Fig. 32. (A) Sagittal MRI (STIR) over the medial compartment. White arrow over the anterior half of the medial tibial plateau showing evidence of chondrogenesis. Red arrow over the posterior half of the medial tibial plateau whereby the "Inkwell" technique was applied showed minimal chondrogenesis. (B) Coronal MRI (STIR) over the posterior half of the medial tibial plateau. White arrow over the medial femoral condyle showing chondrogenesis. Red arrow over the medial tibial plateau showed minimal chondrogenesis.

Histology from the chondral core biopsy of the medial femoral condyle and anterior half of the medial tibial plateau confirmed the regeneration of hyaline cartilage (Fig 33).This case further supports the theory of ideal drilling with abrasion chondroplasty in uncontained lesions (Figs 26 and 28). With ideally placed drill holes and abrasion chondroplasty, there will be a larger volume of blood-clot scaffold for the injected PBPC and HA to form closely integrated individual tufts of cartilage. These closely seeded tufts arising from the subchondral bone will eventually coalesce to cover the bony defect. Chondrogenesis with maturation will result in increasing thickness of the regenerated cartilage covering the entire defect.

In the absence of subchondral drilling over the posterior half of the medial tibial plateau, the "Inkwell" procedure only produces minimal surface coverage as compared to the anterior half of the tibial plateau.

Case 7: A 45-year-old woman underwent right knee arthroscopic lateral patellar release and ideally placed subchondral drilling to the lateral patella facet and lateral trochlear (Fig 34). Beginning one week after surgery, 5 weekly intraarticular injections of HA were given to the operated knee. No PBPC was added to the HA during the intraarticular injections. Radiographs (Fig 35) show improvement of the lateral patellofemoral articulation. In the absence of PBPC in combination with HA, the repair process was only patchy in some areas and the regenerated tissue was found to be of fibrocartilage in nature (Fig 34 and 36).

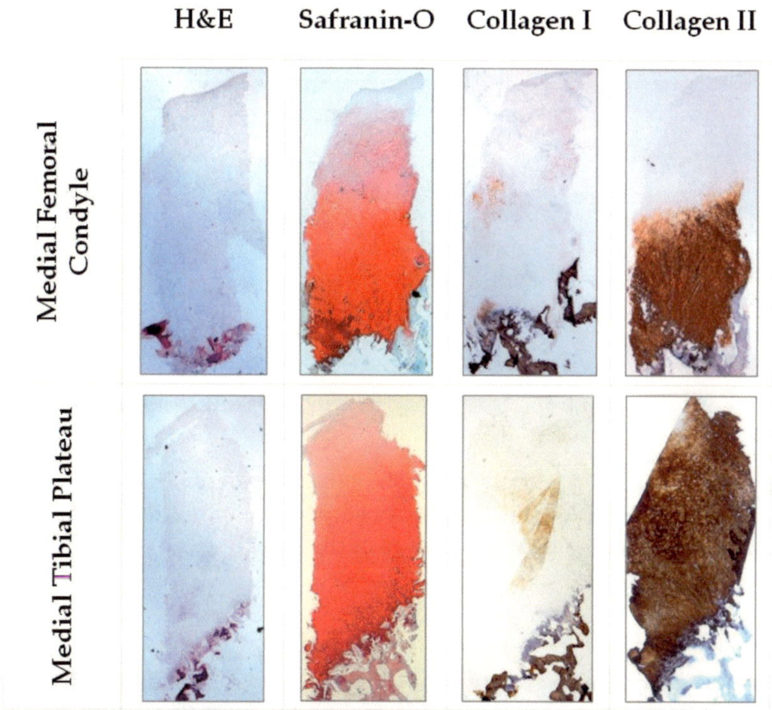

Fig. 33. Case 6 – Histological features showing hyaline cartilage regeneration from the medial femoral condyle and medial tibial plateau biopsies.

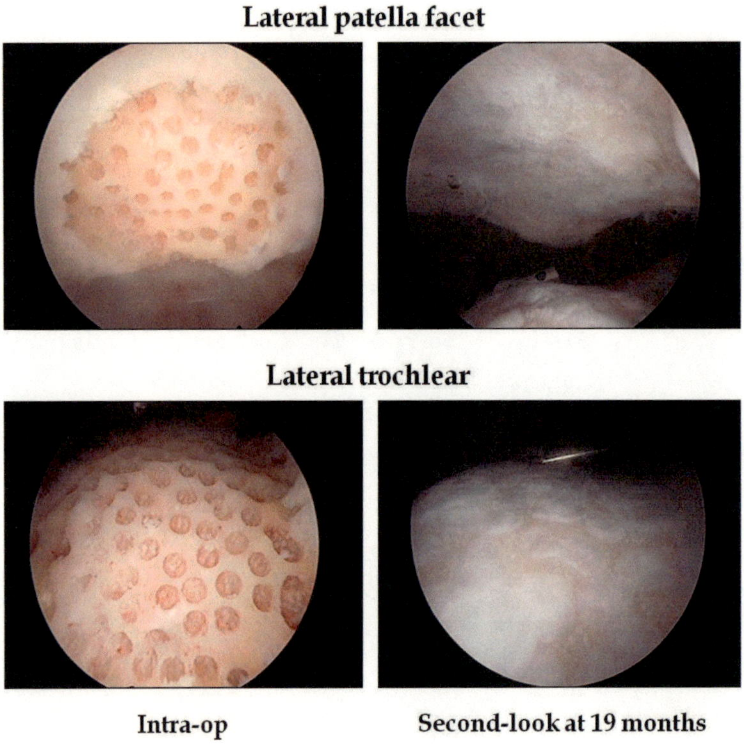

Fig. 34. A 45-year-old woman with intraoperative (Intra-op) and second-look arthroscopy at 19 months. Despite ideal drilling but without postoperative intraarticular injections of PBPC + HA, the end result was only patchy coverage of the bony defects.

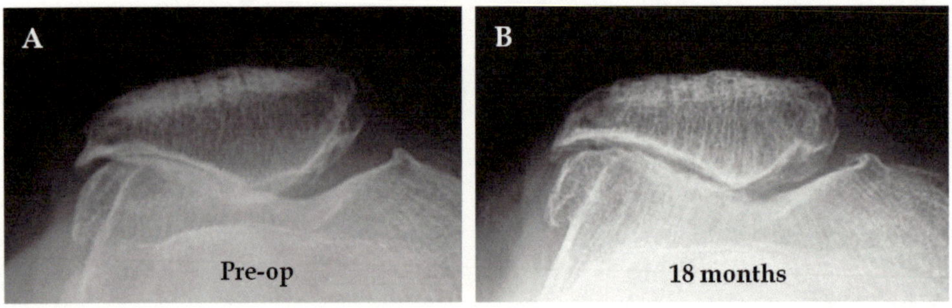

Fig. 35. (A) Preoperative (Pre-op) merchant view showing lateral patellar maltracking with absence of the lateral patellofemoral articulation. (B) XR at 18 months showed improvement of the lateral patellofemoral articulation.

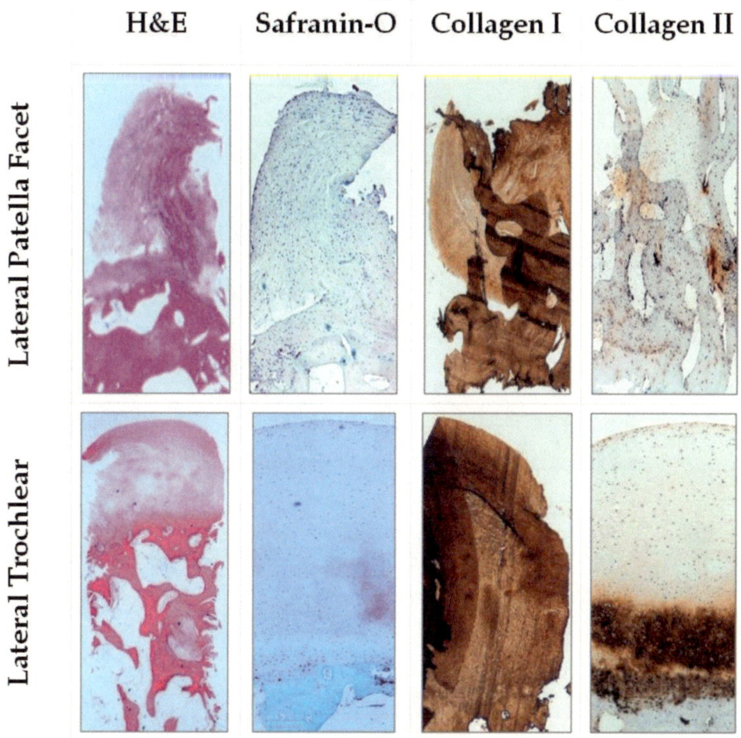

Fig. 36. Case 7 - Histological features showing fibrocartilage repair from the lateral patella facet and lateral trochlear biopsies.

The importance of adjuvant PBPC in combination with HA is well emphasised in this case. In the absence of PBPC, even though ideal subchondral drilling was performed, intraarticular injections of HA alone is ineffective in complete coverage of the bony drill holes and initiate satisfactory articular cartilage repair.

Case 8: A 49-year-old man underwent high tibial osteotomy with Tomofix plate fixation, lateral patellar release and ideal subchondral drilling into the tri-compartmental chondral defects. PBPC in combination with HA were injected intraarticularly into the operated knee 1 week after surgery for a total of five weeks. Postoperative radiographs at 19 months showed reappearance of the lateral patella articulation and improvement of the medial compartment (Fig 37).

Second-look arthroscopy with chondral core biopsy from the lateral trochlear (Fig 38), medial and lateral femoral condyles (Fig 39) showed evidence of hyaline cartilage regeneration (Fig 40). In contrast to case 7 which presented with only chondral defects over the lateral patellofemoral joint, case 8 showed satisfactory chondrogenesis with hyaline cartilage regeneration in all 3 compartments. With the addition of postoperative intraarticular injections of PBPC and HA following subchondral drilling, it is possible to address multiple chondral lesions in addition to the difficult to treat "Kissing" lesions.

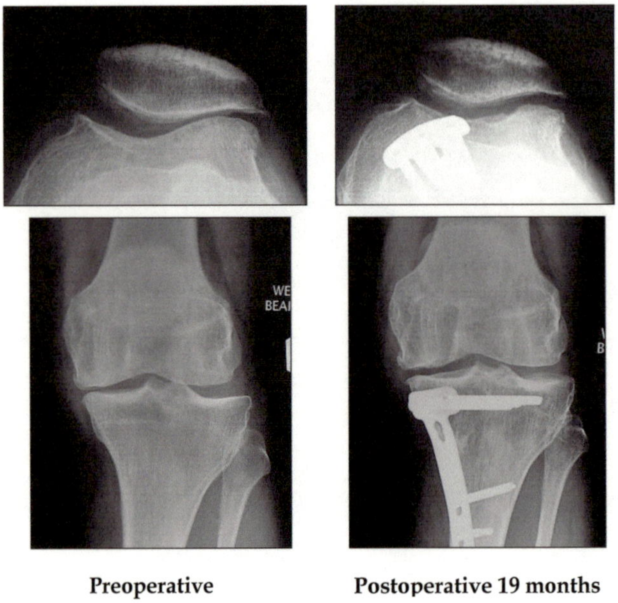

Fig. 37. A 49-year-old man underwent high tibial osteotomy, lateral patellar release and tri-compartmental chondral drilling.

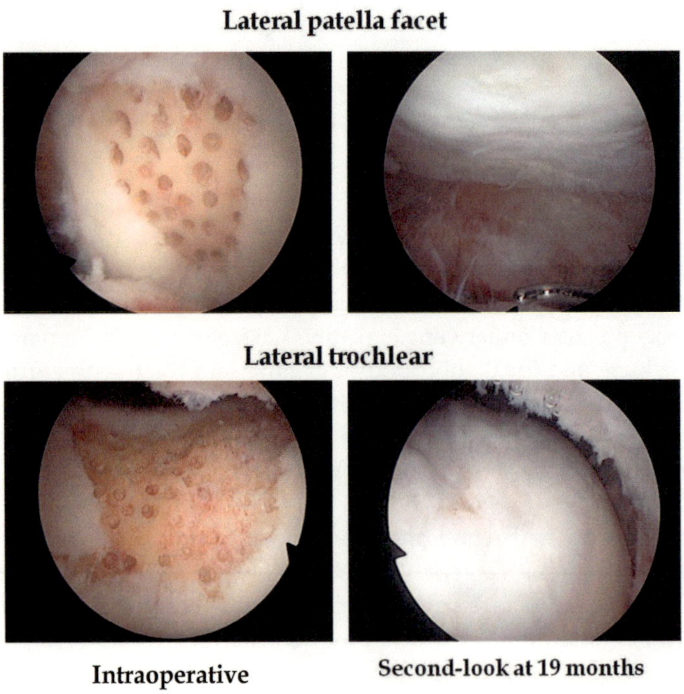

Fig. 38. Second-look at 19 months showed satisfactory coverage of the bony defects by the regenerated tissue.

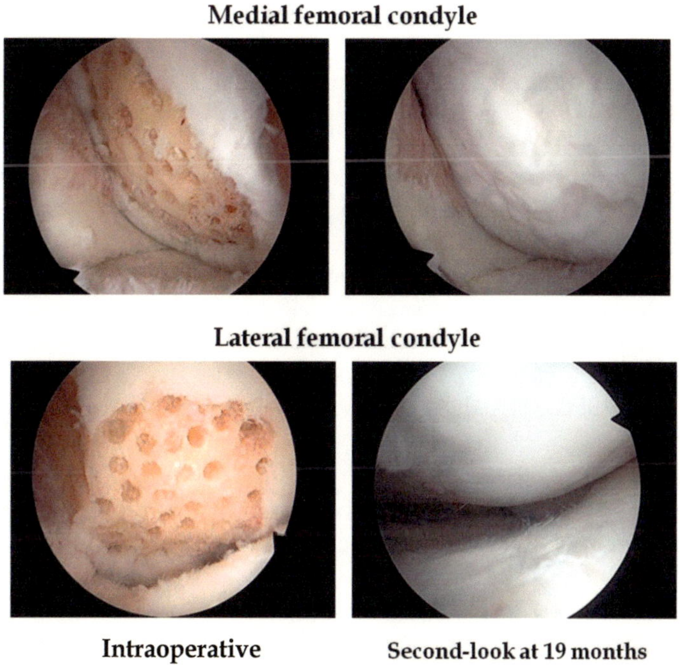

Fig. 39. Second-look at the medial and lateral femoral condyles showed satisfactory chondrogenesis.

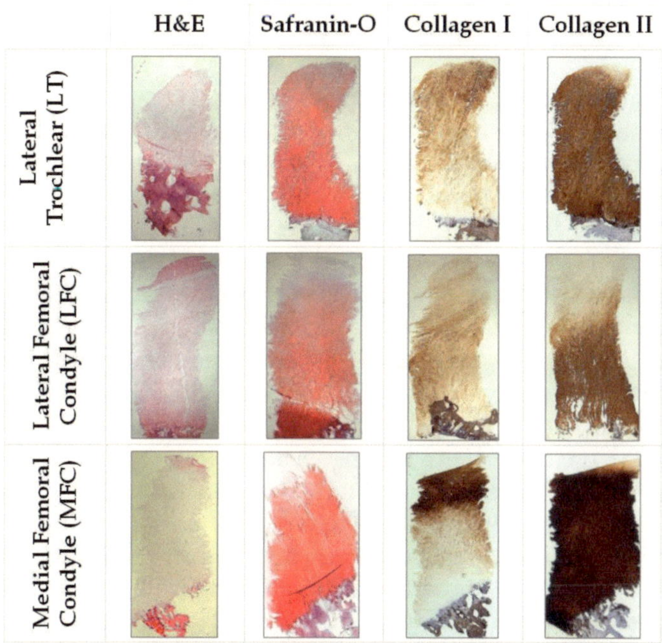

Fig. 40. Case 8 - Histological features showing hyaline cartilage regeneration from the LT, LFC & MFC biopsies.

7.4.8 The importance of PBPC + HA as adjuvant therapy following ideal subchondral drilling

Case 6 emphasizes on the importance of the improved technique of ideal drilling in an uncontained lesion. Cases 7 & 8 illustrates the importance of postoperative intraarticular injections of PBPC + HA.

Possible reasons as to why the microfracture technique has not been successful in achieving consistent coverage with hyaline cartilage can be explained by what is seen on second-look arthroscopy in cases 6, 7 and 8. Firstly, microfractures are usually placed 3 to 5 mm apart and do not penetrate much deeper than the calcified cartilage layer. Microfractures placed more superficially and further apart as compared to ideal subchondral drilling explains one of the possible reasons why the microfracture technique is inconsistent in producing satisfactory articular cartilage repair. Secondly, like the animal model in Fig 9, without postoperative adjunct therapy with PBPC + HA, the regenerated tissue will always be of inferior quality.

7.4.9 Role of weight-bearing

Our biopsy specimens from cases with subchondral drilling followed by postoperative intraarticular injections of PBPC in combination with HA showed histologic features of hyaline cartilage with anti–collagen type I stain (used to highlight collagen type I), anti–collagen type II stain (used to highlight collagen type II), and Safranin-O stain (used to highlight proteoglycans), with the exception of one histologic sample showing mixed cartilage. This biopsy specimen was from an area of abrasion notchplasty, which represented a non–weight-bearing region. Comparison of biopsy specimens from this non–weight-bearing area to those from a weight-bearing area in the same patient has led us to theorize that early partial-weight-bearing is essential for the regeneration and alignment of collagen type II (Fig 18).

7.4.10 Articular cartilage imaging of the knee

Articular cartilage is visible on most standard MRI sequences as a band of intermediate to high signal covering the articular aspect of the bone. Non-injured articular cartilage normally shows a continuous subchondral dark line (low-signal) below the articular cartilage. This dark line likely represents the layer of calcified cartilage and the associated subchondral bone plate. It may be accentuated by chemical shift artifact (of water and fat molecules in the same voxel canceling their respective signals thereby resulting in signal loss). Fig 41 illustrates the articular cartilage and subchondral bone on a sagittal PD image. Evaluating postoperative MRIs, we assessed the restoration of the dark line as evidence of calcified cartilage with subchondral bone healing and fill of the defect as indicative of cartilage regeneration.

Our current imaging preference for assessing chondral lesions of the knee joint utilize 2D PD and PDFS sequences using a high field (1.5T) extremity MRI (GE Medical Systems) - Fig 42. This has the benefits of improved signal to noise and higher resolution. Fig 43 showing examples of chondral lesions seen following MRI scan with arthroscopic correlation (Fig 44). Our earlier cartilage images were obtained by an open MRI system operating at 0.35T (Magnetom C!, Siemens Medical Solutions, Erlangen, Germany) using an extremity receive coil.

MRI scans were utilized preoperatively as part of the diagnostic work up and postoperatively to monitor healing of the chondral defects. We performed MRI scans at shorter intervals for our first 10 patients. Scans were performed on the first postoperative day as a baseline to document the chondral defect after debridement and subchondral drilling. Serial studies were then collected in the postoperative period (at 6, 12, 18, 24 months and beyond) to evaluate the filling of the defect by regenerated cartilage and changes in the subchondral bone.

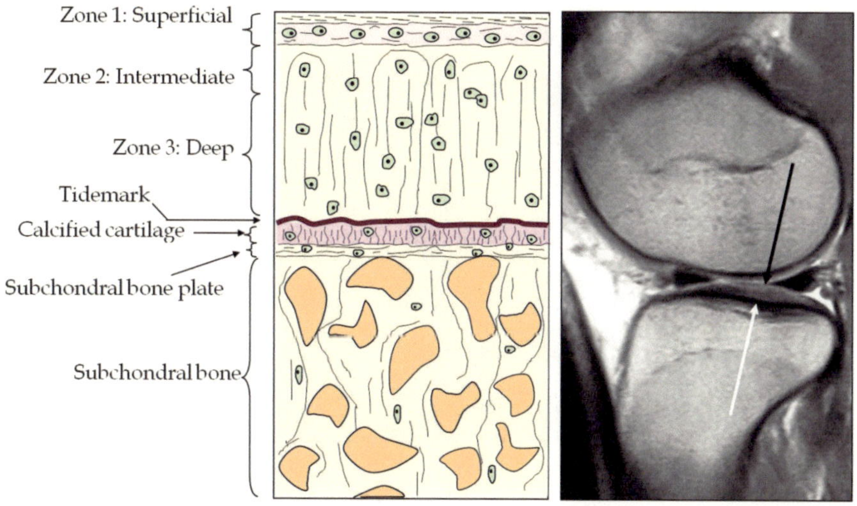

Fig. 41. Articular cartilage as depicted by sagittal PD image at the tibial plateau. Black arrow showing the surface of the tibial plateau articular cartilage and red arrow showing the "Black line" that separates the articular cartilage from the subchondral bone. This layer correlates with the tidemark / calcified cartilage / subchondral bone plate layers.

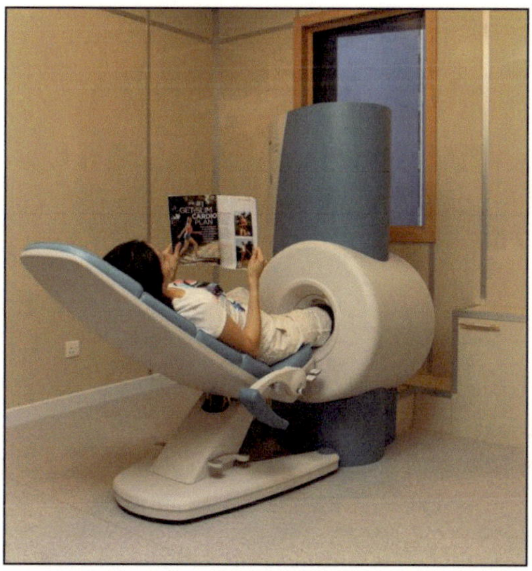

Fig. 42. A patient with her right knee in a high field extremity (1.5T) MRI (GE Medical Systems).

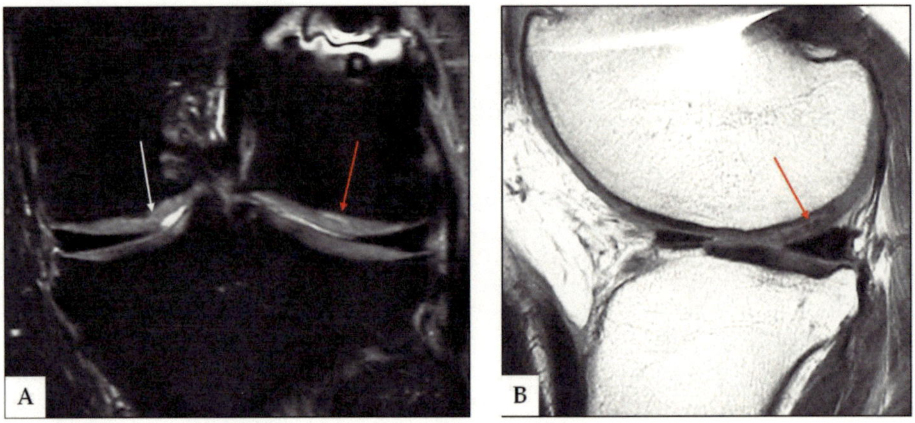

Fig. 43. Images of chondral lesions demonstrated by extremity high field MRI at 1.5T. (A) Chondral flap tear of the medial femoral condyle (white arrow) with red arrow showing a delaminated chondral lesion over the lateral femoral condyle (PDFS). (B) The corresponding chondral lesion of the lateral femoral condyle (red arrow) on a sagittal PD image.

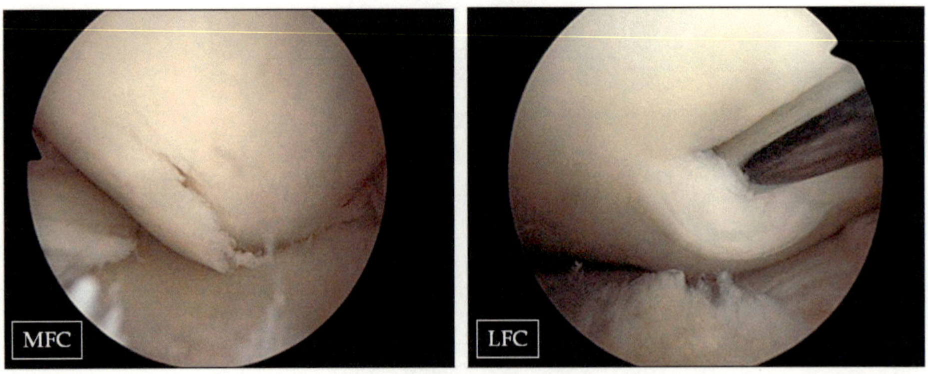

Fig. 44. Corresponding arthroscopic view of the lesions from the medial femoral condyle (MFC) and lateral femoral condyle (LFC) as in Fig 43.

MRI scans performed on the first postoperative day showed the chondral defects as well delineated from surrounding healthy cartilage. The chondral defects were bare or partially filled in with blood clot. Drill tracts and subchondral marrow edema were clearly observed (Figures 45 to 47). Subchondral bone is disrupted, i.e. there is loss of the continuity of the subchondral black line. Over the course of two years, filling-in of the chondral defects by material of similar or same signal as articular cartilage was observed. Re-establishment of subchondral black line paralleled the progressive resolution of marrow edema.

Serial MRI scans of our first patient undergoing this treatment are presented in Figure 45. After full debridement and drilling, the chondral defect is well visualized as a bare area partially filled by clot (Figure 45A). The low signal subchondral bone is disrupted and low signal drill tracts are visualized within the subchondral marrow edema. The disruption of the subchondral dark line represents a conduit through the calcified cartilage layer. Serial scans showed progressive filling of chondral defects by material of similar appearance as articular cartilage, resolution of marrow edema and reappearance of the continuous subchondral dark line (Figure 45B). At one to two years, the calcified cartilage, as depicted by the low signal band, becomes almost as thick at the site of drilling as in the surrounding healthy areas. (Figure 45D). Figures 46 and 47 present an additional patient.

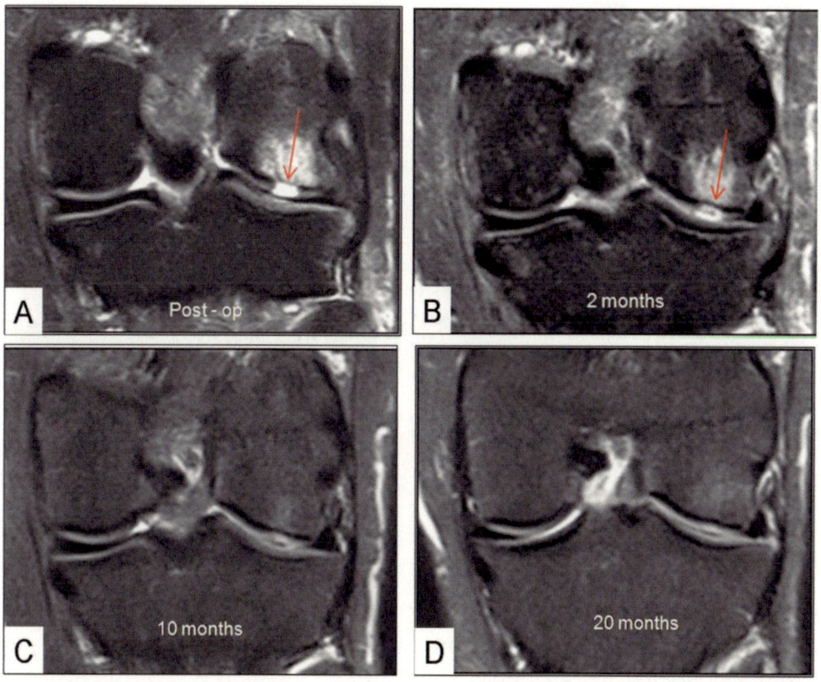

Fig. 45. Serial MRI evaluation (STIR images at 0.35T). Postoperative (Post-op): note the disruption of the subchondral dark line (red arrow). (B) 2 months: partial resolution of marrow edema and reappearance of the continuous subchondral dark line (red arrow). (C) 10 months: almost complete resolution of marrow edema and filling of defect. (D) 20 months: complete healing of defect and re-establishment of subchondral dark line representing healing of the calcified cartilage layer.

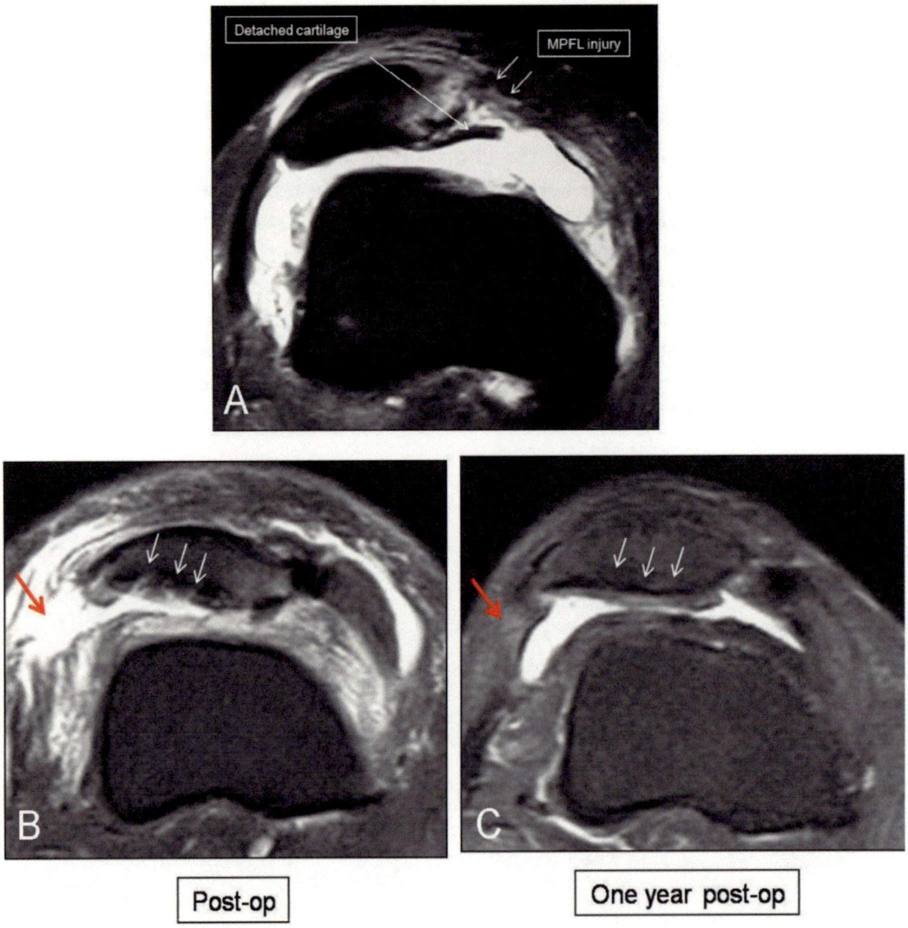

Fig. 46. A 40-year-old woman with patellar dislocation (STIR images at 0.35T). (A) Preoperative MRI with evidence of a delaminating articular cartilage injury and medial patellar femoral ligament (MPFL) injury. The injury was treated with arthroscopic lateral release, subchondral drilling and repair of the MPFL. (B) Postoperative (Post-op) MRI following arthroscopic lateral patellar release (red arrow) and subchondral drilling showing interruption of the low signal subchondral calcified cartilage (white arrows). (C) At one year following surgery, MRI revealed a healed lateral retinaculum (red arrow), re-establishment of the subchondral calcified cartilage (white arrows) and evidence of articular cartilage regeneration at the lateral patella facet.

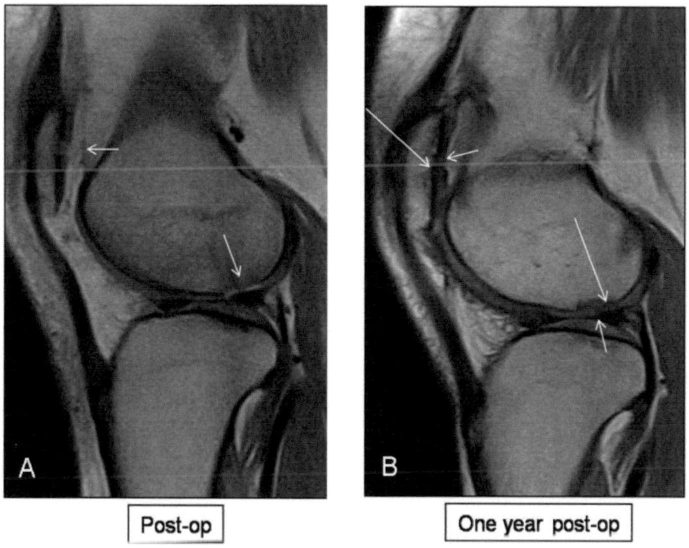

Fig. 47. Sagittal PD MRI (0.35T) of patient in Figure 46. (A) Postoperative (Post-op) MRI: chondral lesions at the lateral patella and lateral femoral chondyle (arrows). Note the disruption to the continous low signal calcified cartilage layer at both sites. (B) MRI at one year after surgery showing the re-establishment of the subchondral calcified cartilage layer (long arrows) together with articular cartilage regeneration (short arrows).

The re-establishment of the calcified cartilage layer and healing of the subchondral bone are important MRI features of articular cartilage regeneration in our series. This is accompanied by filling of the chondral defect. Following arthroscopic subchondral drilling, MRI images revealed extensive marrow edema and interruption of the calcified cartilage layer together with the underlying subchondral bone. This is shown as disruption of the low signal subchondral dark line. As the injected PBPC seed the blood clot scaffold in the presence of HA, chondrogenesis is initiated with the formation of chondrocytes which then occupy the drill holes. This process is gradually replaced by bone resulting in subchondral bone repair. Gradual resolution of marrow edema is observed. The subchondral dark line progressively re-appears on MRI scans indicating the re-establishment of the calcified cartilage layer and healing of the subchondral bone (Figures 45 to 47). This evidence is provided from the histology shown on Figures 20 and 21. Depending on whether the lesion is a contained or uncontained lesion, chondrogenesis follows the gradual re-appearance of this subchondral dark line on serial MRI scans (Figures 24 and 26).

7.4.11 Phase I study clinical outcomes

Since starting clinical trials in 2007, 223 cartilage regeneration cases have been performed on 205 patients. Cases were varied including 38 cases involving isolated cartilage lesions, 92 cases involving multiple cartilage lesions, 54 cases involving patellofemoral cartilage lesions, 7 cases involving concomitant lower limb realignment procedures, and 32 cases involving ligament reconstruction. When evaluating two-year clinical outcomes, 24 months has passed for 155 of these 223 cases. Within this group, 52 cases have preoperative, 12-month, and 24-month IKDC values available for clinical outcome evaluation. This group had a preoperative IKDC average of 50.5, a 12-month IKDC average of 70, and a 24-month IKDC average of 70. 30 patients had 30-month data available and illustrated a 30-month IKDC average of 71 (Fig 48).

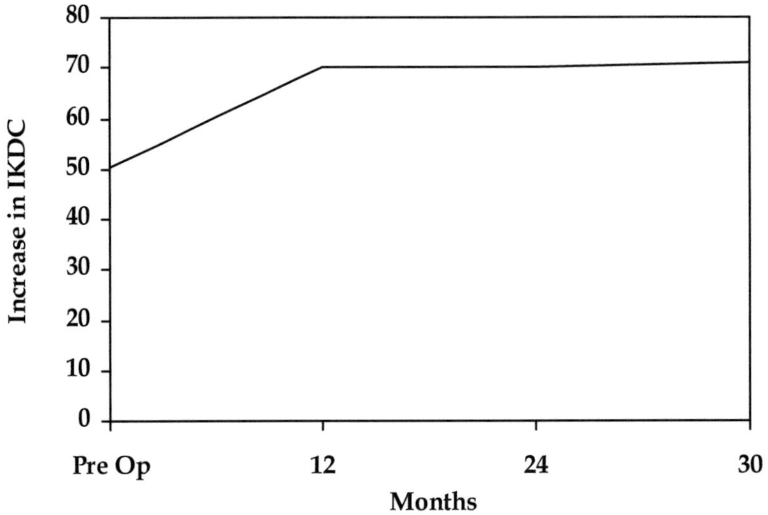

Fig. 48. International Knee Documentation Committee (IKDC) outcomes.

Our IKDC results illustrated a significant increase similar to studies documenting overall outcomes in the literature with marrow stimulation and chondrocyte implantation. Historically, microfracture has shown a peak functional outcome at 24 months (Blevins et al, 1998; Peterson et al, 2000; Steadman et al, 2003; Gobbi et al, 2005, Mithoefer et al, 2005; Knutsen et al, 2007). Two studies have illustrated a decline after the first 18 to 24 months with microfracture, including Mithoefer et al (2005) documenting 69% of their patients reporting lower IKDC scores after 24 months. Conversely, two outcome studies have found sustained improvement at the 24-month time interval (Steadman et al, 2003; Kneutsen et al, 2004). In comparison of these four studies, the average age of the study groups documenting decline was 39.5 years and 41 years. In contrast, the average age of the studies documenting sustained improvement was 30.4 years and 31.1 years (Steadman et al, 2003; Mithoefer et al, 2005; Kruez et al, 2006; Knutsen et al, 2004). In a group with an average age of 47.1 years, our IKDC scores showed sustained improvement at 24 months with 30 cases documenting continued improvement at 30 months.

Comparing microfracture and chondrocyte implantation, decisive superiority has not been established. Two randomized studies have sought to directly compare outcomes with differing results. Saris et al. (2009) found significantly better outcomes with ACI at 36 months. They found a continued increase in Knee Injury and Osteoarthritis Outcome Scores (KOOS) from 6 to 36 months with ACI and a plateau in scores at 18 months with microfracture (Saris et al, 2009). However, Knutsen et al. found no significant clinical or radiographic difference between microfracture and ACI at 60 months utilizing four clinical outcome scoring systems and 2 radiologic outcome systems (Knutsen et al,2007). Zeifang et al. (2010) in comparison of conventional methods of ACI with refined methods of ACI for treatment of femoral chondral lesions found an increase from a baseline IKDC (51.1) by 21 points and 25 points respectively. This series had an average age of 29.3 years (Zeifang et al, 2010). At 24 months, this rise declined slightly in the conventional method to 19 points above baseline and remained stable in the refined method at 25 points above baseline (Zeifang et al, 2010). This compares to our rise above a baseline IKDC of 50.5 by 20 points at 12 months, 20 points at 24 months, and 21 points at 30 months (Fig 48). Of note, our patient group has a mean age of 47.1 years and included patients with multiple chondral lesions, while Zeifang et al. (2010) evaluated isolated defects of the femoral condyle.

Our clinical results indicate that the regenerated tissue is resilient and coincide with histological results suggesting that this technique produces hyaline cartilage. However, evaluating phase I data has weaknesses. As this portion of the clinical trial has included evolution in technique and cell processing, there is some inherent variation. Additionally, IKDC collection was inconsistent in the initial phases. Also, when attempting to evaluate this early data, there is no control group available for comparison. Currently a randomized controlled trial is underway under the direction of the first author.

7.4.12 Complications

Specific complications are mild bone pain associated with Neupogen injections, and discomfort of PBSC harvesting and localized pain following intraarticular injections with PBPC and HA. One male patient in his mid-forties had a previous infection from Anterior Cruciate Ligament (ACL) surgery, multiple microfractures and subsequent ACL revision surgery with postoperative PBPC and HA. He had recurrence of intercondylar osteophytes and reactive arthritis and eventually chose a total knee replacement. Three other patients had secondary procedure for persistent osteophytes and treatment for further areas of chondral degeneration.

It is evident that with adjuvant PBPC and HA therapy, chondrogenesis is possible with hyaline cartilage, but a small proportion of patients may return for further treatment because of newly diagnosed areas of chondral degeneration in the treated knee.

7.5 Current control randomized trial

A randomized controlled trial comparing a group with PBPC and HA injections with a group with HA injection alone following arthroscopic subchondral drilling is currently under way, being supervised by the first author. The early results seem to support the benefit of adjuvant postoperative intraarticular injections of PBPC in combination with HA.

7.6 Summary of theory

Our theory is that providing a high percentage of immature multipotent progenitor cells into the right environment allows these cells to populate areas of subchondral drilling and regenerate hyaline cartilage. Our histologic findings of chondrocytes below the calcified cartilage layer at a subchondral drill hole (Figs 20 and 21) and the porcine model (Lee et al, 2007) illustrating mesenchymal stem cells at the base of newly formed cartilage support the idea that injected progenitor cells are attracted to the site of marrow injury, proliferate into chondrocytes, and regenerate hyaline cartilage from the subchondral base. We theorize that the addition of matrix substance, in the form of HA and passive stimulating kinetic movement of the involved joint (continuous passive motion), provides chemical and cellular signals for regeneration. Partial to full weight-bearing in the early phase of rehabilitation provides the essential environment to assist in the remodelling of the collagen fibrils to align along the axis of weight transmission.

8. Conclusion

It is evident that for ideal chondrogenesis with hyaline cartilage in contained or uncontained lesions, the correct surgical technique with attention to detail, a postoperative adjuvant therapy with a high percentage of viable PBPC in combination with HA, and the importance of a postoperative rehabilitation program are important. Failure to adhere to these three important basic principles will result in inferior repair tissue which will inevitably deteriorate with time.

Articular hyaline cartilage regeneration is possible with arthroscopic subchondral drilling followed by postoperative intraarticular injections of autologous PBPC in combination with HA.

9. References

Asik, M.; Ciftci, F.; Sen, C.; Erdil, M.; and Atalar, A. (2008). The microfracture technique for the treatment of full-thickness articular cartilage lesions of the knee: midterm results. *Arthroscopy,* Vol 24, No 11, pp 1214-20.

Blevins FT, Steadman JR, Rodrigo JJ, Silliman. (1998). Treatment of articular cartilage defects in athletes: an analysis of functional outcome and lesion appearance. *Orthopedic,* Vol 21, No 7, pp:761-768.

Brittberg M, Aglietti P, Gambardella R, et al. (2000). The ICRS clinical cartilage injury evaluation system-2000. *Presented at the 3rd Meeting of the International Cartilage Repair Society, Goteborg, Sweden,* 2000, April 27-28.

Cesselli D, Beltrami AP, Rigo S, et al. (2009) Multipotent progenitor cells are present in human peripheral blood. *Circulation Research* . Vol 104, No 10, pp1225-34.

Chen et al (2006). Mesenchymal stem cells in immunoregulation. *Immunology Cell Biology.* Vol 84, pp413-421.

Chung C.A., T.W. Yang, Chen C.W. (2006). Analysis of cell growth and diffusion in a scaffold for cartilage tissue engineering *Biotechnol. Bioeng.* Vol94, No6, pp1138–1146

Dominici M., K.Le Blanc, I. Mueller, I. Slaper-Cortenbach, F.C. Marini, D.S. Krause, R.J. Deans, A. Keating, D.J. Prockop and E.M. Horwitz (2006). Position Paper: Minimal criteria for defining multipotent mesenchymal stromal cells. The International Society for Cellular Therapy position statement. *Cytotherapy.* Vol8, No 4, pp315 317.

Flanigan, D. C.; Harris, J. D.; Trinh, T. Q.; Siston, R. A.; and Brophy, R. H. (2010). Prevalence of chondral defects in athletes' knees: a systematic review. *Med Sci Sports Exerc,* Vol42, No10, pp1795-801.

Fortier, L. A., Potter, H.g., Rickey, E.J., Schnabel, L.V., Foo, L.F., Chong, L.R., Stokol, T., Cheetham, J., and Nixon, A.J., (2010) Concentrated bone marrow aspirate improves full-thickness cartilage repair compared with microfracture in the equine model. *Journal of Bone Joint Surgery America.* Vol92, No 10, pp1927-1937.

Freedman, K. B.; Fox, J. A.; and Cole, B. J. (2004) Knee Cartilage: Diagnosis and Decision Making. In *Textbook of Arthroscopy.* Edited by Miller, M., and Cole, B., Philadelphia, PA, Eslevier, 2004.

Gill, T. J. (2000) The treatment of articular cartilage defects using microfracture and debridement. *Am J Knee Surg,* Vol13, No1, pp33-40.

Gobbi A, Nunag P, Malinowski K. (2005). Treatment of full thickness chondral lesions of the knee with microfracture in a group of athletes. Knee Surg Sports Traumatology *Arthroscopy*. Vol 13, No 3, pp213-215.

Gooding, C. R.; Bartlett, W.; Bentley, G.; Skinner, J. A.; Carrington, R.; and Flanagan, A. (2006) A prospective, randomised study comparing two techniques of autologous chondrocyte implantation for osteochondral defects in the knee: Periosteum covered versus type I/III collagen covered. *Knee*, Vol13, No3, pp203-10.

Holig K, Kramer M, Kroschinsky F, et al. (2009) Safety and efficacy of hematopoietic stem cell collection from mobilized peripheral blood in unrelated volunteers: 12 years of single-center experience in 3928 donors. *Blood.* Vol114, No18, pp3757-63.

Horvai, A. (2011) Anatomy and Histology of Cartilage. In *Cartilage Imaging*. Edited by Link, T., NY, Springer, 2011.

Jakobsen, R. B.; Engebretsen, L.; and Slauterbeck, J. R. (2005) An analysis of the quality of cartilage repair studies. *J Bone Joint Surg Am*, Vol87, No10, pp 2232-9.

Johnson, L. L. (1986) Arthroscopic abrasion arthroplasty historical and pathologic perspective: present status. *Arthroscopy*, Vol2, No1, pp 54-69.

Kang, S. W.; Bada, L. P.; Kang, C. S.; Lee, J. S.; Kim, C. H.; Park, J. H.; and Kim, B. S. (2008) Articular cartilage regeneration with microfracture and hyaluronic acid. *Biotechnol Lett*, Vol30, No3, pp 435-9, 2008.

Kaplan, L. D. et al. (2009) The effect of early hyaluronic acid delivery on the development of an acute articular cartilage lesion in a sheep model. *Am J Sports Med*, Vol37, No12, pp 2323-7, 2009.

Knutsen G, Engebretsen L, Ludvigsen TC, et al. (2004). Autologous chondrocyte implantation compared with microfracture in the knee. A randomized trial. *Journal of Bone and Joint Surgery (American)*. Vol 86-A, No 3, pp:455-464.

Knutsen G, Drogset JO, Engebretsen L, et al. (2007) A randomized trial comparing autologous chondrocyte implantation with microfracture. Findings at five years. *Journal of Bone and Joint Surgery (American)*. Vol 89, No 10, pp:2105-2112

Koch TG, Berg LC, Betts DH.(2008) Concepts for the clinical use of stem cells in equine medicine. *Can Vet J*. Vol49, No10, Oct 2008, pp1009-17.

Kreuz PC, Steinwachs MR, Erggelet C, et al. (2006). Results after microfracture of full-thickness chondral defects in different compartments in the knee. *Osteoarthritis Cartilage*. Vol 14, No 11, pp: 1119-1125.

Kujawa, M. J., and Caplan, A. I. (1986) Hyaluronic acid bonded to cell-culture surfaces stimulates chondrogenesis in stage 24 limb mesenchyme cell cultures. *Dev Biol*, Vol114, No2, pp504-18.

Kuroda R et al (2007). Treatment of a full-thickness articular cartilage defect in the femoral condyle of an athelete with autologous bone marrow stromal cells. *Osteoarthritis Cartilage*. Vol15, pp226-231.

Lee, K. B.; Hui, J. H.; Song, I. C.; Ardany, L.; and Lee, E. H.(2007) Injectable mesenchymal stem cell therapy for large cartilage defects--a porcine model. *Stem Cells*, Vol25, No11, pp2964-71.

Legovic, D. et al. (2009) Microfracture technique in combination with intraarticular hyaluronic acid injection in articular cartilage defect regeneration in rabbit model. *Coll Antropol*, Vol33, No2, pp619-23.

Lubowitz, J. H.; Appleby, D.; Centeno, J. M.; Woolf, S. K.; and Reid, J. B., 3rd (2007) The relationship between the outcome of studies of autologous chondrocyte implantation and the presence of commercial funding. *Am J Sports Med*, Vol35, No11, pp1809-16.

Magnussen, R. A.; Dunn, W. R.; Carey, J. L.; and Spindler, K. P. (2008) Treatment of focal articular cartilage defects in the knee: a systematic review. *Clin Orthop Relat Res*, Vol466, No4, pp952-62.

Mankin, H. J.; Mow, V. C.; Buckwalter, J. A.; Iannotti, J. P.; and Ratcliffe, (2000) A.: Articular Cartilage Structure, Composition, and Function. In *Orthopaedic Basic Science 2nd Edition*. Edited by Buckwalter, J. A.; Einhorn, T. A.; and Simon, S. R., AAOS, 2000.

McCarty R.C., C.J. Xian, S. Gronthos, A.C.W. Zannettino and B.K. Foster (2010). Application of autologous bone marrow derived mesenchymal stem cells to an ovine model of growth plate cartilage injury. *The Open Orthopaedics Journal*, Vol4, pp204-210.

McGuire, D. A.; Carter, T. R.; and Shelton, W. R. (2002) Complex knee reconstruction: osteotomies, ligament reconstruction, transplants, and cartilage treatment options. *Arthroscopy*, Vol18, No9 Suppl 2, pp 90-103.

Menche, D. S.; Frenkel, S. R.; Blair, B.; Watnik, N. F.; Toolan, B. C.; Yaghoubian, R. S.; and Pitman, M. I.(1992): A comparison of abrasion burr arthroplasty and subchondral drilling in the treatment of full-thickness cartilage lesions in the rabbit. *Arthroscopy*, Vol12, No3, pp280-6.

Messner, K., and Maletius, W. (1996) The long-term prognosis for severe damage to weight-bearing cartilage in the knee: a 14-year clinical and radiographic follow-up in 28 young athletes. *Acta Orthop Scand*, Vol67, No2, pp165-8.

Mithoefer K, Williams RJ 3rd, Warren RF, et al. (2005) The microfracture technique for the treatment of articular cartilage lesions in the knee. A prospective cohort study. *Journal of Bone and Joint Surgery (American)*. Vol 87, No 9, pp: 1911-1920.

Murphy et al (2003). Stem cell therapy in a caprine model of osteoarthritis. *Arthritis Rheumotology*. Vol48, pp3464-3474.

Nakamura, N.; Miyama, T.; Engebretsen, L.; Yoshikawa, H.; and Shino, K. (2009) Cell-based therapy in articular cartilage lesions of the knee. *Arthroscopy*, Vol25, No5, pp 531-52.

Nöth U., Steinert A.F. and S.T. Rocky (2008). Technology Insight: Adult Mesenchymal Stem Cells for Osteoarthritis Therapy. *Nature Clinical Practice Rheumatology*, Vol4, No7, pp371-380.

Noyes, F. R.; Bassett, R. W.; Grood, E. S.; and Butler, D. L. (1980) Arthroscopy in acute traumatic hemarthrosis of the knee. Incidence of anterior cruciate tears and other injuries. J *Bone Joint Surg Am*, Vol62, No5, pp687-95, 757.

Ordemann R, Holig K, Wagner K, et al. (1998) Acceptance and feasibility of peripheral stem cell mobilisation compared to bone marrow collection from healthy unrelated donors. *Bone Marrow Transplant*, Vol 21, No Suppl 3, ppS25-8.

Ossendorf, C.; Kaps, C.; Kreuz, P. C.; Burmester, G. R.; Sittinger, M.; and Erggelet, C. (2007) Treatment of posttraumatic and focal osteoarthritic cartilage defects of the knee with autologous polymer-based three-dimensional chondrocyte grafts: 2-year clinical results. *Arthritis Res Ther*, Vol9, No2, ppR41.

Panagiota A.S., Sonia A. P., Maria S., Constantin N.B., Michael P. (2005). Characterization of the Optimal Culture Conditions for Clinical Scale Production of Human Mesenchymal Stem Cells. *Stem Cells Express* :DOI: 10.1634/stemcells.2004-0331

Pacini S, Spinabella S, Trombi L, Fazzi R, Galimberti S, Dini F, Carlucci F, Petrini M. (2007) Suspension of bone marrow-derived undifferentiated mesenchymal stromal cells for repair of superficial digital flexor tendon in race horses. *Tissue Eng.* Vol13, No12, December 2007, pp2949-55.

Peterson L, Minas T, Brittberg M, Nilsson A, Sjogren-Jansson E, Lindahl (2000). A. Two- to 9-year outcome after autologous chondrocyte transplantation of the knee. *Clinical Orthopaedics Related Research.* Vol 374, pp: 212-234.

Pridie, K. H. (1959): A method of resurfacing osteoarthritic knee joints. *J Bone Joint Surg [Br]*, Vol41, pp 618-19.

Sanchez, M.; Anitua, E.; Azofra, J.; Aguirre, J. J.; and Andia, I. (2008) Intra-articular injection of an autologous preparation rich in growth factors for the treatment of knee OA: a retrospective cohort study. *Clin Exp Rheumatol*, Vol26, No5, pp910-3, 2008.

Saris DB, Vanlauwe J, Victor J, et al. (2009). Treatment of symptomatic cartilage defects of the knee: characterized chondrocyte implantation results in better clinical outcome at 36 months in a randomized trial compared to microfracture. *American Journal of Sports Medicine.* Vol 37, No Suppl 1, pp:10S-19S.

Saw KY, Hussin P, Loke SC, Azam M, Chen HC, Tay YG, Low S, Wallin KL and Ragavanaidu K. (2009) Articular cartilage regeneration with autologous marrow aspirate and hyaluronic acid: an experimental study in a goat model. *Arthroscopy*, Vol25, No12, pp1391-1400.

Saw KY, Anz A, Tay YG, Ragavanaidu K, Jee CSY and McGuire DA (2011) *Arthroscopy: The Journal of Arthroscopic and Related Surgery*, Vol 27, No 4, April 2011, pp 493-506

Steadman JR, Rodkey WG, Briggs KK, Rodrigo JJ. (1999) The microfracture technique in the management of complete cartilage defects in the knee joint. *Orthopade* , Vol28, No1, pp26-32.

Steadman, J. R.; Briggs, K. K.; Rodrigo, J. J.; Kocher, M. S.; Gill, T. J.; and Rodkey, W. G. (2003) Outcomes of microfracture for traumatic chondral defects of the knee: average 11-year follow-up. *Arthroscopy*, Vol19, No5, pp 477-84.

Steinert, A. F.; Ghivizzani, S. C.; Rethwilm, A.; Tuan, R. S.; Evans, C. H.; and Noth, U. (2007) Major biological obstacles for persistent cell-based regeneration of articular cartilage. *Arthritis Res Ther*, Vol9, No3, pp213.

Steinwachs, M. R.; Guggi, T.; and Kreuz, P. C. (2008) Marrow stimulation techniques. *Injury*, Vol39, No Suppl 1,pp S26-31.

Strauss, E.; Schachter, A.; Frenkel, S.; and Rosen, J. (2009) The efficacy of intra-articular hyaluronan injection after the microfracture technique for the treatment of articular cartilage lesions. *Am J Sports Med*, Vol37, No4, pp720-6.

Taylor SE, Smith RK, Clegg PD. (2007) Mesenchymal stem cell therapy in equine musculoskeletal disease: scientific fact or clinical fiction? *Equine Vet J.* Vol39, No2 March 2007, pp172-80

Tuan, R. S. (2007) A second-generation autologous chondrocyte implantation approach to the treatment of focal articular cartilage defects. *Arthritis Res Ther*, Vol9, No5, pp109.

Tytherleigh-Strong, G.; Hurtig, M.; and Miniaci, A. (2005) Intra-articular hyaluronan following autogenous osteochondral grafting of the knee. *Arthroscopy*, Vol21, No8, pp999-1005.

Uccelli et al (2007). Mesenchymal Stem cells: a new strategy for immunosuppression. *Trends in Immunology*. Vol28, pp219-226.

Violini S, Ramelli P, Pisani LF, Gorni C, Mariani P (2009) Horse bone marrow mesenchymal stem cells express embryo stem cell markers and show the ability for tenogenic differentiation by in vitro exposure to BMP-12. *BMC Cell Biol*. Vol22, April 2009, pp10:29.

Wakitani S et al (2004). Autologous bone marrow stromal cell transplantation for repair of full thickness articular cartilage defects in human patellae: two case reports. *Cell transplantation*. Vol13,pp 595-600.

Zeifang F, Oberle D, Nierhoff C, Richter W, Moradi B, Schmitt, H. (2010). Autologous Chondrocyte Implantation Using the Original Periosteum-Cover Technique Versus Matrix-Associated Autologous Chondrocyte Implantation: A Randomized Clinical Trial. *American Journal of Sports Medicine*. Vol 38, No 5, pp:924-933.

8

Traumatic Chondral Lesions of the Knee Diagnosis and Treatment

Masoud Riyami
Sultan Qaboos University, Oman
Sultanate of Oman

1. Introduction

1.1 Anatomy and knee joint function

The knee joint is classified as a modified hinge joint, with its structure providing a highly mobile and complex joint (fig.1). It consists of two condylar joints between the medial and lateral condyles of the femur and the corresponding plateaus of the tibia, and anteriorly a synovial plane patellofemoral joint. The articular surface of the knee is covered by Hyaline cartilage that is supported by subchondral bone. This Hyaline cartilage is very soft and yields its interstitial water easily when compressed yet it is very stiff in tension along planes parallel to the articular surface (Buckwalter and Mow, 2003). Intact cartilage provides a smooth, lubricated gliding surface with a coefficient of friction better than most man-made bearing materials (Buckwalter and Mow, 2003). In the knee articular cartilage distributes the loads of articulation, thereby minimizing peak stresses acting on the subchondral bone whilst the tensile strength of the tissue maintains its structural integrity under loading. These biomechanical properties make the tissue remarkably durable and wear resistant, enabling it to last many decades, even under high and repetitive stresses (Buckwalter and Mow, 2003).

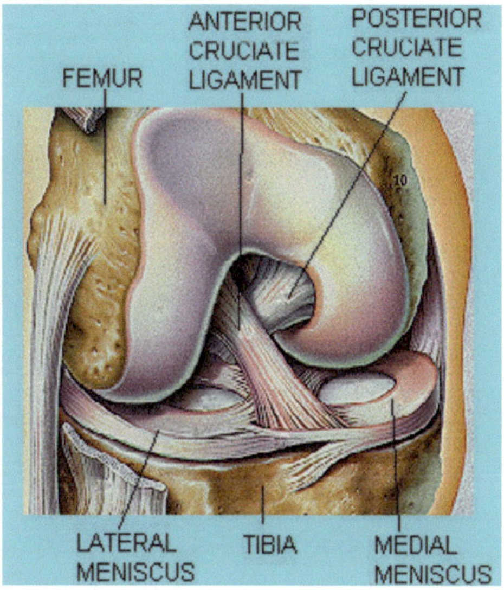

Fig. 1. Structure of knee joint (www.arthroscopy.com)

Flexion and extension are the primary movements of the knee. When the knee is flexed a small amount of rotation can occur. The patella glides along the distal portion of the femur during movements of flexion to extension.

Semi-lunar shaped fibrocartilage discs, triangular in cross-section, form the menisci that are found between the tibia and femur. They deepen the articular surface, improve joint congruency and assist in shock absorption. The medial meniscus is attached to the joint capsule and the deep fibres of the medial collateral ligament. The lateral meniscus does not have these attachments, resulting in increased mobility (Marieb, 1992).

The intra-articular ligaments consist of the anterior cruciate ligament (ACL) and the posterior cruciate ligament (PCL). The ACL provides stability to anterior translation, and prevents the posterior displacement of the femur on the tibia. The PCL prevents anterior displacement of the femur on the tibia.

The main extra-articular ligaments comprise of the medial and lateral collateral ligament and provide side-to-side stability.

Stability of the knee joint is therefore provided by two menisci, intra and extra-capsular ligaments, and the dense muscular structures surrounding the joint. Injuries frequently occur to one or more of these stabilizing structures.

1.2 Structure of articular cartilage

Articular cartilage consists of various substances, each of which contribute to its overall integrity, durability, deformability and ability to repair itself (Hayes et al, 2001).

From embryological life articular cartilage is derived from mesenchymal cells and develops at the future end of epiphyseal bone (Hayes et al, 2001). Cartilage is composed of a matrix of collagen surrounded by proteins and negatively charged proteoglycans (fig.2). The roll of collagen is to serve as an anchor to the proteoglycan matrix protecting chondrocytes. Articular cartilage consists mainly of types II, IX, and XI collagen. Collagen helps to resist extrinsic forces during loading (Vigarita, 1999; cited by Hayes et al, 2001).

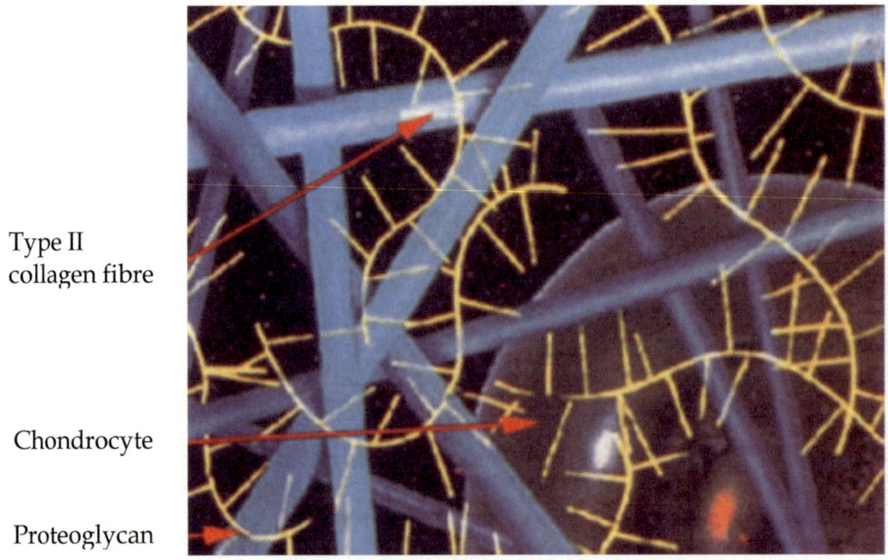

Fig. 2. Spatial relations of collagen, proteoglycans and cells in cartilage (Kocheta and Toms, 2004)

Cartilage has an organized layered structure that can be functionally and structurally divided into four zones (fig.3): Superficial zone, the middle (transitional) zone, the deep zone and a calcified cartilage zone. The superficial zone is the articulating surface that provides a smooth gliding surface and resists sheer. This zone makes up approximately 10 to 20 percent of articular cartilage thickness. It has the highest collagen contents of the zones. The collagen fibrils in this zone are densely packed and have a highly ordered alignment parallel to the articular surface (Mow, 1989; cited by Pearle et al, 2005). This superficial zone has the lowest compressive modulus and will deform approximately 25 times more than the middle zone (Pearle et al, 2005).
The middle zone encompasses 40 to 60 percent of the articular cartilage volume. This zone has a higher compressive modulus than the superficial zone and a less organized arrangement of the collagen fibers. The deep zone makes up 30 percent of the cartilage, and consists of large diameter collagen fibril layers perpendicular to the articular surface. This layer has the highest compressive modulus. The tide mark separates the deep zone from the calcified cartilage, which rests directly on the subchondral bone. The calcified cartilage contains small cells in a chondral matrix speckled with apatitic salts (Mow, 1989; cited by Pearle et al, 2005).
Normal adult cartilage is composed of 75 percent water and 25 percent solids. The solids consist of collagen and proteoglycan, and a fluid phase composed of water and ions (Eichellberger, 1951; cited by Hayes et al, 2001).

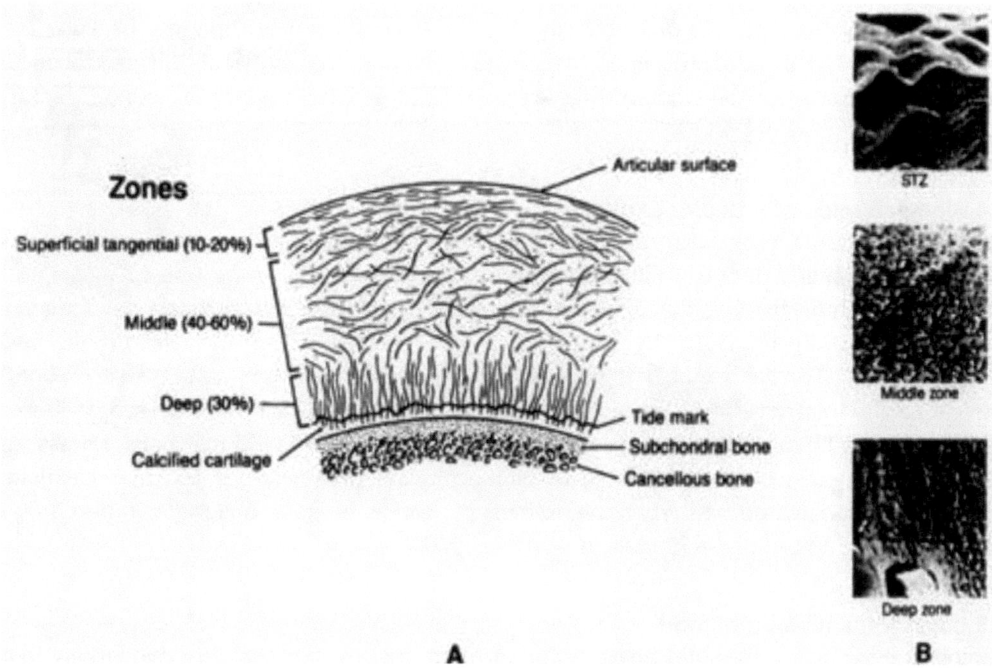

Fig. 3. Articular cartilage zones (Buckwalter and Mow, 2003)

1.3 Metabolism of articular cartilage

A high level of metabolism exists in articular cartilage. Historically, one of the factors that led to the impression that articular cartilage was inert was the early demonstration that, although articular cartilage had a well-defined glycolytic system, oxygen use was considerably lower in articular cartilage than in other tissues. This difference subsequently was found to be related to the spares cell (*sic*) population rather than to a lack of metabolic activity per cell. Nevertheless, articular cartilage chondrocytes rely principally on the anaerobic pathway for energy production (Oegema and Thompson, 1989).

Chondrocytes synthesize and assemble the cartilaginous matrix components and direct their distribution within the tissue. These synthetic and assembly processes are complex. They involve synthesis of proteins; synthesis of glycosaminoglycan chains, and their addition to the appropriate cores; and secretion of the completed molecules into the extra-cellular matrix (Guilak et al, 1997).

Chondrocytes are responsible for the synthesis, assembly and sulfation of the proteoglycan molecule. However, in normal tissue, in repair and degradation processes proteoglycans of articular cartilage are continually being broken down and released from the cartilage. This activity is a normal event in the maintenance of the tissue and can occur at an accelerated rate. The rate of catabolism can be affected by soluble mediators and by various types of joint loading (Mankin et al, 2005b).

Collagen is much more stable than the proteoglycan components. However, the collagen network is subject to metabolism, and in osteoarthritic or injured cartilage the collagen turnover increases, but as yet little is known about the mechanism of collagen breakdown (Mankin et al, 2005b).

The source of nutrients for articular cartilage is somewhat of an enigma. Because the tissue is avascular in adult life most investigators believe that nutrients diffuse through the matrix, either from the surrounding synovial fluid or from underlying bone (Mankin et al, 2005b).

1.4 Biomechanics of articular cartilage

The articular cartilage of diarthrodial joints is subject to high loads applied statically and repetitively for many decades. Thus, the structural molecules, which include collagens and proteoglycans must be organized into a strong, fatigue-resistant and tough solid matrix capable of sustainig the high stresses and strains developed within the tissue (Soltz and Ateshian, 2000). The solid matrix is porous and permeable, and very soft. Water, 65 to 80 percent of the total weight of normal articular cartilage, resides in the microscopic pores. This water may be caused to flow through the porous-permeable solid matrix by a pressure gradient or by matrix compaction. The biomechanical properties of articular cartilage therefore are understood best when the tissue is viewed as biphasic material composed of a solid phase and a fluid phase (Soltz and Ateshian, 2000).

1.5 Local transmission of load

Although it is porous, the solid phase of the cartilage has low permeability due largely to a high frictional resistance to fluid flow. This causes a high interstitial fluid pressurization in the fluid phase, which contributes more then 90 percent of the load transmission function of cartilage (Soltz and Ateshian, 2000). The high pressurization of the fluid phase and the Low permeability of the solid phase establish both the stiffness and the visco-elastic properties of cartilage (Felson et al, 2000).

This hydraulic pressure provides a significant component of the load support of the cartilage, which protects and stress shields the solid phase of the matrix from much of the load burden (Pearle et al, 2005).

1.6 Mechanism of articular cartilago injury

Direct blunt trauma, indirect impact loading, or torsional loading of a joint can damage articular cartilage and the calcified cartilage-subchondral bone region without disrupting the surrounding soft tissue. Examples of direct blunt trauma to articular cartilage of the knee include a shoe kick, knees colliding in games such as football and rugby, and falling on a hard surface. Examples of indirect impact and torsional loading include a blow to a bone that forms the subchondral part of a joint, and severe twisting of a joint that is loaded (Williams and Wilkins, 1998).

1.7 Age related chondral lesions

Clinical experience suggests that there are age-related differences in the risk and patterns of articular surface injuries. High energy bone or joint trauma causes intra-articular osteochondral fractures in people of all age, but older people and people with more osteopenic bone tend to have more severely comminuted fractures (Buckwalter et al, 1993; Buckwalter and Lane, 1996). Chondral fractures associated with participation in sports generally occur in skeletally mature people, whilst osteochondral fractures associated with participation in sports typically occur in skeletally immature people or young adults. This difference may result from age-related changes in the mechanical properties of the articular surface, including the uncalcified cartilage, the calcified cartilage zone, and the subchondral bone (Buckwalter et al, 1993; Buckwalter and Lane, 1996). That is, age-related alteration in the articular cartilage matrix decreases the tensile stiffness and strength of the superficial zone, and the calcified cartilage zone. The subchondral bone region minimizes fully following completion of skeletal growth, presumably creating a marked difference in mechanical properties between the uncalcified cartilage and the calcified cartilage-subchondral bone region (Williams and Wilkins, 1998).

1.8 Response of articular cartilage to blunt impact

Articular cartilage can withstand single or multiple moderate and occasionally high impact loads. However, a number of studies have addressed the effects of either a single excessive high-impact force causing injury to the cartilage without a break in the surface, or repetitive below-trauma threshold loads causing an accumulation of damage to the cartilage by repeated application of the load. Both can lead to chondrocyte death, matrix damage, fissuring of surface, injury to underlying bone, and thickening of the tide mark region. At a certain threshold of impact loading, the cartilage may be sheared off the subchondral bone (Mankin et al, 2005).

Excessive impact or torsional joint loading causes three types of articular cartilage injury: chondral damage without visible tissue disruption; disruption of articular cartilage alone (chondral fractures and flaps); and disruption of articular cartilage and subchondral bone (osteochondral fractures) (Buckwalter et al, 1988). Intensity and rate of loading, muscle contractions that affect the transmission of force to the articular surface, age, and genetically determined differences in articular cartilage may influence the type of articular surface injury in a given individual (Buckwalter et al, 1988).

1.9 Healing of articular cartilage

More than a century ago articular cartilage was documented as lacking regenerative power; it had been observed that wounds in articular cartilage healed with fibrous tissue and fibrocartilage (Chen et al, 1999). As cartilage is avascular its reparative process differs significantly from the three-phase response of necrosis, inflammation and repair that occurs in vascularized tissue. Cartilage undergoes the initial phase of necrosis in response to injury, but there is less cell death, given its relative insensitivity to hypoxia (Chen et al, 1999). The second phase, inflammation, is largely absent as this response is primarily mediated by the vascular system. No fibrin clot or network is developed to act as a scaffold for the in growth of repair tissue, and no mediators or cytokines are released to stimulate cellular migration and proliferation. The third phase, repair, is also severely limited due to the lack of a preceding inflammatory response and recruitment of undifferentiated mesenchymal cells that normally proliferate and modulate the repair response. The burden of repair thus falls on the existing chondrocytes in a process termed intrinsic repair (Chen et al, 1999).

1.10 Role of chondrocytes in healing

Chondrocytes near the injured part may proliferate and form clusters or clones and synthesize new matrix, but the chondrocytes do not migrate into the lesion. The new matrix they produce remains in the immediate region of the chondrocytes, and their preoperative and synthetic activity fails to provide new tissue to repair the damage. This repair phase is initially brisk. It is, however, limited in scope and duration, disappearing within a matter of weeks (Mankin et al, 2005). Results from experimental studies of injuries limited to cartilage clearly demonstrate the inability of chondrocytes to repair cartilage defects. The results also show that limited experimental injuries to normal articular surfaces in normal synovial joints generally do not progress to full thickness loss of cartilage (Mankin et al, 2005).

1.11 Incidence of articular cartilage injuries

The incidence of articular cartilage injuries to the knee, determined arthroscopically, has been most frequently reported as part of a large series of assessment for haemarthrosis. Noyes et al (1980) reported a 20 percent incidence, Gillquist et al (1977) a 10 percent occurrence, and DeHaven (1980) a 6 percent incidence of chondral or osteochondral injuries. In a review of 1,000 knee arthroscopies Hjelle et al (2002) reported chondral or osteochondral occurrence in 61 percent of the patients, but focal chondral or osteochondral defects were found in 19 percent of the patients. With the increasing age of the patients the incidence of articular cartilage injury increased. Characteristic injury depth patterns have been found to be associated with the degree of skeletal maturity (Hopkinson et al, 1985 and Johnson-Nurse et al, 1985; cited by Speer et al, 1991). In children and adolescents osteochondral fractures are more frequent than full-thickness or partial-thickness chondral injuries. It has been suggested that the bond between articular cartilage and subchondral bone is stronger than the bone itself. With increasing age and skeletal maturity the basal layers of articular cartilage become calcified and the tide mark develops. This provides a plan of weakness through which separation may occur. Full thickness chondral lesions are most frequently seen in patients in their 30s. Beyond this age the plane of weakness moves further from the subchondral bone into more superficial cartilage, with subsequent increasing incidence of partial thickness chondral injuries (Johnson-Nurse et al, 1985; cited by Speer et al, 1991). In a multicentral study conducted in the USA, between 1991 and 1995, Walton found the prevalence of chondral injuries in 31,516 knee arthroscopies to be 19,827 (63 %). A total of 53,569 hyaline cartilage lesions were found during these 19,827 arthroscopies, an average of 2.7 lesions per knee. The average age of the patient with lesions was 43 years. More male than female patients had lesions (61.6 and 38.4 percent, respectively). The lesions consisted of osteochondritis dissecans (0.7 %), articular fractures (1.3 %), grade I lesions (9.7 %), grade II lesions (28.1 %), grade III lesions (41.0 %), and grade IV lesions (19.2 %). Grade III lesions were the most common in patients over 30 years of age. The most common locations for grade III lesions were patella and medial femoral condyle. The medial femoral condyle was the most common location for single grade IV lesions. The patella and lateral femoral condyle were the next two most common sites (Walton et al, 1997).

1.12 Grading of articular cartilage lesions

Although there are several different classification systems for the description of articular cartilage damage, each has certain limitations and deficiencies that can lead to confusion (Noyes and Stabler, 1989). Some systems combine the surface appearance of the articular cartilage lesion and the depth of involvement under a single description category, and then make no distinction as to the depth of involvement (Noyes and Stabler, 1989). According to the Outerbridge classification Grade II and III are identical in appearance (fragmentation and fissuring). The classification does not specify the extent of involvement from surface to bone in either stage. Rather, the distinction between the grades is based on the diameter of involvement (Noyes and Stabler, 1989). In the classification system of Bentley there is no category reserved for lesions with an intact surface. Furthermore, grades I, II and III all described as fibrillation or fissuring, and the distinction between grades is based on the area of damage (Noyes and Stabler, 1989). Ficet and Hangerford distinguished between closed (grade I) and open (grade II) lesions, but do not separate lesions within each category according to severity. Grade I describes varying degrees of softening from simple to pitting oedema. Grade II distinguishes between fissures and ulcerations, but either can be superficial and localized or can extend to subchondral bone (Noyes and Stabler, 1989). The classification systems of Casscells and Insall both describe lesions that become more extensive as one moves from grade I to grade IV. Casscell's system makes no allowance for a lesion without surface changes (Noyes and Stabler, 1989). Insall's system is problematic because the specification for grade II (Fissuring) and grade III (fibrillation) are somewhat qualitative and may or may not be applied similarly by observers (Noyes and Stabler, 1989). Although according to Noyes and Stabler (1989) Goodfellow differentiates between surface degeneration and basilar degeneration, the terms fasciculation I, blister, and fasciculation II, under the general category of basilar degeneration, can cause some confusion. Most other authors seem to use the term fasciculation when referring to disruption of an intact surface (Noyes and Stabler, 1989).

1.12.1 Outerbridge classification

The Outerbridge classification system (Outerbridge, 1961) was originally designed to classify chondromalacia patellae. Over the years it has been extrapolated for use in classifying chondral lesions throughout the body (Noyes et al, 1977). The accuracy and reproducibility of this classification system was addressed by Cameron et al, (2003) when they determined the intraobserver reliability, interobserver reproducibility and the accuracy of the system for grading chondral lesions in knees viewed arthroscopically. They compared the results obtained by using the system with observations at arthrotomy of six cadaveric donors. The accuracy rate ranged from 22 to 100 percent, with lower grade lesions diagnosed with less accuracy than higher-grade lesions (Cameron et al, 2003). The Outerbridge grading system is given in table.1 and figure 4.

1.12.2 International Cartilage Repair Society (ICRS) classification

This system classifies Hyaline cartilage lesion after debridement of loose bodies, and defines a lesion as a superficial, partial thickness, or full thickness defect (Brittberg and Winalski, 2003). The ICRS classification system focuses on the lesion depth (graded 0 to 4) and the area of damage (graded from normal to severely abnormal with use of the IKDC system) (www.cartilage.org).

Figure 5 shows the ICRS system. This classifies macroscopically normal cartilage without a notable defect as ICRS 0. If the cartilage has an intact surface but fibrillation and/or slight softening is present, it is classified as ICRS 1a, and if additional superficial lacerations and fissures are found, it is classified as ICRS 1b (nearly normal). Defects that extend deeper but involve less than 50 percent of the cartilage thickness are classified as ICRS 2 (abnormal). Lesions that extend to more than 50 percent of the cartilage thickness are classified as ICRS 3 (severely abnormal). However, there are four subgroups of this grade: 3a, 3b, 3c, and 3d depending on the involvement of a calcified layer. Joint trauma may create cartilage defect that extend into the subchondral bone. These full thickness osteochondral injuries are classified as ICRS 4 (severely abnormal). Excluded from this grade are defects that are classified as osteochondritis dissecans (OCD), which have a classification system of their own (Brittberg and Winalski, 2003).

Grade	Surface description	Lesion diameter
I	Softening and swelling	None
II	Fragmentation and fissuring	Less than half inch
III	Fragmentation and fissuring	More than half inch
IV	Exposed subchondral bone	None

Table 1. Outerbridge grading system

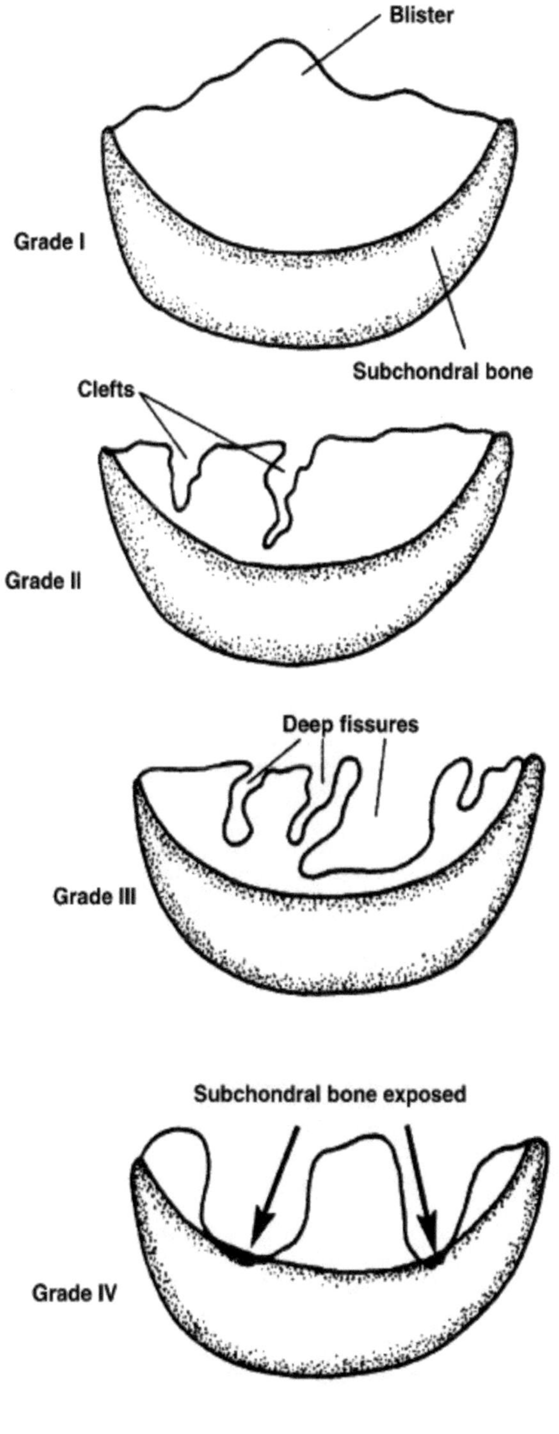

Fig. 4. Outerbridge system for grading chondral defects (Kocheta and Tomes, 2004)

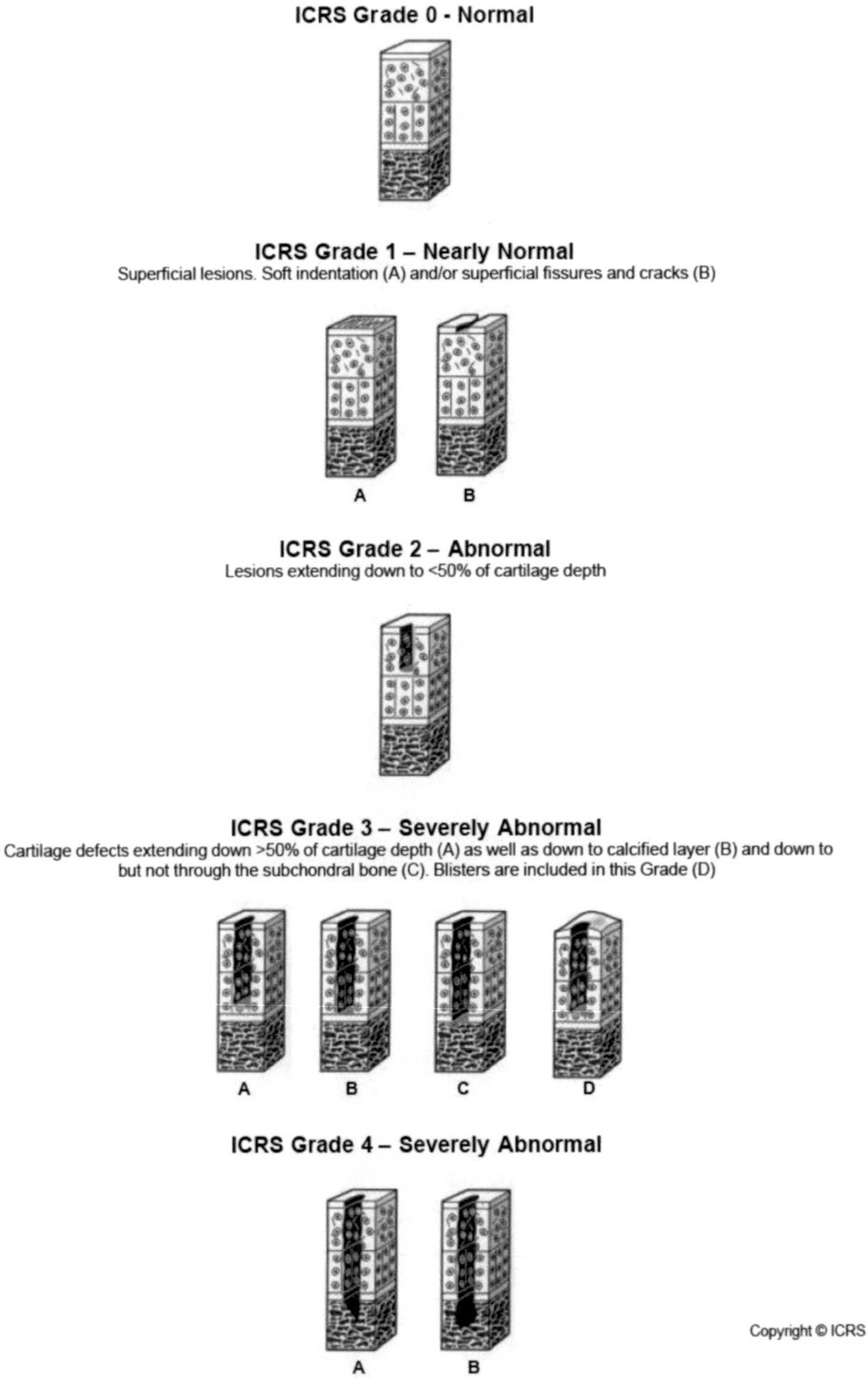

Fig. 5. ICRS classification (www.cartilage.org)

2. Diagnosis of articular surface damage

The clinical diagnosis of a chondral injury by history and physical examination can be difficult, and may be a source of confusion (Speer et al, 1991).
The initial symptoms of this injury are often obscure, and the immediate disability may be slight. The symptoms are very suggestive of a torn meniscus because of catching, locking, and giving way of the knee (Gilley, 1981; cited by Speer et al, 1991). An accurate diagnosis of traumatic articular cartilage injury is essential as individuals with these lesions have a poor prognosis for rapid recovery. Their mean rehabilitation time is almost triple that of a routine knee meniscal injury (Speer et al, 1991).

2.1 Conventional radiographic technique

Conventional radiographic techniques have proved to be of limited value in the imaging of articular cartilage as such techniques only allows the indirect assessment of cartilage (Lund, 1980; cited by Recht et al, 1993). Plain radiographs, in general, significantly underestimate the extent of cartilage damage (Blackburn et al, 1994). However, plain X-ray may reveal osteochondral lesions, including osteochondritis dissecans and loose bodies (Morelli et al, 2002).
Scintigraphy and computerized tomographic evaluations are limited because of their lack of sensitivity and requirement for ionizing radiation (Blackburn et al, 1994). Computed tomography combined with arthrography improves both the visualization of cartilage and the detection of abnormalities, but this method is relatively insensitive in the delineation of small cartilage lesions (Handelberg et al, 1990). Bone scans may indicate osteochondral injuries, but is not specific and does not necessarily indicate pure chondral lesions or their size (Morelli, et al. 2002).

2.2 Arthroscopy

The most accurate diagnostic modality for traumatic knee articular cartilage injury is arthroscopy (DeHaven, 1980). However, even with this "Gold Standard" modality the posterior tibial and femoral lesions can be difficult to identify and may be missed (Terry, 1988; cited by Speer 1991). Although arthroscopy treatment can be performed on a chondral fracture discovered unexpectedly, it would be advantageous to know before arthroscopy whether a chondral injury is present. The surgeon then could advise the patient before surgery about treatment options and expected outcome, and decide on the type and timing of surgery (Rubin, 1998).

2.3 Magnetic resonance imaging

The MR imaging appearance of chondral fractures is analogous to their arthroscopic appearance (Rubin et al, 1997). Chondral separations manifest as a defect in the articular surface extending down to the subchondral plate, with vertically oriented walls and sharp demarcation from the surrounding cartilage. When a flap is present a fragment will be seen, attached on one side (Rubin et al, 1997). Lesion conspicuity can be increased by performing MR arthrography, especially if the patient is examined some time after the acute insult (Rubin, 1998). The presence of a joint effusion could alleviate the need for iatrogenic introduction of intra-articular contrast agents. The theory is that this would offer an

"arthrogram" effect, and allow indirect visualization of chondral lesions as well (Beltran, 1980; Spritzer 1988; cited by Speer 1991).
In a comparison study between MR and anatomic section Hodler et al (1992) concluded that standard MRI does not consistently allow detection of focal articular cartilage defects. Commonly used MRI sequences are not reliable enough to be effective in the diagnostic evaluation of degenerative changes of articular cartilage.

2.4 Can MRI replace arthroscopy in diagnosis?

The role of MRI for the diagnosis of chondral lesions of the knee joint is still unclear, and the sensitivity of the method ranges from 15 to 96 percent (Friemert et al, 2003). In a prospective study by Friemert et al (2003) of how MRI can replace arthroscopy in the routine diagnosis of cartilage damage, they found that the MRI cartilage specific sequences have a sensitivity of 33 percent and specificity of 99 percent and positive and negative prediction values of 75 and 98 percent respectively. With gadolinium enhanced MRI the sensitivity was 53 percent and the specificity was 98 percent. The positive prediction value was 48 percent and the negative prediction value was 98 percent. They concluded that the MRI examination techniques recommended in the literature are not able to replace arthroscopy for the diagnosis of cartilage damage of the knee joint, and in view of the high specificity (97 to 98 %) MRI is suitable for identifying cartilage lesions. In view of the low sensitivity of MRI to cartilage injury, a cautious attitude towards an operative cartilage treatment is justified. Because that MRI can not replace arthroscopy for the diagnosis of cartilage damage and so arthroscopy still has to be seen as the method of choice for the evaluation of cartilage damage (Friemert et al, 2003).

2.5 Best MRI sequences to visualize articular cartilage

Currently the most widely used techniques for articular cartilage imagining by MR are fat suppressed proton-density weighted fast spin-echo sequences, and fat suppressed spoiled gradient recalled echo (SPGR) sequences (Kornaat et al, 2005). SPGR sequences are often chosen for cartilage volume and thickness estimation because the 3D acquisition, along with higher intensity cartilage signal, provides robust visualization of cartilage and detection of cartilage pathology. However, new MR imaging pulse sequences, specifically steady-state free precession (SSFP), have recently attracted attention for their optimal visualization of cartilage. The new sequences give greater cartilage intensity, increased cartilage and contrast-to-noise ratio and reduced imaging time than conventional pulse sequences (Kornaat et al, 2005).

2.6 Comparison between 3-D SPGR and conventional MR imaging

Fat suppressed 3-D spoiled gradient recalled acquisition in the steady state (SPGR) MRI technique was compared with 2-D SPGR images and conventional T1 and T2 weighted spin-echo and multiplanar by Disler et al (1994). They studied ten healthy volunteers and concluded that fat-suppressed 3-D SPGR imagining is an improvement over fat-suppressed spin-echo imagining because the fluid signal is diminished relative to cartilage. As the sequence essentially suppresses all stationary tissue, it is not useful in evaluating the fibrocartilage, ligaments or soft tissues of the knee. However the technique shows cartilage as an object of high signal intensity relative to adjacent tissues, giving the technique great potential for evaluating this structure.

2.7 Advantages of 3-D SPGR

Fat-suppressed 3-D SPGR imagining has several advantages over conventional sequences. It generates positive contrast between cartilage and adjustment structures, making joint infusion unnecessary to show the cartilage margin (Kornaat et al, 2005).
Fat-suppression maximizes the contrast between cartilage and adjacent marrow, an improvement over T2–weighted spin-echo imagining, and minimizes chemical- shift artifact. Three-dimensional acquisition can generate very thin slices without loss of information.
In summary, fat-suppressed 3-D SPGR imagining of the knee provides a striking positive contrast between hyaline cartilage and adjacent structures, and may improve the accuracy of MR diagnosis of hyaline cartilage abnormalities (Disler et al, 1994).
The sensitivity of fat-suppressed 3-D SPGR imaging was compared with that of standard MR imaging for detecting hyaline cartilage defects of the knee, using arthroscopy as the standard of reference. Disler et al (1994) assessed 114 consecutive patients for hyaline cartilage defects of the knee with both standard MR imaging sequences and a sagittal fat-suppressed 3-D SPGR sequences. Forty eight patients with meniscal or ligament injury or persistent symptoms underwent subsequent arthroscopy. The standard MR and SPGR images of these 48 patients were then retrospectively analyzed for articular defects in a blinded fashion by two independent observers. Sensitivity, specificity, and intra-observer and inter-observer agreement were determined for the different imaging techniques. A quarter of the patients who went on to arthroscopy were found to have isolated hyaline cartilage lesions. The SPGR imaging sequences had a significantly higher sensitivity than the standard MR imaging sequences for detecting hyaline cartilage defects (75 to 85 % and 29 to 38 % respectively, $p < 0.001$, for each component). Significant differences in sensitivity were found for each surface except the trochlear and lateral tibial surfaces. No difference in specificity were found (97 % and 97 % respectively, $p > 0. 99$). Combined evaluation of standard MR and SPGR images gave no added diagnostic advantage (sensitivity 86 %; specificity 97 %; $p > 0.42$). Except for the lateral tibial surface, reproducibility among readings and between readers was excellent. The conclusion from the study was that fat-suppressed 3-D SPGR imaging is more sensitive than standard MR imaging for the detection of hyaline cartilage defects of the knee (Disler et al, 1996). In day-to-day practice a routine clinical MRI scan has low sensitivity in diagnosing chondral damage when compared with arthroscopic findings (Bobic, 2005).
Levy et al (1996) reported that preoperative MRI scans correctly identified 21 percent of the chondral lesions seen at arthroscopic examination. However, since 1996 the new awareness of the significance of chondral problems, due to extensive laboratory and clinical research, and various attempts to repair hyaline articular surface, has resulted in an increased interest in magnetic resonance imaging as a diagnostic and evaluation tool (Bobic, 2005).
Development of refined MRI techniques and recent advantages in MRI technology appear to be very promising. Magnetic resonance imaging has the potential to replace the more conventional invasive techniques, like arthroscopy and biopsy, in the evaluation of articular cartilage damage and repair (Bobic, 2005).

2.8 Significant of focal subchondral oedema

Rubin et al (2000) retrospectively reviewed the MR studies of 18 knees with arthroscopically proven acute articular cartilage defects, noting the associated subchondral oedema.

Subchondral oedema was defined as the focal region of high signal intensity in the bone immediately underlying an articular surface defect on a T2 weighted or short inversion time inversion recovery (STIR) images. In their study the subchondral oedema was found to be associated with chondral surface defects in 83 % (Observer 1) and 72 % (observer 2) of subjects. Focal subchondral oedema is commonly visible on MR images of treatable, traumatic chondral lesions in the knee. This MR finding may prove to be an important clue to assist in the detection of these traumatic chondral defects (Rubin et al, 2000). They postulate three possible mechanisms for the generation of this marrow oedema: the injury to the subchondral bone can (1) precede the articular cartilage injury, (2) occur at the same time as the cartilage injury, or (3) follow the cartilage injury. Support for the first possibility comes from animal studies of experimentally created chondral injuries that show injury to the overlaying cartilage by several weeks (Radin et al, 1973 and 1984; cited by Rubin et al, 2000). Marrow oedema shown on MR images is thought to reflect the initial injury to the overlaying cartilage by several weeks (Thompson et al, 1993; cited by Rubin et al, 2000). The support for the second possibility is that the initial force responsible for the cartilage fracture produces a transient depression of the articular surface that is transmitted to the subchondral plate. In this instance, the subchondral marrow oedema would represent a direct contusion, or true bone "bruise". The support for the third hypothesis is that the initial insult produces a cartilage defect large enough to expose the underlying bone to direct compression against the opposing articular surface once joint loading recommences (Minas et al, 1997; cited by Rubin et al, 2000).
Characteristic subchondral oedema revealed on fat-suppressed STIR images may alert the radiologist to the presence of a defect in the overlaying chondral surface that otherwise may have been overlooked (Rubin et al, 2000).

3. Treatment of articular surface lesions

Articular cartilage injuries are notorious for their inability to produce a healing response. The management of symptomatic lesions must take into consideration several patient factors before initiating a long-term treatment plan. Most, if not all, patients should have a trial of nonoperative measures in an attempt to alleviate symptoms (Morelli et al, 2002). Patients' not responding to treatment should be considered for surgical management (Morelli et al, 2002). Although a rapid development of diagnostic and therapeutic methods of articular cartilage lesions has been made, a problem of choosing the best treatment still persists. Isolated, particularly symptomatic, deep chondral lesions seem to be problematic (Widuchowski et al, 2007).
Experimental studies have shown that variations in the treatment of articular cartilage lesions can restore some form of cartilaginous articular surface, but formation or transplantation of cartilaginous tissue in an animal model does not prove that a given method has the potential to relieve joint symptoms, or improve joint function in humans (Buckwalter, 1999). The effort to restore cartilaginous articular surfaces has now reached the point where investigators should evaluate the results of experimental methods to restore cartilaginous articular surfaces, and identify the most promising approaches to the solution of clinical problems (Buckwalter, 1999). Important issues concerning the experimental models include the types of articular surface defects studied, the age of the animal, and differences in articular cartilage among species. Important considerations in assessing the outcome of procedures designed to restore an articular surface include the overall function

of the animal or patient, the function of the joint, the structure of the joint, and the structure, composition and mechanical properties of the new tissue (Buckwalter, 1999). This approach to evaluating methods of restoring a cartilaginous articular surface assumes that the goal of any of these methods is to provide sustained improved joint function, and decrease joint symptoms in people with traumatic or degenerative joint damage. Tissues that differ from normal articular cartilage may achieve this goal (Buckwalter, 1999).

There are several choices for the treatment of articular cartilage defects. For the last few years new techniques that aim to reestablish hyaline cartilage have been introduced. They include the use of cultured cells, bone mesenchymal stem cells, as well as tissue engineering (Morcacci et al, 2002). On the other hand, there are papers suggesting that minimum invasive, simple method, or even willful negligence of a surgical treatment, might also be effective in achieving good function of the joint (Morcacci et al, 2002). Messner and Maletius (1996) showed that without treatment 22 of the 28 patients had good to excellent function 14 years after surgery. Another study, Shelbourne et al (2003), showed that at ten years follow-up there was no significant difference between the outcomes of patients with ACL-associated untreated cartilage injury and patients with no cartilage injury. It is suggested that in certain conditions conservative treatment of cartilage defects should be also considered (Aroen et al, 1998).

During the last decade, novel surgical techniques have been introduced and the mid-to long-term functional results of those procedures are awaited (Morelli et al, 2002).

3.1 Objectives of treatment

The main objective of any treatment regimen is pain modulation, with secondary objective consisting of the restoration of joint function. Non-operative treatment attempts to achieve these goals, yet long-term follow-up reveal decreased objective knee function scores whilst patients' subjective scores remain favorable (Messner and Maletius, 1996).

3.2 Indications of operative treatment

Operative management should be considered for patients who present with symptomatic partial thickness or deep chondral lesions, and for patients with intact osteochondral fragments, as commonly encountered in the skeletally immature and young adult. In the decision-making process of any treatment option, several factors must be taken into consideration, including defect size and location, acuteness of injury, age, desired activity level, alignment, arthritis, joint stability, and severity of symptoms (Minas, 2000).

3.3 Nonoperative treatment

3.3.1 Physiotherapy

The goal of physiotherapy is to reduce swelling and maintain or improve knee function by focusing on quadriceps and hamstring strengthening. It may prove beneficial in the prevention and treatment of associated morbid conditions such as joint stiffness and patellofemoral symptoms subsequent to surgery or injury (Morelli et al, 2002).

3.3.2 Nonsteroidal anti-inflammatory drugs (NSAIDs)

NSAIDs act by inhibition of prostaglandin synthesis and thereby function as modulators of pain and inflammation. Earlier works suggest that some NSAIDs may actually promote cartilage degeneration and progression to arthritis by its inhibitory action on proteoglycan synthesis (Brandt, 1991).

3.3.3 Intraarticular viscosupplementation and oral supplements

Some preliminary studies suggest that hyaluronic acid, glucosamine, and chondroitine sulfate may have beneficial effects on articular cartilage. Hyaluronan appears to have two effects in the short-term: pain modulation and improved clinical function in early arthritis, and a reduction in the size of the chondral lesions (Evanich et al, 2001; Rolf et al, 2005). Similar results have been reported in trials using glucosamine, chondroitin sulfate, and manganese ascorbate. Glucosamine appears to exert its action by stimulating glycosaminoglycan synthesis, whereas chondroitin sulfate and manganese ascorbate inhibit protease activity thereby delaying progression of cartilage degeneration (Lippiello et al, 2000). However, before definitive conclusion can be drawn with respect to these substances, large-scale randomized controlled trials are warranted.

4. Reference

Aroen A., Deryk G., Jones DG. and Fu FH. (1998). Arthroscopic diagnosis and treatment of cartilage injuries. Sports Med. Arthrosc. Rev. 6: 31-40.

Blackburn WD., Berneuter WK. and Rominger M. (1994). Arthroscopic evaluation of the knee articular cartilage: A comparison with plain radiograph and magnetic resonance imaging. J. Rheumatol. 21: 675-679.

Bobic V. (2005). Magnetic resonance imaging of articular cartilage defects and repair. Int. Soc. Arth. Knee Surg. Orth. Current concepts. Published on line 7th June (www.isakos.com).

Brandt KD. (1991). Mechanism of action of non-steroidal anti-inflammatory drugs. Rheumatol Suppl. 27: 120-121.

Brittberg M. and Winalski CS. (2003). Evaluation of cartilage injuries and repair. J. of Bone and joint surgery Am. 85A: 58-68.

Buckwalter JA. (1999). Evaluation methods of restoring cartilaginous articular surfaces. Clin Orthop Relat Res. 367 suppl: 224-238.

Buckwalter JA. And Lane NE. (1996). Aging, sports and osteoarthritis. Sports Med. Arth. Rev. 4: 276-287.

Buckwalter JA. and Mow VC. (2003). Basic science and injury of articular cartilage, menisci, and bone. Orthopaedic sports medicine principles and practice, second edition. pp: 67-87.

Buckwalter JA., Rosenberge LC., Coutts R., Hunziker E., Reddi AH. and Mow VC. (1988). Articular cartilage: Injury and repair. Am Academy of Orthopaedic Surgeons. pp: 465-482.

Buckwalter JA., Woo SL-Y., Goldberg VM., Hadley EC., Booth F., Oegma TR. And Eyre DR. (1993). Soft tissue aging and musculoskletal function. J. Bone Joint Surg. (Am). 75A: 1533-1548.

Cameron ML., Briggs KK. and Steadman JR., (2003). Reproducibility and reliability of the Outerbridge classification for grading chondral lesions of the knee arthroscopically. Am J Sport Med. 31: 83-86.

Chen FS., Frenkel SR., and DiCesare PE. (1999). Repair of articular cartilage defects: Basic science of cartilage healing. Am J Ortho. 28: 31-33.

DeHaven KE, (1980). Diagnosis of acute knee injuries with haemarthrosis. Am. J. Sports Med. 8: 9-14.

Disler DG., McCauley TR., Kelman CG., Fuchs MD., Ratner LM., Wirth CR. and Hospodar PP. (1996). Fat-suppressed three-dimensional spoiled gradient-echo MR imaging of hyaline cartilage defects in the knee. Am J Radol. 167: 127-132.

Disler DG., Peters TL., Muscoreil LM., Wagle WA., Cousins JP. And Rifkin MD. (1994). Fat-suppressed spoiled GRASS imaging of knee hyaline cartilage: technique optimization and comparison with conventional MR imaging. Am. J. Radol. 163: 887-892.

Evanich JD., Evanich CJ., Wright MB. and Rydlewicz, JA. (2001). Efficacy of intraarticular hyaluronic acid injections in knee osteoarthritis. J. Clin Ortho. 390: 173-181.

Felson DT., Lawrence RC. and Dieppe PA. (2000). Osteoarthritis: new insight. Part I: the disease and its risk factors. J. Ann Intern Med. 8: 635-646.

Friemert B., Oberlander Y., Schwarz W., Habele HJ., Baren W., Gerngrob H. and Danz B. (2003). Diagnosis of chondral lesions of the knee joint: Can MRI replace arthroscopy?. Knee Surg. sports Traum. Arthro. Published on line 5th August. (www.ingentaconnect.com).

Gillquist J., Hagberg G., Oretrop N. (1977). Arthroscopy in acute injuries of the knee joint. Acta Ortho Scand. 48: 190-196.

Guilak F., Sah R. and Setton LA. (1997). Physical regulation of cartilage metabolism. Basic Orthopaedic Biomechanics. Second edition. pp: 179-207.

Handelberg F., Shahapour M. and Casteleyn P. (1990). Chondral lesion of patella evaluated with computed tomography, magnetic resonance imaging and arthroscopy. J. Arthroscopy. 6: 24-29.

Hayes DW., Brower RL., and John KJ. (2001). Articular cartilage anatomy, injury, and repair. J. Clin Pod. Med. Surg. 18: 35-53.

Hjelle K., Solheim E., Strand T., Muri R. and Brittberg M. (2002). Articular cartilage defects in 1,000 knee arthroscopies. J. Arthroscopy and related Surg. 18: 730-734.

Hodler J., Berthiaume MJ. and Resnick D. (1992). Knee joint hyaline cartilage defects: a comparative study of MR and Anatomic sections. J Comp. Ass. Tom. 16: 597-603.

Kornaat PR., Reeder SB., Koo S., Brittain JH., Yu H., Andriacchi TP. and Gold GE. (2005). MR imaging of articular cartilage at 1.5 T and 3.0 T: Comparison of SPGR and SSFP sequences. J. Osteo. and Cart. 13: 338-344.

Levy A., Lohnes J., Sculley S., LeCroy M. and Garrett W. (1996). Chondral delamination of the knee in soccer players. Am. J. Sports Med. 24(5): 634-639.

Lippiello L., Woodward J., Karpman R., and Hammad TA., (2000). In vivo chondroprotection and metabolic synergy of glucosamine and chondroitin sulfate. J. Clin. Orthop. 381: 229-240.

Mankin HJ., Mow VC. and Buckwalter JA. (2005b). Articular cartilage repair and osteoarthritis. Am. Acad. Orth. Surg. Orthopedic Basic Science. Ch 18:471-488.

Mankin HJ., Mow VC., Buckwalter JA., Iannotti JP. and Ratcliffe A. (2005a). Articular cartilage structure, compositition, and function. Am. Acad. Orth. Surg. Orthopedic Basic Science. Ch 17: 443 - 469.

Marieb EN. (1992). Joints. Human anatomy and physiology. 2nd Edition. The Benjamin/Cummings Publishing Company,Inc. pp. 222-245.

Messner K. and Maletius W. (1996). The long term prognosis for sever damage to weight-bearing cartilage in the knee: A 14 years clinical and radiographic follow-up in 28 young athletes. J. Acta Orth . Scand. 67: 165-168.

Minas T. (2000). A practical algorithm for cartilage repair. Op. Tech. Sports Med. J. 8: 141-143.
Morcacci M., Zaffangnini S., Kon E., Visani A., Iacono F. and Loreti I., (2002). Arthroscopic autologous chondrocyte transplantation: technical note. J. Knee Surg. Sorts Traumatol. Arthrosc. 10: 154-159.
Morelli M., Nagamori J. and Miniaci A. (2002). Articular lesions in the knee: evaluation and treatment options. Curr Openion in Ortho. J. 13: 155-161.
Morelli M., Nagamori J. and Miniaci A. (2002). Articular lesions in the knee: evaluation and treatment options. Curr Openion in Ortho. J. 13: 155-161.
Noyes FR., Bassset FW. and Grood ES. (1980). Arthroscopy in acute traumatic haemarthrosis of the knee. J. Bone Joint Surg (Am). 62A: 687-696.
Noyes FR., Grood ES. and Nusshaum NS. (1977). Effect of intraarticular corticosteroids on ligament properties: a biomechanical and histological study in Rhusus knees. J. Clin. Orthop. 123: 197-207.
Oegema TR. and Thompson RC. (1986). Metabolism of chondrocytes derived from normal and osteoarthritic human cartilage. Articular Cartilage Biochemistry. NY, Raven press. pp: 257-271.
Pearle AD., Warren RF. and Rodeo SA. (2005). Basic science of articular cartilage and osteoarthritis. J. Clin Sports Med. 24: 1-12.
Recht MP., Kramer J. and Marcelis S. (1993). Abnormalities of articular cartilage in the knee: Analysis of available MR techniques. J. Radiol. 187: 473-478.
Rolf CG., Engstrom B., Ohrvik J., Valentin A., Lilja B. and Levin, DW. (2005). A comparative study of the efficacy and safety of Hyaluronan Viscosupplements and placebo in patients with symptomatic and arthroscopy-verified cartilage pathology. J. Clin. Res. 8: 15-32.
Rubin DA. (1998). Magnetic resonance imaging of chondral and osteochondral injuries. J. Topics. Mag. Res. Imag. 9: 348-359.
Rubin DA., Harner CD. and Costello JM. (1997). Chondral fractures in the knee: MR imaging diagnosis without cartilage specific pulse sequences. J Radiol. 205: 364.
Rubin DA., Harner CD. and Costello JM. (2000). Treatable chondral injuries in the knee: Frequency of associated focal subchondral edema. Am. J. Radiol. 175: 1099-1106.
Shelbourne KD., Jari S. and Gray T. (2003). Outcome of untreated traumatic articular defects of the knee: A natural history study. J. Bone Joint Surg. (Am). 85: 8-16.
Soltz MA. and Ateshian GA. (2000). Interstitial fluid pressurization during confined compression cyclical loading of articular cartilage. Ann. Biomed. Eng. 2: 150-159.
Speer KP., Spritzer CE., Goldner JL. and Garrett WE. (1991). Magnetic resonance imaging of traumatic knee articular cartilage injuries. Am. J. Sports Med. 19: 396-402.
Walton W., Jonathan K., Stanly G., Julia R., Beth PS. and Gary GP. (1997). Cartilage injuries: A review of 31,516 knee arthroscopies. J. Arthroscopy. 13: 456-460.
Widuchowiski W., Widuchowiski J. and Trazaska T. (2007). Articular cartilage defects: study of 25,124 knee arthroscopies. Knee J. 14(3): 177-182.
Williams L. and Wilkins I. (1998). Articular cartilage: injuries and potential for healing. J. of Ortho. sports Therapy. 28: 192-202.

9

Contemporary Anterior Cruciate Ligament Reconstruction

P. Christel[1] and W. Boueri[2]
[1]*Habib Medical Center, Riyadh*
[2]*Bellevue University Medical Center, Mansourieh - El metn*
[1]*Saudi Arabia*
[2]*Lebanon*

1. Introduction

The modern era of anterior cruciate ligament (ACL) reconstruction started in the early 1990's with the development of arthroscopic knee reconstruction procedures. Early on, graft fixation issues and, graft choice have been extensively debated. Then, the transtibial technique appeared (Rosenberg & Deffner, 1997; Chen et al., 2003). This was an easy and quick way to reconstruct the ACL which became soon adopted by most surgeons. However, the outcome was not always as good as expected (Freedman et al.,2003, Lewis et al., 2008) and with the re-discovery of the ACL anatomy and biomechanics, deep changes have been introduced in the way to reconstruct the ACL. This chapter reviews the main features related to ACL reconstruction and focus on the current state of the art in this field

2. ACL anatomy

The reader will find all the necessary details in the numerous articles which have been recently published in this field (Colombet et al.,2006; Edwards et al., 2006; Giron et al. 2006; Harner et al.,1999; Mochizuki et al., 2007; Petersen & Zantop, 2007; Purnell et al.,2008; Takahashi et al., 2006; Zantop et al., 2006,). We will summarize the main relevant points for surgical reconstruction of the ACL.
The ACL consists of at least two functional bundles, anteromedial (AMB) and posterolateral (PLB). The AMB is about twice long and big as compared to the PLB. The AM bundle is more sagitally oriented, limiting the anterior tibial translation while the more oblique PLB (Fig 1), limits the internal rotation of the tibia (Zantop et al.,2007).
Both bundles are parallel in full knee extension and, due to the location of their attachments, they cross each other when the knee bends. During knee flexion, the PLB shortens by more than 30%, while the AMB elongates by 15%. The PLB is tight when the knee is close to extension whereas the AMB is tensed when the knee bends. The range of length variation for the AMB varies between 1-3mm while the PLB exhibits a much widerrange, 4-7mm. In order to reproduce the ACL anatomy several studies have assessed and quantify the footprints.

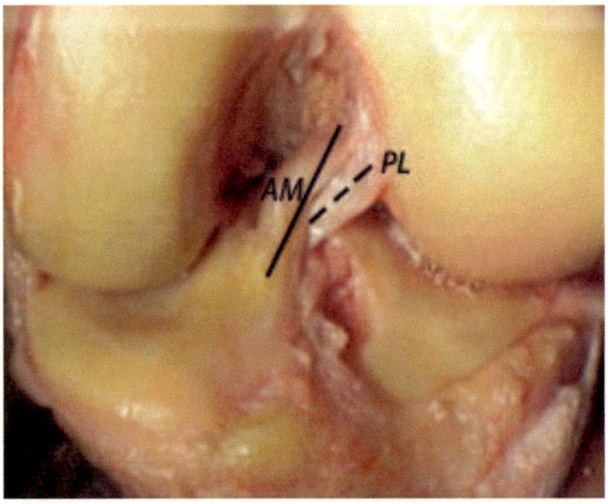

Fig. 1. ACL bundles. Solid line: anteromedial bundle (AM), dotted line; posterolateral bundle (PL)

2.1 ACL femoral foot print

In Western subjects, the length of the foot print is 18.3mm ± 2.3mm, the width 10.3mm ± 2.7mm (Colombet et al., 2006). The distance between the bundle centers is 8.2mm ± 1.2mm. In anatomic position, the most anterior fibers of the foot print are located behind the lateral intercondylar ridge (Fu & Jordan, 2007). There are no ACL fibers located in front of the lateral intercondylar ridge (Fig. 2). The most posterior fibers are located at 2-3mm from the lateral femoral condyle articular cartilage limit, following its curvature. The bifurcate ridge, perpendicular to the lateral intercondylar ridge separates the AMB from the PLB attachment.

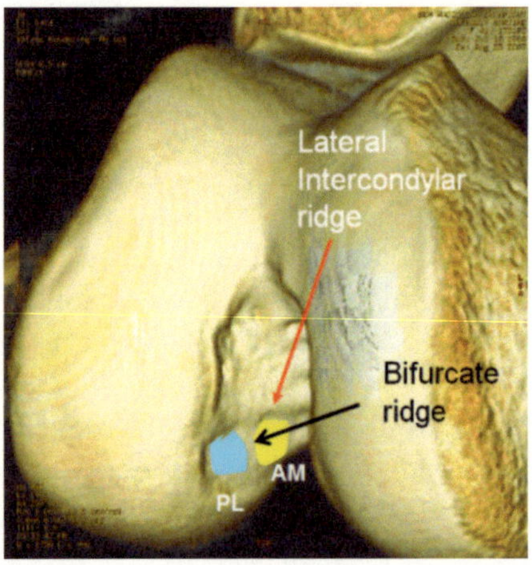

Fig. 2. Three-dimensional CT view of the intercondylar notch in "endoscopic" position (femoral shaft horizontal). The ACL bundle attachment sites are shown in relation with the lateral intercondylar- and the bifurcate ridges.

On a lateral X-ray it is possible to locate the lateral intercondylar ridge (Farrow et al, 2008). When the femur is in the endoscopic position, i.e. horizontal, the ridge originates at the posterior part of the Blumensaat's line (80% from anterior) and the mean Blumensaat's-ridge angle is 75.5°. In this position, the whole ACL femoral footprint becomes posterior to the ridge. The center of the femoral bundles can be also located using the quadrants method described by Bernard et al (Bernard et al, 1997). The position of the centers is illustrated on Fig. 3.

2.2 Tibial footprint

It is larger than on the femoral side with a 17.6mm ± 2.1mm length and 12.7mm ± 2.8mm witdth. The distance between the bundle centers is 8.4 mm ± 0.4mm (Colombet et al., 2006). The most anterior point of the tibial footprint is located right behind the posterior edge of the anterior inter-meniscal ligament. The most posterior fibers of the footprint are located at 10.3mm ± 1.9mm in front of the retro eminence ridge which corresponds to the ridge limiting the anterior attachment of the posterior cruciate ligament on the tibia. The center of the ACL tibial footprint is thus located 20-22mm in front of the PCL attachment. The distribution and the surface area of the bundle attachments is variable (Colombet et al., 2006; Edwards et al., 2007) and there is no visible ridge separating the bundles as on the femoral side.

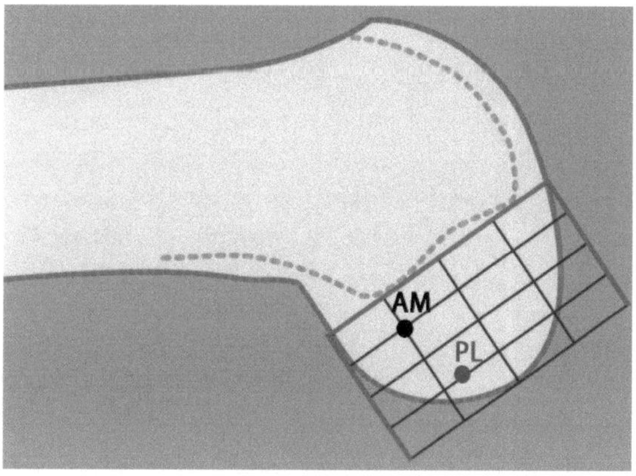

Fig. 3. Location of the femoral bundle centers according to the quadrant's method of Bernard.

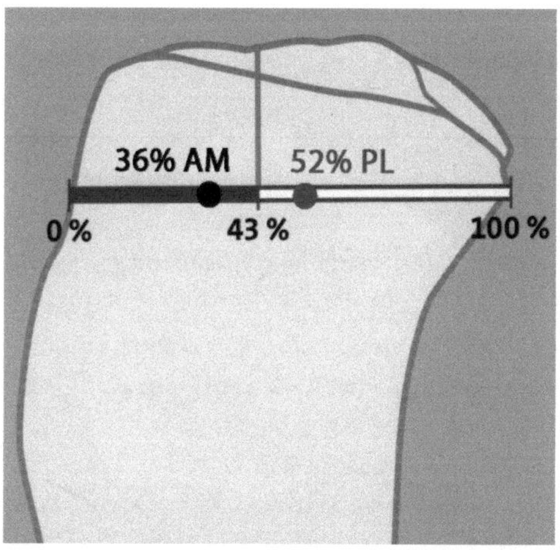

Fig. 4. Position of the tibial bundle centers projected on the Staubli & Rauschning line. The center of the ACL is located at 43% of the AP diameter

On lateral X rays it is possible to locate the various centers of the tibial ACL foot print. Using the Stäubli and Rauschning technique (Fig. 4), the footprint center is located at 43 % of the antero-posterior diameter of the tibia (Stäubli & Rauschning, 1994) while the center of the AMB is located at 36% and the center of the PLB at 52% (Colombet et al., 2006).

3. Graft selection

3.1 Autografts

Contrary to a common belief, the bone-patellar-tendon-bone (BPTB) remains the most frequently used autograft (Shelton and Fagan, 2011), but hamstring and quadriceps tendon grafts are common alternative.

Graft type	Anterior knee pain	Anterior knee Numb-ness	Failure rate	Knee Tight-ness	Residual Weak-ness	Exten-sion deficit	Patient Satis-faction
BPTB	High	High	Low	High	Quadri-ceps muscle	High	High
Ham-string	Low	Low	Slightly Higher	Slightly lower	Ham-strings	Low	High
Quadri-ceps	Low	Low	Low	High	Quadri-ceps mucle	Low	High

Table 1. This table summarizes the factors to be considered in ACL autograft selection (from Shelton and Fagan, 2011).

All three graft types exhibit strength values above 2,000 N.

3.1.1 BPTB autograft, which has two bone plugs at each of its extremities, affords the most secure fixation, a low failure rate and high rate of patient satisfaction. This is the graft of choice among team physicians dealing with high level professional athletes (Pandarinath et al., 2011). However, it is associated with increased anterior knee pain and numbness with a greater incidence of extension loss and long term osteoarthritis of the knee. Residual anterior knee pain can be decreased by filling the bony defects of the harvesting sites, and numbness can be prevented by saving the infrapatellar branch of the saphenous nerve during harvesting.

3.1.2 Hamstring grafts are associated with less harvesting morbidity than BPTB, however, they exhibit a slighter degree of laxity, especially in females. Their harvesting weakens flexion strength of the knee and may account in the reported incidence of graft failure. They are usually fashioned in a quadrupled stranded graft using both gracilis and semitendinosus tendons.

3.1.3 Quadriceps tendon has a low incidence of anterior knee pain and almost no residual numbness. It can be fashioned with or without bone plug. After harvesting, quadriceps deficit is temporary. Clinical outcome is excellent with residual laxity similar to BTB both in males and females, without extension deficit. For many, this is the graft of choice for ACL revision or posterior cruciate ligament reconstruction.

Most studies which have reported results of ACL reconstruction show no significant difference in residual anterior laxity, functional results and International Knee Documentation Committee (IKDC) scores regardless the autograft which is used (Aune et al., 2001; Beynnon et al., 2002; Freedman et al., 2003; Maletis et al., 2007; Yunes et al., 2001)

3.2 Allografts

Allografts avoid harvesting tendons with their drawbacks, i.e anterior knee pain or numbness. In countries where legal issues are important, especially the United States (USA), allografts became the graft of choice for ACL reconstruction.

3.2.1 Currently, three kinds of allografts are available: chemically treated, irradiated and/or fresh frozen. Due to their poor mechanical properties, chemically treated or irradiated allografts are gradually abandoned (Krych et al., 2008). Currently, fresh frozen allografts are the most widely used. Tissue banks insure the proper donor selection as well as bacterial and viral screening. With the current infection control protocols, the incidence of viral or bacterial contamination is null. Graft quality is an issue and donor age must be known. Thus the choice of the tissue bank is critical.

3.2.2 Fresh frozen tibialis anterior or posterior tendons, Achilles' tendon with bone plug and BPTB are the most widely used. The outcome is similar to autografts (Foster et al., 2010) however, allografts have significantly lower normal stability rates than autografts (Bach et al.,2005; Prodromos et al., 2007).

Most of the US authors do not recommend the use of allografts in young and high demanding athletes. Also the use of allografts add a significant cost to the procedure (c.a. $ 3,000 in the USA). Thus, for the authors, the use of allografts which lead to inferior results compared to autografts at an increased cost remains questionable

4. Graft fixation issues

4.1 Composite grafts with bone plugs are commonly fixed in the tunnels either with absorbable or metal interference screws.. This method provides the highest strength and rigidity. However there is concern that a too rigid construct may alter the full range of knee motion and some surgeons prefer suspensory fixation with sutures tied on post or buttons or buttons with build in tissue loops. Soft tissue grafts fixation relies on numerous different methods: interference screws, suspensory devices, cross pins. On the femoral side suspensory devices with build in tissue loop, like the Endobutton® Continuous Loop provides the strongest and stiffest fixation. With hamstring grafts, graft slippage at the tibial fixation site may occur explaining the slight increase in laxity compared to BTB.

4.2 Tunnel enlargement

Following ACL reconstruction, tunnel enlargement occurs regardless the graft choice and the fixation system (L'Insalata et al., 1997). This is an early phenomenon which occurs during the first-three post operative months. Biomechanical (bungee cord and wiper windshield effects) as well as biological factors (local cytokine release) may account for this enlargement (Wilson et al., 2004). Until now, one important factor might have been underestimated: the graft positioning. With anatomic placement of the ACL grafts tunnel enlargement is less (Chhabra et al., 2006).

5. The evolution of ACL reconstruction

Before the early 1990's most of the ACL reconstruction were performed through medial arthrotomy which became with time mini arthrotomy. However, arthroscopic reconstruction (Paulos et al., 1991) undergone rapid development. Although achievement of stability has been well-documented in open ACL reconstructive procedures, it quickly appeared arthroscopically assisted ACL reconstruction offered significantly diminished morbidity, and more predictable rehabilitation after surgery. Improvements in instrumentation allowed refining the precision of the technique.

5.1 The transtibial technique

Rosenberg is the surgeon who introduced the transtibial technique for ACL reconstruction (Rosenberg & Deffner, 1997; Rosenberg & Brown, 1997; Chen et al., 2003). We will briefly summarize the technique. In a first step, regardless the nature of the graft, a specific tibial drill guide is used to insert a 2.4mm guide wire in the foot of the ACL tibial footprint. In the sagittal plane, a 55° angle orientation with regard to the plane of the tibial plateau is recommended (Fig. 5A). In the coronal plane the guide wire is inserted 1.5cm medial to the tibial tubercle (Fig. 5B), above the pes anserinus tendons, and oriented at 25° with regard to the tibial axis (75° with regard to the tibial plateau surface). The guide wire is then used to guide a cannulated drill bit which diameter corresponds to the graft diameter (Fig.5C).

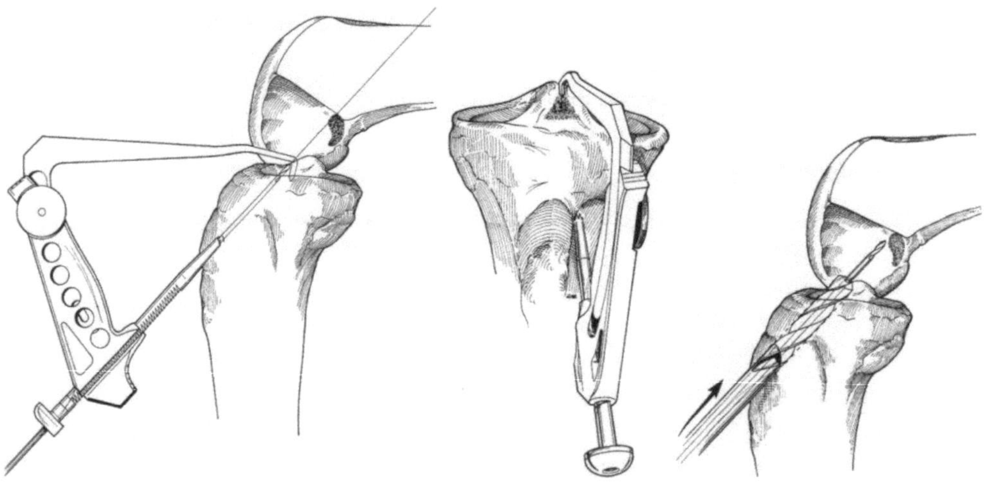

A B C

Fig. 5. Transtibial technique, tibial steps. A: insertion of the tibial guide wire at 55 degree inclination with regard to the tibial plateau plane. B: the starting point of the guide wire is just medial to the tibial tubercle. C: a cannulated drill, which size corresponds to the graft diameter is passed on the guide wire. The knee is maintained at 90 degree of flexion.

In a second step, with the knee bent at 90° of flexion, a femoral guide is introduced through the tibial tunnel inside the intercondylar notch region. The femoral guide has a hook at its intra articular tip which offset (3-9mm) is chosen according to the size of the knee and where the surgeon decides to drill the femoral tunnel in relation with the ACL femoral footprint

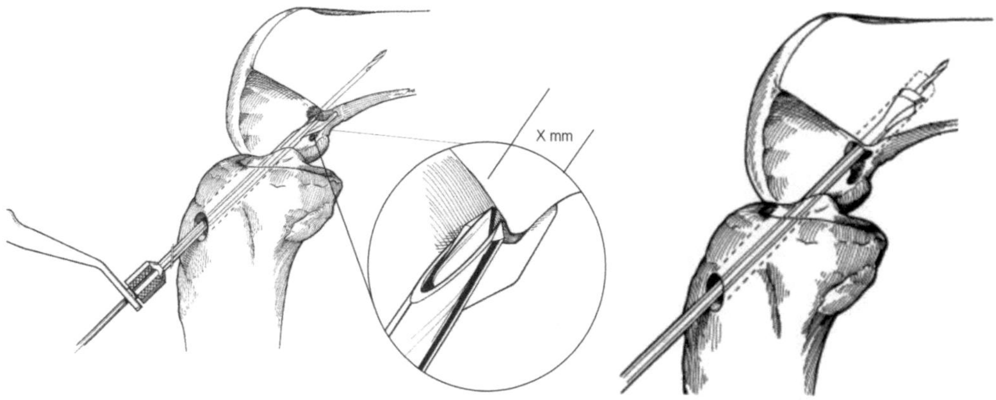

A B

Fig. 6. Transtibial technique, femoral steps. A: An endofemoral guide wire is introduced through the tibial tunnel. The knee remains bent at 90 degree. The hook located at the proximal tip has variable offset with regard to the shaft of the aimer (X mm). An eyelet needle is drilled through the lateral femoral condyle. This drawing perfectly illustrates the fact one can't reach the center of the ACL femoral footprint with the transtibial technique. B: An endoscopic cannulated drill is passed on the on the guide wire drilling a femoral socket at the desired depth. During drilling, the tibial tunnel is widened by the drill.

(Fig. 6). A long guide wire with an eyelet is inserted with the help of the femoral guide, through the lateral femoral condyle, breaching the lateral cortex until it passes through the skin of the lateral side of the thigh. The femoral guide is removed keeping the guide wire in the condyle. Then, maintaining the knee at 90° of flexion, a cannulated endoscopic drill, which head is the cutting part and the shaft smaller, is threaded on the guide wire through the tibial tunnel, the intercondylar notch, the lateral femoral condyle at a depth which depends on graft type and fixation type. The diameter of the endoscopic drill is chosen according to the graft diameter. The eyelet of the guide wire is used to pull a loop suture through the tibial tunnel, the intercondylar notch and the tibial tunnel exiting on the lateral side of the thigh. The loop stitch is use do pull the graft until it settles in the femoral tunnel and fixed appropriately either with an interference screw, an Endobutton or with cross pins. Then the graft is put under Manual tension; the knee is cycled from full extension to full flexion at least 20 times. The length variation of the graft at the exit of the tibial tunnel is measured and the graft fixed in the tibia either with an interference screw or using extra cortical fixation: button or screw post and washer. The knee flexion at fixation depends on the graft length variation: the larger is the length variation, closer to extension the fixation must be done in order to avoid extension deficit.
As the reader will notice the "clock-face" reference do determine the tunnel position is not used in this chapter. Although this reference has been widely accepted in the literature to describe femoral tunnel positioning it has generated more confusion than clarification (Fu, 2008; Van Eck et al., 2010). The "clock-face" system is based on radiographs of the knee in extension while ACL reconstruction is performed at 90 degree of flexion or more. Therefore

the orientation of the clock face is no longer valid as the ACL femoral insertion site moves from vertical to horizontal when the knee bends. Furthermore the intercondylar notch is a 3-dimensional structure while the clock-face refers to a 2-diemnsional structure which is neglectful of the depth of the notch.

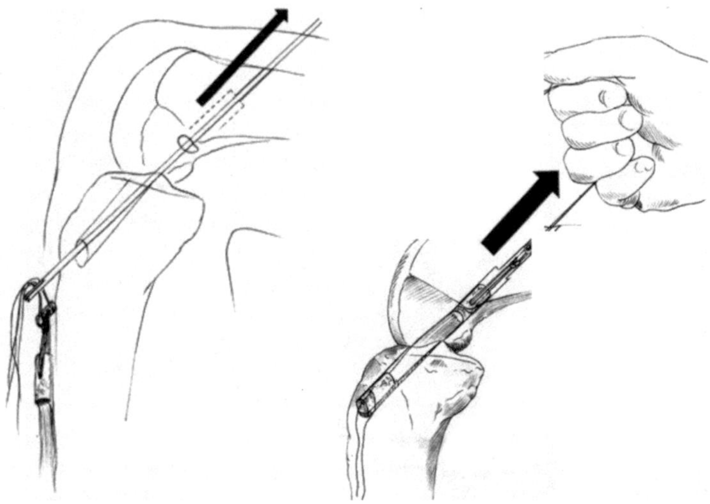

A B

Fig. 7. Passing the graft. A: the leading stiches of the graft are first pulled through the tibial and femoral tunnel with the help of the eyelet guide wire. B: the graft is then pulled through the tunnels until it fills the femoral tunnel.

As the whole reconstruction procedure is performed through a small tibial incision which is used for harvesting and drilling, the transtibial technique is also called "one-incision" technique. Alternatively, "two-incision" technique has been developed. With this technique a lateral thigh incision is performed in order to settle, behind the lateral femoral condyle, a rear entry femoral guide, which position is arthroscopically controlled. The guide wire and the tunnel drilling are then performed from outside in. With the "two-incision" technique, the position of the femoral guide wire is independent from the tibial tunnel. However, due to the lateral thigh incision and its associated morbidity, the "two-incision" technique has never known a large development. On the contrary, the one-incision technique has quickly spread worldwide. With appropriate instruments "one-incision"ACL reconstruction with quadrupled hamstring tendons can be performed in less than 30 minutes in skilful hands.

5.2 Outcome of transtibial ACL reconstruction

5.2.1 Systematic review

There are many articles which address the outcome of single bundle transtibial reconstruction. We will summarize one of the most recent systematic review of single-bundle ACL reconstruction outcomes by Lewis et al. (Lewis et al.,2008). The authors reported a systematic review of 11 randomized, controlled trials comparing patellar tendon and hamstring tendon grafting. The respective outcomes of each group were combined to assist the orthopaedic surgeon in assessing the current success of single-bundle reconstruction. The primary factors assessed were tibial subluxation and side-to-side differences in laxity. Secondary outcomes included concomitant injuries and treatments, complications, graft failure, range of motion, and radiographic evidence of degenerative changes. In this review of 1024 single-bundle anterior cruciate ligament reconstructions, including HS and BTPB autografts, 495 concomitant meniscal tears, 95 chondral injuries, and 2 posterior cruciate ligament tears were noted. The complication rate was 6%, and graft failure 4%. Reported pivot-shift test results were negative in 81% of cases; reported Lachman tests were negative in 59% cases; and KT-1000 arthrometer side-to-side differences were ≤ 5 mm in 86% of cases. Flexion and extension deficits were reported in 9 of 11 studies through mean range of motion or deficit ranges. Radiographic changes of articular surface were observed in 7% of the knees at follow-up. The authors concluded this systematic review of a significant body of unbiased outcome data on single-bundle ACL reconstruction demonstrates it to be a safe, consistent surgical procedure affording reliable results. On the other hand, there was still 19%persisting positive pivot shift tests (5-32%), 41% positive Lachman tests (14-76%), and 29% KT1000 side-to-side difference ≥ 3mm (10- 54%). It appears the range of the values is quite variable from one publication to another. This is related to subjective bias when evaluating the patients. If one considers the persistence of a positive pivot shift test as a criterion for anatomic failure, single bundle transtibial ACL reconstruction has failed to restore a normal knee kinematic in 5 to 32% of the cases. The KT1000 arthrometer, which is certainly the most objective test method, showed almost 30% of anatomical failures. Accordingly one may questions the validity of single bundle transtibial ACL reconstruction which lead to 30% of anatomic failures.

5.2.2 Factors influencing the outcome

Regardless the graft types (allograft vs autograft), graft source (bone patellar tendon bone, hamstring or Achilles tendon), some significant factors influence the outcome (Kowalchuk et al., 2009) of single bundle reconstruction: lower patient-reported outcome is strongly associated with obesity (BMI>30), smoking, meniscectomy and severe chondrosis at time of surgery. Also, a more vertical orientation of the graft influences the occurrence of a residual pivot shift test (Pinczewski et al., 2008).

In the long term range, following BPTB, good results are maintained at 15 years after surgery with respect to ligamentous stability, subjective outcomes, and range of motion while kneeling pain remains a significant problem. Concern remains regarding the incidence of further anterior cruciate ligament injury (24% sustained contralateral ACL ruptures, and 8% ruptured the graft). Graft rupture was associated with a graft inclination angle <17°. Contralateral anterior cruciate ligament rupture was associated with age<18 years at time of primary injury. There is increasing number of patients (51%) with radiographic and clinical signs of osteoarthritis despite surgical stabilization (Hui et al., 2011). The joint degeneration seems to be more frequently met after BPTB graft than after HS grafts.

6. The move toward anatomy

Several surgeons, who early recognized the need to further improve the outcome of ACL reconstruction, moved towards a more anatomic way to reconstruct the ACL. This was mostly based on the drawbacks of the transtibial technique

- When the tibial tunnel was drilled through the tibial ACL footprint, the resulting femoral tunnel is too high in the notch (Fig. 8) inducing an impingement with the anterior part of the intercondylar notch leading to the necessity to widen the notch during surgery to avoid the impingement (notch plasty).
- It became obvious the femoral tunnel could not be drilled through the ACL footprint using the transtibial technique (Arnold et al., 2001; Gougoulias et al., 2008; Heming et al., 2007; Kaseta et al., 2008). In order to overcome this issue Howell proposed to shift the tibial tunnel posteriorly in order to reach, at least partially, the ACL femoral footprint and also avoid impingement with the roof of the intercondylar notch (Howell& Clark, 1992; Howell, 1998; Howell et al. 2001). However, this resulted in a vertical graft placement (posterior on the tibia and high in the notch) which was able to control the anterior tibial translation but not the tibial rotation. This explains the high rate of residual positive pivot shift. Many clinical and experimental studies have supported this issue (Boden et al., 1996; Herbort et al., 2010; Jepsen et al., 2007; Khalfayan et al., 1996; Lee et al., 2007; Markolf et al., 2002; Muneta et al., 1995; Mushal et al., 2005; Ristanis et al., 2003; Rue et al., 2008; Sommer et al., 2000; Scopp et al., 2004).
- However, contrary to all the studies which have demonstrated the influence of the femoral tunnel aperture location and orientation on the knee stability, tibial tunnel position has fewer influence on knee laxity (Morgan et al., 1995; Romano et al., 1993).

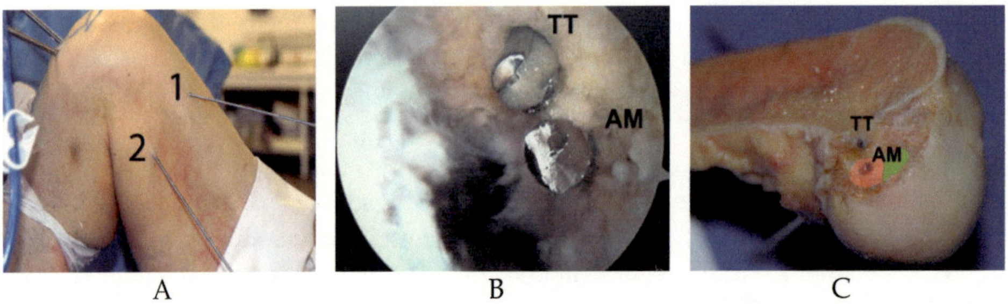

Fig. 8. Position of the femoral guide wire inserted eiher transtibial or transportal in cadaver. All the three illustrations are from the same right knee. A: 1 transtibial guide wire inserted at 90 degree of flexion, 2 transportal guide wire inserted at 110 degree of knee flexion. B: intra-articular visualization of the guide wires from the medial side (TT transtibial, AM transportal). C: The medial femoral condyle has been removed. The TT guide wire is located in the roof of the intercondylar notch out of the ACL foot print. The AM guide wire is right in the center of the AMB attachment sire (pink). The PL footprint is colored in green.

7. Transportal technique

Drilling the femoral tunnel through an anteromedial (AM) portal has been described early on (Clancy, 1985; Cain & Clancy, 2002; Deehan & Pinczewski, 2002). These authors recognized the best and easiest way to reach the femoral ACL footprint was to drill through an AM portal. Transportal technique allows positioning the femoral tunnel lower in the notch, where the ACL is attached, with a more horizontal tunnel, offering in addition to the tibial translation control a better rotational control compared to the transtibial technique (Alentorn-Geli et al., 2009; Bedi et al., 2010; Bedi et al., 2011; Bottoni, 2008; Dargel et al., 2009; Gavriilidis et al., 2008; Loh et al.,2003; Rue et al., 2008; Sohn & Garrett, 2009; Zantop et al., 2008). Also, drilling the femoral tunnel through an AM portal allows obtaining tunnel aperture which overlaps with the native ACL footprint, while drilling through the tibial tunnel hardly covers part of the AM footprint (Abebe et al., 2009). Modifying the tibial tunnel orientation to overcome this issue has been proposed (Chhabra et al., 2004; Heming et al., 2007; Kopf et al., 2010; Miller et al., 2010). When drilling a more horizontal tunnel, and starting more medial it becomes possible to target the native ACL footprint. However, the resulting tunnel becomes very short, with a quite oval intra-articular tunnel aperture, putting the medial tibial plateau at risk for fracture, rising concerns for tibial graft fixation, and compromising graft stability at the tunnel aperture. Nevertheless, transportal drilling technique has pearls and pitfalls which have been described in the literature (Basdekis et al., 2008; Harner et al., 2008; Lubowitz, 2009; Zantop et al., 2008).

7.1 Portals

The location of the instrumental anteromedial (AM) portal, also called accessory AM- or far medial portal is critical (Fig. 9). The best way to locate it is to use a spinal needle, keeping the scope through the anterolateral (AL) portal in order to optimize its placement under direct vision. The needle must sit above the anterior segment of the medial meniscus, far enough from the medial femoral condyle not to damage the cartilage when using endoscopic drills. Single fluted endoscopic drills reduce the risk for cartilage damages. If the portal is close to the patellar tendon the drill will be oriented at sharp angle with regard to the lateral wall of the intercondylar notch resulting in an oval femoral tunnel aperture. If the portal is more medial, the orientation of the drill will result in a more circular aperture.

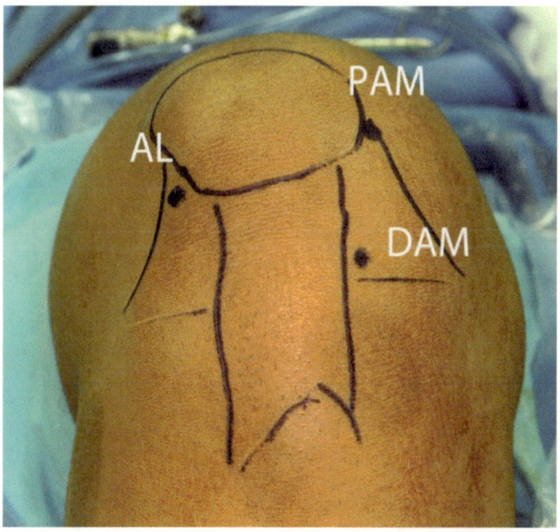

Fig. 9. Portal location for transportal drilling technique. Anterolateral portal (AL) is high in the soft spot above the fat pad. Proximal anteromedial portal (PAM) is located at the junction betwwen the patella and the medial femoral condyle. Distal anteromedial (DAM) portal is located above the anterior segment of the medial meniscus

7.2 Drilling

During drilling, the knee must be bent at least at 110 degree of flexion in order to avoid blowing up the posterior wall of the lateral femoral condyle (Fig. 10). The more the knee is bent the longer is the femoral tunnel (Basdekis et al., 2008). It might be necessary to resect part of the fat pad in order to obtain an appropriate vision of the lateral wall of the notch. Keeping the scope through the AL portal provides a tangential view of the lateral wall of the notch and the ACL footprint. So, in order to insure a good visualization of the footprint it is better to view the notch from the medial side of the knee. Placing the scope through a proximal AM portal and the instruments through an accessory AM portal is also called three-portal technique (Cohen & Fu, 2007) as it combines one AL portal with 2 AM portals. Watching the lateral wall of the intercondylar notch from medial provides a full view of the ACL foot print from the anterior cartilage margin to the posterolateral outlet and allows precise visualization of the lateral intercondylar ridge.

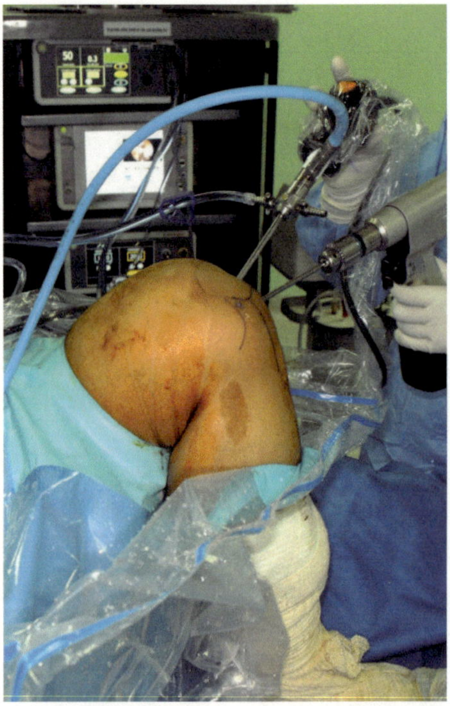

Fig. 10. Drilling the femoral tunnel transportal. The knee is bent at least at 110 degree of flexion. The scope is through the PAM portal and the drill through the DAM portal (Right knee).

7.3 Transportal drilling limitations

- intra-articular visualization of the notch may be restricted so that the surgeon must be confident with the arthroscope and eventually needs to remove soft tissues around the notch
- cross-pin graft fixation techniques require guide instruments that are designed for transtibial insertion only
- As the femoral tunnel is more horizontal when drilled through an AM portal, the graft – tunnel angulation may increase resulting in higher contact pressures at the anterior aspect of the graft with full extension and might cause bone tunnel enlargement.

However, Chhabra et al (Chhabra et al., 2006) comparing transtibial femoral tunnel expansion vs AM drilling found significantly less enlargement with the transportal technique

8. Development of anatomic double-bundle ACL reconstruction

Anatomic ACL reconstruction is defined as the functional restoration of the ACL to its native dimensions, collagen orientation, and insertion sites (Van Eck et al., 2010). The concept and development of double-bundle ACL reconstruction comes from the rediscovery of the ACL bundles anatomy and biomechanics of ACL reconstruction. Several studies have shown that rotational control of the tibia as well as anterior tibial translation were much improved when the PLB was reconstructed in addition to the AMB (Colombet et al., 2007; Kanaya et al., 2009; Markolf et al., 2009; Sbihi et al., 2004; Yagi et al., 2002; Zaffagnini et al., 2008; Zantop et al., 2007).

Already in his original transtibial technique, T Rosenberg was mentioning the possibility to reconstruct 2 bundles, if the femoral footprint size was big enough, by drilling 2 sockets in the femur and one tunnel in the tibia. This idea was further developed in Japan (Hara et al., 2000; Hamada et al., 2001; Mae et al., 2001;Munetta et al., 1999), then in France (Franceschi et al, 2002; Bellier et al., 2004) and finally in the USA. While few authors persisted in the use of transtibial technique (Yasuda et al., 2004), it appeared rapidly to most surgeons that double bundle ACL reconstruction which necessitates drilling 2 femoral sockets and 2 tibial tunnels could be only performed either with transportal technique or two-incision technique.

8.1 Following is a brief summary of the principles of anatomic double-bundle ACL reconstruction technique. We will describe transportal technique with four tunnels, which is the most widely used. Few surgeons are using alternative techniques like two-incision- (Aglietti et al., 2005) or modified transtibial technique (Yasuda et al., 2004). Most of the authors use autogenous hamstring tendons. Usually the AMB is reconstructed with a double-stranded semitendinosus tendon, while the gracilis is used for the PLB. According to their size or length, tendons can be doubled, tripled or even quadruple-stranded. Allografts are used mostly in the USA. In Western patients, with autogenous hamstrings, the average AMB diameter is 7mm (6-9mm) and PLB 6mm (5-7mm). Most of the authors use Endobutton® CL for the femoral fixation. Others are using interference screws. On the tibial side, various fixation methods have be described: interference screws, plate and screw, screw post and washer. As femoral tunnels are drilled independently one may start either by drilling tibial- or femoral tunnels.

8.1.1 Femoral tunnels

The femoral footprint is visualized through an AM portal and carefully identified according to the landmarks previously described (Cha et al., 2005). Identifying the intercondylar ridge is a key issue and fluoroscopy may help. Through an accessory AM portal two sockets are drilled through the center of each bundle attachment with the knee bent at least at 110° of flexion (Basdekis et al., 2008; Basdekis et al., 2009; Hoshino et al., 2009). Specific instruments allow proper positioning of the tunnels, keeping a 2-3 mm bone bridge (Fig. 11) between them in order to insure independent fixation of each bundle (Bellier et al., 2004; Christel et al., 2005; Christel et al., 2008 a-c). Three-dimensional CT studies (Fig 12 A) have validated the accuracy of the instruments (Basdekis et al., 2009a). The resulting cortical bone bridge separating the tunnel apertures remains stable with time (Hantes et al., 2010). When the knee is at 90° of flexion, PLB tunnel is located in front and lower compared to AMB tunnel. The axis going through the center of both tunnels should make a 30° angle with the long axis of the femur.

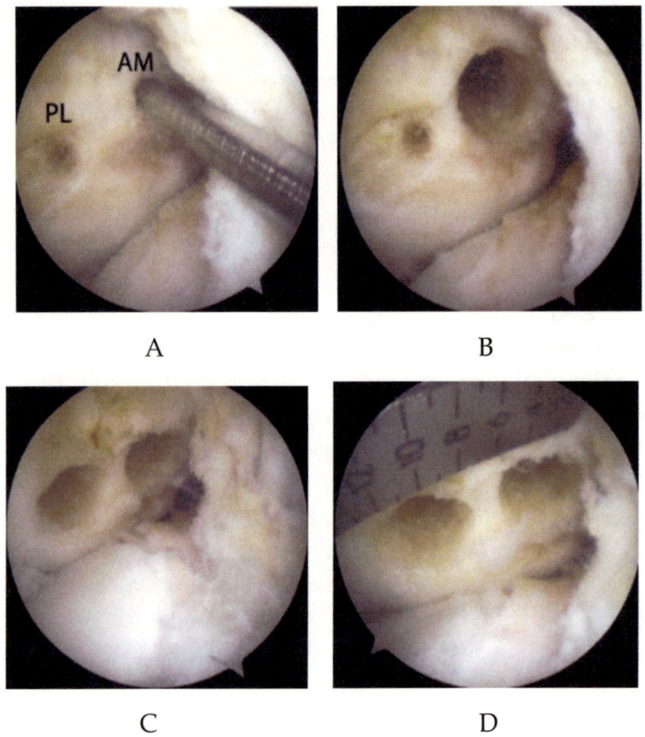

Fig. 11. Double bundle ACL reconstruction, left knee, drilling of the femoral sockets. The lateral wall of the intercondylar notch is viewed from medial. A: the centers of both bundles are marked. A guide wire is inserted through the center of the AMB, knee bent at 110 degree. B: the AM socket is drilled at a diameter equal to the bundle graft. C: both sockets are drilled, knee views from medial at 90 degree of flexion. D: there is a 2mm bone bridge between the 2 sockets.

8.1.2 On the tibial side, the AMB tunnel starts along the medial side of the tibial tubercle and opens in the center of the AMB footprint. The PLB tunnel starts more medially, in front of the anterior edge of the medial collateral ligament. Specific instrumentation allows drilling the PLB tunnel through the center of the PLB footprint, 8-9mm behind and slightly lateral to the AMB aperture, saving a 2-3mm bone bridge between the two tunnels (Christel et al., 2005; Christel et al., 2008 a-c). Three-dimensional CT studies (Fig.12B) have validated the accuracy of the instruments (Saharsrabudhe et al., 2010). The diameters of the tunnels correspond to the graft diameters.

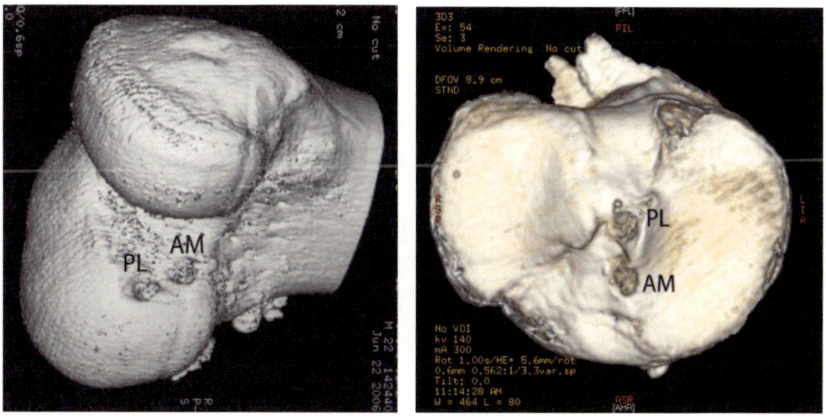

A B

Fig. 12. Three-dimensional CT scan views of the tunnels after double-bundle AC reconstruction. A: femoral sockets, B: intra-articular aperture of the tibial tunnels.

As for single-bundle ACL, several authors have shown tunnel position is highly critical for proper tension and bundles efficacy (Forsythe et al., 2010; Giron et al., 2007, Nishimoto et al., 2009; Silva et al., 2010). Unfortunately most of the publications related to double-bundle ACL reconstruction outcome do not document the position of the tunnels. In order to document tunnel position after surgery, 3-dimensional CT scan is the method of choice (Basdekis et al., 2009a; Forsythe B et al., 2010; Saharsrabudhe et al., 2010). Accordingly, if many publications relate to double-bundle ACL reconstruction, it is hard to distinguish between those which perform anatomical reconstruction, i.e. with tunnels drilled within the ACL footprints, and those with non-anatomical reconstructions where tunnels are drilled outside the ACL footprints.

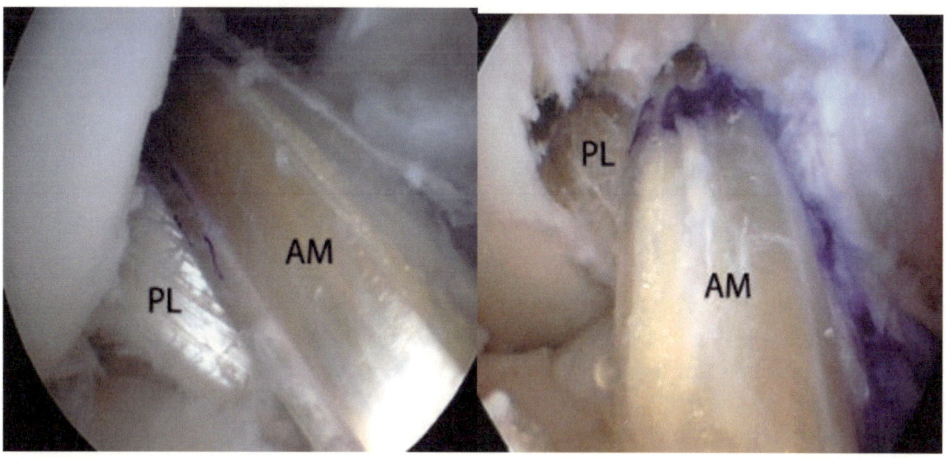

A B

Fig. 13. Intra-articular view of a double bundle ACL graft. The AMB is reconstructed with a double-stranded semitendinosus while the PLB is reconstructed with a double stranded gracilis. A: grafts viewed through the AL portal, B: grafts viewed through an AM portal

8.2 Outcome of anatomic double-bundle ACL reconstruction
8.2.1 Review study

Authors Year of publication	Level of evidence	Technique	N	KT 134 N(mm)	Pivot shift %> glide
Yagi et al, 2007	2	SB AM	20	1.9	35
		SB PL	20	1.7	20
		A2B	20	1.9	15
Aglietti et al, 2007	2	SB	25	2.4	42
		2B transtibial	25	1.6	24
		2B 2-incision	25	1.4	16
Yasuda et al, 2006	2	SB	24	2.8	50
		A 2B	24	1.1	12.5
Jarvela, 2007	1	SB	52	1.8	36
		A2B	25	1.4	3.3
Muneta et al, 2007	1	SB	34	2.4	41.2
		A2B	105	1.4	14.7
Asagumo et al, 2007	3	SB	52	1.9	19.2
		A2B	71	1.7	12.7
Kondo et al, 2008	2	SB	157	2.5	49
		A2B	171	1.2	19
Siebold et al, 2008	1	SB	35	1.6	31.4
		A2B	35	1.0	0.04
Streich et al, 2008	1	SB	25	0.94	25
		A2B	24	1.1	24
Kim et al, 2009	3	SB	28	2.6	11
		A2B	31	1.8	0
Aglietti et al, 2010	1	SB	35	2.1	26
		A2B	35	1.2	14

Table 2. Summary of the main studies comparing the outcome of single-bundle (SB) with anatomic double-bundle (A2B) ACL reconstruction. N is the number of patients in the study groups. Mean KT 1000 arthrometer results are given for a 134N load. Positive pivot shift test corresponds to pivot shift glide or more. All studies have at least a 2-year minimum follow up.

The above table summarizes 15 comparative studies, 6 level 1, 7 level 2, 2 level 3, all with follow up > 2 years and effective follow up, single-bundle 96.2 %, anatomic double-bundle 93.4 %. There is total number of 455 single-bundle patients and, 520 anatomic double-bundle. There is no statistical difference regarding the KT 1000 outcome. However, there is clearly less residual pivot shift after anatomic double-bundle reconstruction (12% vs 33%).

8.2.2 Meta-analysis
Meredick et al. (Meredick et al., 2008) have conducted a meta-analysis where they systematically identified randomized controlled trials (RCTs) comparing single-bundle versus doublebundle ACL reconstruction.

Two outcome measures were reported (in a manner permitting meta-analysis) in at least 3 of 4 trials: KT-1000 arthrometer and pivot-shift testing. On average, KT-1000 arthrometer side-to-side difference was 0.52 mm closer to normal in patients treated with double-bundle reconstruction. This difference is demonstrated to be clinically insignificant. The odds of a normal or nearly normal pivot shift is higher in the patients treated with double-bundle ACL reconstruction than in those treated with single bundle. However, this finding is not statistically significant because the 95% confidence intervals include 0. The authors concluded double-bundle reconstruction does not result in clinically significant differences in KT-1000 arthrometer or pivot shift testing. One may argue the authors grouped together normal and nearly normal knees, while the goal of ACL surgery is to restore a normal knee. When considering the figures of this study and separating normal- from nearly normal knees it appears that following single-bundle (293 patients) 63.5 % of them had no pivot shift while following double bundle (318 patients), 87.7% had no pivot shift ($p<0.001$). In fact all the single-bundle versus double-bundle studies have compared anatomic with non-anatomic reconstructions. Single bundle technique was based on a transtibial approach (with a femoral tunnel almost entirely located outside the ACL footprint) while, double-bundle tunnels were located within the ACL footprints.

9. Anatomic double bundle reconstruction limitations

If one wish to maintain a sufficient graft size (7mm for AMB and 6mm for PLB), small ACL footprints (less than 14mm long) do not allow drilling independent tunnels with a sufficient bone bridge in between. In this case single bundle reconstruction must be used. Also narrow intercondylar notch is a severe limitation as it does not leave enough space for the graft.
The concept of anatomic double bundle ACL reconstruction was further applied to partial tears of the ACL when one bundle only has been ruptured. In these particular cases it has been proposed to reconstruct only the damaged bundle, performing an ACL augmentation (Borbon CA et al., 2011; Serrano-Fernandez JM et al., 2010).

10. The anatomic single bundle ACL reconstruction

Taking into account technical difficulties for drilling 4 independent tunnels with consistent bone bridges and the renewed knowledge of ACL anatomy, anatomic single bundle ACL reconstruction was a logic development. The basis for this technique is to drill the femoral tunnel in the center of the femoral foot print, between the centers of both bundles, behind the intercondylar ridge, in such way that it includes part of both AMB and PLB fibers (Ho et al., 2009; Rue et al., 2008; Shino et al., 2008, Steiner, 2009; van Eck et al., 2011; Yamamoto et al., 2004).

10.1 Technical principles

In order to perform an optimal anatomic single-bundle ACL reconstruction the transportal technique must be used. As stated before, with the lens from the medial side it is easy to identify the femoral ACL stump, the intercondylar ridge and the centers of the AMB and PLB. The center of the anatomic femoral tunnel is located in at mid distance from the bundle centers. It can be drilled right in the middle of the footprint and will contain 50% of AMB fibers and 50% of PLB fibers. I can also be drilled more proximally to contain more AMB fibers or more distally, containing more PLB fibers. However a single tunnel in the middle of the foot print will contain less fiber than 2 tunnels drilled in the center of each bundle attachment. On the tibial side the tunnel is drilled in the center of the ACL foot print, slightly medial. As the femoral tunnel is much lower than with the transtibial technique, the resulting graft has a more oblique orientation and is able to resist anterior tibial translation and tibial internal rotation (Fig. 14).

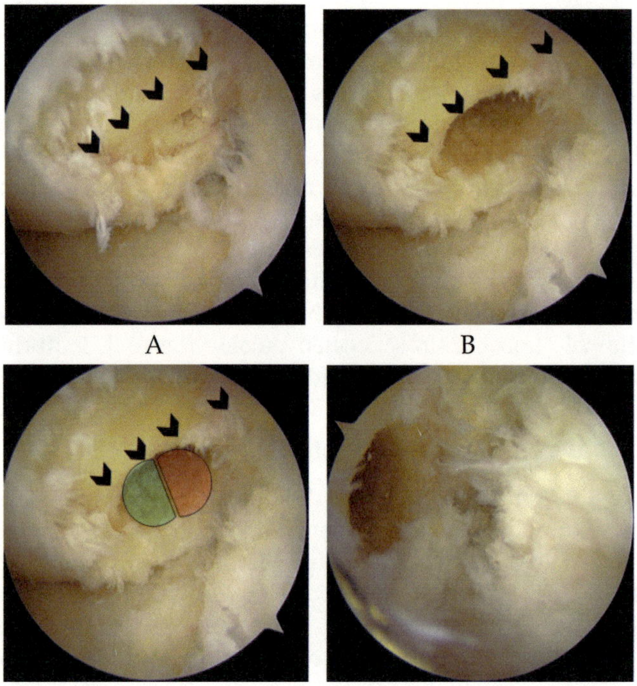

A B

Fig. 13. Femoral socket for single bundle anatomic reconstruction. A: the lateral wall of the intercondylar notch has been gently cleaned with a curette to locate the lateral intercondylar ridge (arrows). B: position of a 9mm socket, right behind the intercondylar ridge. C: the socket aperture is positioned in such a way that it overlaps 50% of the PLB- and 50% of the AMB attachment sites. A,B, and C views are taken from the medial side. D: view of the socket from the AL portal.

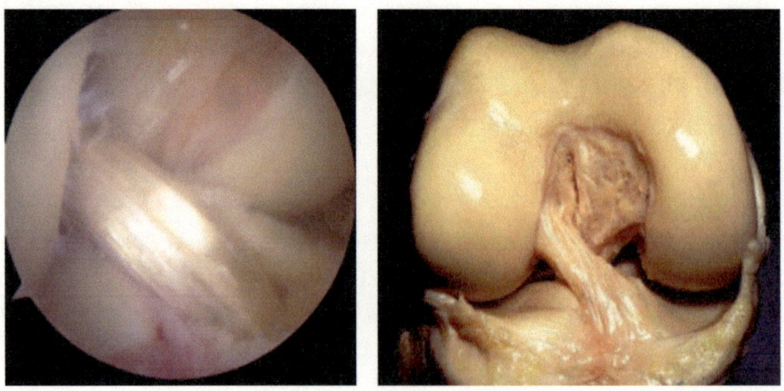

A B

Fig. 14. Comparison of the obliquity of an anatomic single bundle ACL (A) with a native ACL (B). Note the similarity in orientation of both reconstructed and native ACL.

10.2 Outcome of anatomic single-bundle ACL

Currently, only few published papers deal with comparison of the outcome of anatomic single- with anatomic double-bundle (Gobbi et al., 2011; Park et al., 2010; Song et al., 2009). On the clinical stand point these studies show no statistical differences between the objective and subjective outcomes of the two techniques. Thus it seems that reconstructing the ACL with anatomic single-bundle technique is a valid option with improved results compared to single-bundle transtibial. Further publications and longer follow-up should confirm these preliminary results.

11. Conclusion

There is still much to learn about ACL reconstruction. The old transtibial technique which does not reconstruct the ACL where it is attached has progressively evolved toward anatomical ACL reconstruction. Currently anatomic single- and double-bundle ACL reconstruction are well established and well described. However, if the outcome of these techniques has considerably improved with regard to the transtibial technique, the results are still far to be perfect. There are still small percentages of fair results for which improvements have to be made. Only long term results will tell if the restoration of ACL anatomy is going to decrease knee joint degeneration which remains the major issue of long term outcome of ACL reconstruction

12. References

Abebe ES, Moorman III CT, Dziedzic TS, Spritzer CE, Cothran RL, Taylor DC, William E. Garrett WE Jr, DeFrate LE. (2009) Femoral Tunnel Placement During Anterior Cruciate Ligament Reconstruction : An In Vivo Imaging Analysis Comparing Transtibial and 2-Incision Tibial Tunnel -Independent Techniques. *Am J Sports Med,* 37, No.10 (October), pp 1904-1911

Aglietti P, Cuomo P, Giron F, Boerger TO. (2005). Double-bundle anterior cruciate ligament reconstruction: surgical technique. *Operative Techniques in Orthopaedics,* F Fu (Ed), WB Saunders Pub, Philadelphia. Vol 15, No.2 (April), pp 111-115

Aglietti P, Giron F, Cuomo P, Losco M, Mondanelli N. (2007). Single- and doubleincision double-bundle ACL reconstruction. *Clin Orthop Relat Res.* 454, pp 108-113.

Aglietti P, Giron F, Losco M, Cuomo P, Ciardullo A, Mondanelli N. (2010). Comparison between single-and double-bundle anterior cruciate ligament reconstruction: a prospective, randomized, single-blinded clinical trial. *Am J Sports Med,* 38, No.1 (January), pp 25-34.

Alentorn-Geli E, Lajara F, Samitier G, Cugat R (2010) The transtibial versus the anteromedial portal technique in the arthroscopic bone-patellar tendon-bone anterior cruciate ligament reconstruction. *Knee Surg Sports Traumatol Arthrosc.* 18, No. 8 (August), pp 1013-1037.

Arnold MP, Kooloos J, van Kampen A (2001) Single-incision technique misses the anatomical femoral anterior cruciate ligament insertion: a cadaver study. *Knee Surg Sports Traumatol Arthrosc,* 9, pp 194–199

Asagumo H, Kimura M, Kobayashi Y, Taki M, Takagishi K. (2007) Anatomic reconstruction of the anterior cruciate ligament using double-bundle hamstring tendons: surgical techniques, clinical outcomes, and complications. Arthroscopy 23:602–609

Aune AK, Holm I, Risberg MA, Jensen HK, Steen H (2001) Four-strand hamstring tendon autograft compared with patellar tendon-bone autograft for anterior cruciate ligament reconstruction. A randomized study with two-year follow-up. *Am J Sports Med*, 29, pp722–728

Bach BR Jr. Aadalen KJ, Dennis MG. et al.(2005). Primary anterior cruciate ligament reconstruction using fresh-frozen, nonirradiated patellar tendon allograft: Minimum 2-year follow-up. *Am J Sports Med*, 33, pp284-292.

Basdekis G. Abisafi C. Christel P. (2008). Influence of knee flexion angle on femoral tunnel characteristics when drilled through the anteromedial portal during anterior cruciate ligament reconstruction. *Arthroscopy*, 24, pp 459-464.

Basdekis G, Christel P, Anne F. (2009a). Validation of the position of the femoral tunnels in anatomic double-bundle ACL reconstruction with 3-D CT scan. *Knee Surg Sports Traumatol Arthrosc*, 17, pp 1089-1094

Basdekis G, Abisafi C, Christel P. (2009b). The effect of knee flexion angle on the length and orientation of posterolateral femoral tunnel drilled through the anteromedial portal during anatomic double-bundle ACL reconstruction. *Arthroscopy*, 25, pp 1108-111.

Bedi A, Raphael B, Maderazo A, Pavlov H, Williams RJ III. (2010). Transtibial versus anteromedial portal drilling for anterior cruciate ligament reconstruction: A cadaveric study of femoral tunnel length and obliquity. *Arthroscopy*, 26, No 3 (March), pp 342-350.

Bedi A, Musahl V, Steuber V, Kendoff D, Choi D, Allen AA, Pearle AD, Altchek DW. (2011). Transtibial versus anteromedial portal reaming in anterior cruciate ligament reconstruction: An anatomic and biomechanical evaluation of surgical technique. *Arthroscopy*, 27, No 3 (March), pp 380-390

Bellier G, Christel P, Colombet P, Djian P, Franceschi JP, Sbihi A. (2004). Double Stranded Hamstring Graft For Anterior Cruciate Ligament Reconstruction. *Arthroscopy*, 20, pp 890-894

Bernard M, Hertel P, Hornung H, Cierpinski T. (1997). Femoral insertion of the ACL: radiographic quadrant method. *Am J Knee Surg*, 10, pp 14–21

Beynnon BD, Johnson RJ, Fleming BC, Kannus P, Kaplan M, Samani J, Renstrom P (2002) Anterior cruciate ligament replacement: comparison of bone-patellar tendon-bone grafts with two-strand hamstring grafts. A prospective, randomized study. *J Bone Joint Surg Am*, 84A, pp 1503–1513

Boden B, Migaud H, Gougeon F, Debroucker MJ, Duquennoy A. (1996). Effect of graft position on laxity after anterior cruciate ligament reconstruction. Stress radiography in 90 knees 2 to 5 years after autograft. *Acta Orthopaedica Belgica*, 62, pp 2-7

Borbon CA, Mouzopoulos G, Siebold R. (2011). Why perform an ACL augmentation? Knee Surg Sports Traumatol Arthrosc. 17, Jun 9. [Epub ahead of print]

Bottoni CR. (2008). Anterior cruciate ligament femoral tunnel creation by use of anteromedial portal. *Arthroscopy* 24,No. 11 (November), pp 1319 (letter to the editor).

Cain EL Jr, Clancy WG Jr. (2002). Anatomic endoscopic anterior cruciate ligament reconstruction with patella tendon autograft. *Orthop Clin North Am*, 33, No.4, pp 717-725.

Cha PS, Brucker PU, West RV, et al. (2005). Arthroscopic double bundle anterior cruciate ligament reconstruction: An anatomic approach. *Arthroscopy,* 21, pp1275.e1-1275.e8.

Chen L, Cooley V, Rosenberg T. (2003).ACL reconstruction with hamstring tendon. *Orthop Clin North Am,* 34, No. 1 (January), pp 9-18.

Chhabra A, Diduch DR, Blessey PB, Miller MD. (2004). Recreating an acceptable angle of the tibial tunnel in the coronal plane in anterior cruciate ligament reconstruction using external landmarks. *Arthroscopy,* 20, pp 328-330.

Chhabra A, Kline AJ, Nilles KM, Harner CD. (2006).Tunnel expansion after anterior cruciate ligament reconstruction with autogenous hamstrings: A comparison of the medial portal and transtibial techniques. *Arthroscopy,* 22, pp 1107-1112.

Christel P, Franceschi JP, Sbihi A, Colombet P, Djian P, Bellier G. (2005). Anatomic ACL Reconstruction: the French Experience. *Operative Techniques in Orthopaedics,* F Fu (Ed), WB Saunders Pub, Philadelphia. Vol 15, No.2 (April), pp 103-110.

Christel P, Basdekis G, Abisafi C. (2008a). Double-bundle ACL reconstruction technique: France. In: *Current concepts in ACL reconstruction,* Fu FH, Cohen SB, eds. Thorofare, NJ: Slack, pp 275-286.

Christel P, Sahasrabudhe A, Basdekis G. (2008b). Anatomic double-bundle anterior cruciate ligament reconstruction with anatomic aimers. *Arthroscopy,* 24, No. 10 (October), pp 1146-1151

Christel P, Sahasrabudhe A, Basdekis G. (2008c). Double-bundle ACL reconstruction with the Anatomic Director set. *Operative Tech in Sports Med,* 16, pp 131-137

Clancy WG Jr. Intra-articular reconstruction of the anteriorcruciate ligament. *Orthop Clin North Am.* 1985; 16:181 -189.

Cohen SB, Fu FH. (2007). Three-portal technique for anterior cruciate ligament reconstruction: Use of a central medial portal. *Arthroscopy,* 23, No 3 (March), pp 325.e1-325.e4

Colombet P, Robinson J, Christel P, et al. (2006).Morphology of anterior cruciate ligament attachments for anatomic reconstruction: A cadaveric dissection and radiographic study. *Arthroscopy,* 22, pp984-992.

Colombet P, Robinson J, Christel P, Franceschi JP, Djian P. (2007).Using navigation to measure rotation kinematics during ACL reconstruction. *Clin Orthop Relat Res,* 454, (Januray), pp59-65.

Dargel J, Schmidt-Wiethoff R, Fischer S, Mader K, Koebke J, Schneider T. (2009). Femoral bone tunnel placement using the transtibial tunnel or the anteromedial portal in ACL reconstruction: A radiographic evaluation. *Knee Surg Sports Traumatol Arthrosc,* 17, pp 220-227.

Deehan DJ, Pinczewski LA. (2002). Endoscopic anterior cruciate ligament reconstruction using a four strand hamstring tendon construct.J R Coll Surg Edinb. 2002 Feb;47(1):428-36

Edwards A, Bull AM, Amis AA. (2007). The attachments of the anteromedial and posterolateral fibre bundles of the anterior cruciate ligament: Part 1: tibial attachment. *Knee Surg Sports Traumatol Arthrosc.* Dec;15, No.12 (Dec), pp 1414-1421.

Edwards A, Bull AM, Amis AA. (2008).The attachments of the anteromedial and posterolateral fibre bundles of the anterior cruciate ligament. Part 2: Femoral attachment. *Knee Surg Sports Traumatol Arthrosc,* 16, pp 29–36

Farrow LD, Gillespie RJ, Victoroff BN, Cooperman DR. (2008). Radiographic location of the lateral intercondylar ridge its relationship to Blumensaat's line. *Am J Sports Med,* 36, No. 10 (October), pp 2002-2006

Forsythe B, Kopf S, Wong AK, Martins CAQ, Anderst W, Tashman S, Fu FH. (2010). The Location of Femoral and Tibial Tunnels in Anatomic Double-Bundle Anterior Cruciate Ligament Reconstruction Analyzed by Three-Dimensional Computed Tomography Models. *J Bone Joint Surg Am,* 92, pp 1418-1426.

Foster TE, Wolfe BL, Ryan S, Silvestri L, Krall Kaye E. (2010). Does the graft source really matter in the outcome of patients undergoing anterior cruciate ligament reconstruction? : An evaluation of autograft versus allograft reconstruction results: A systematic review *Am J Sports Med,* 38, No.1 (January), pp 189-199.

Franceschi JP, Sbihi A, Champsaur P. (2002). Dual arthroscopic reconstruction of the anterior cruciate ligament using anteromedial and posterolateral bundles. *Rev Chir Orthop,* 88, pp 691-697

Freedman KB, D'Amato MJ, Nedeff DD, Kaz A, Bach BR Jr (2003) Arthroscopic anterior cruciate ligament reconstruction: a metaanalysis comparing patellar tendon and hamstring tendon autografts. *Am J Sports Med,* 31, pp 2–11.

Fu FH, Jordan SS. (2007). The lateral intercondylar ridge- a key to anatomic anterior cruciate ligament reconstruction. *J Bone Joint Surg Am,* 89, pp 2103-2104.

Fu FH. (2008). The clock-face reference: Simple but nonantomic. *Arthroscopy,* 24, 1433, author reply 1434.

Gavriilidis I, Motsis EK, Pakos EE, Georgoulis AD, Mitsionis G, Xenakis TA. (2008). Transtibial versus anteromedial portal of the femoral tunnel in ACL reconstruction: a cadaveric study. *Knee* 15, pp 364–367.

Giron F, Cuomo P, Aglietti P, Bull RJ AM, Amis AA (2006) Femoral attachment of the anterior cruciate ligament. *Knee Surg Sports Traumatol Arthrosc* 1, pp 250–256.

Giron F, Cuomo P, Edwards A, Bull AM, AmisAA, Aglietti P. (2007). Double-bundle "anatomic" anterior cruciate ligament reconstruction: A cadaveric study of tunnel positioning with a transtibial technique. *Arthroscopy,* 23, pp 7-13.

Gobbi A, Mahajan V, Karnatzikos G, Nakamura N. (2011). Single- versus Double-bundle ACL Reconstruction: Is There Any Difference in Stability and Function at 3-year Followup? *Clin Orthop Relat Res.* 469, No.6, On line June 11. [Epub ahead of print]

Gougoulias N, Khanna A, Griffiths D, Maffulli N. (2008). ACL reconstruction: can the transtibial technique achieve optimal tunnel positioning? A radiographic study. *Knee,* 15, pp 486–490.

Hamada M, Shino K, Horibe S, et al. (2001). Single- versus bi-socket anterior cruciate ligament reconstruction using autogenous multiple-stranded hamstring tendons with Endobutton femoral fixation: A prospective study. Arthroscopy, 17, pp 801-807

Hantes ME, Liantsis AK, Basdekis GK, Karantanas AH, Christel P, Malizos KN. (2010) Evaluation of the bone bridge between the bone tunnels after anatomic double-bundle anterior cruciate ligament reconstruction: a multidetector computed tomography study. *Am J Sports Med,* 38, No.8 (August), pp1618-1625.

Hara K, Kubo T, Suginoshita T , et al. (2000). Reconstruction of the anterior cruciate ligament using a double-bundle. *Arthroscopy,* 16, pp 860-864

Harner CD, Baek GH, Vogrin TM, Carlin GJ, Kashiwaguchi S, Woo SL. (1999). Quantitative analysis of human cruciate ligament insertions. *Arthroscopy,* 15,pp741–749

Harner CD, Honkamp NJ, Ranawat AS. (2008). Anteromedial portal technique for creating the anterior cruciate ligament femoral tunnel. *Arthroscopy,* 24, No. 1 (January), pp 113-115.

Heming JF, Rand J, Steiner ME. (2007). Anatomical limitations of transtibial drilling in anterior cruciate ligament reconstruction. *Am J Sports Med,* 35, pp 1708-1715.

Herbort M, Lenschow S, Fu FH, Petersen W, Zantop T. (2010). ACL mismatch reconstructions: influence of different tunnel placement strategies in single-bundle ACL reconstructions on the knee kinematics. *Knee Surg Sports Traumatol Arthrosc,* 18, pp1551–1558

Ho JY, Gardiner A, Shah V, Steiner ME (2010) Equal kinematics between central anatomic single-bundle and double-*bundle Knee Surg Sports Traumatol Arthrosc,* 18, No. 12 (December), pp 1551–1558

Hoshino Y, Nagamune K, Yagi M, Araki D, Nishimoto K, Kubo S, Minoru D, Kurosaka M, Kuroda R. (2009). The effect of intraoperative knee flexion angle on determination of graft location in the anatomic double-bundle anterior cruciate ligament reconstruction. *Knee Surg Sports Traumatol Arthrosc,* 17, No.9 (September), pp 1052–1060

Howell SM. Clark JA. (1992). Tibial tunnel placement in anterior cruciate ligament reconstructions and graft impingement. *Clin Orthop,* 283, pp 187-195.

Howell SM.(1998). Principles for placing the tibial tunnel and avoiding roof impingement during reconstruction of a tom anterior cruciale ligament. *Knee Surg Sports Traumatol Arthrosc,* 6(suppl I), pp S49-S55.

Howell SM. Gittins ME. Gottlieb JE, Traina SM. ZoellnerTM. (2001). The relationship between the angle of the tibial tunnel in the coronal plane and loss of flexion and anterior laxity after anterior cruciate ligament reconsu-uction. *AmJ Sports Med,*29, pp 567-574.

Hui C, Salmon LJ, Kokb A, Maeno S, Linklater J, Pinczewski LA. (2011). Fifteen-Year Outcome of Endoscopic Anterior Cruciate Ligament Reconstruction With Patellar Tendon Autograft for "Isolated" Anterior Cruciate Ligament Tear. Am J Sports Med, 39, No. 1(January), pp 89-97

Jarvela T. (2007). Double-bundle versus single-bundle anterior cruciate ligament reconstruction: a prospective, randomized clinical study. *Knee Surg Sports Traumatol Arthrosc.* 15, pp 500-507.

Jepsen CF, Lundberg-Jensen AK, Faunoe P. (2007). Does the position of the femoral tunnel affect the laxity or clinical outcome of the anterior cruciate ligament reconstructed knee.' A clinical, prospective, randomized, double-blind study. *Arthroscopy,* 23, pp 1326-1333.

Kanaya A, Ochi M, Deie M, Adachi N, Nishimori M, Nakamae A (2009) Intraoperative evaluation of anteroposterior and rotational stabilities in anterior cruciate ligament reconstruction: lower femoral tunnel placed single-bundle versus double-bundle reconstruction. *Knee Surg Sports Traumatol Arthrosc* 17:907–913

Kaseta MK. DeFrate LE. Charnock BL. Sullivan RT. Garrett WE Jr. (2008). Reconstruction technique affects femoral tunnel placement in ACL reconstruction. *Clin Orthop,* 466, pp 1467-1474.

Khalfayan EE, Sharkey PF, Alexander AH, Bruckner JD, Bynum EB. (1996). The relationship between tunnel placement and clinical results after anterior cruciate ligament reconstruction. *Am J Sports Med,* 24, pp 335-341.

Kim SJ, Jo SB, Kumar P, Oh KS. (2009). Comparison of single- and double-bundle anterior cruciate ligament reconstruction using quadriceps tendon-bone autografts. *Arthroscopy,* 25, No. 1 (January), pp:70-77

Kondo E, Yasuda K, Azuma H, Tanabe Y, Yagi T. (2008). Prospective clinical comparisons of anatomic double-bundle versus single-bundle anterior cruciate ligament reconstruction procedures in 328 consecutive patients. Am J Sports Med, Sep;36, No.9 (September), pp1675-1687.

Kopf S, Martin DE, Tashman S, Fu FH. (2010). Effect of tibial drill angles on bone tunnel aperture during anterior cruciate ligament reconstruction. *J Bone Joint Surg Am,* 92,pp 871-881.

Kowalchuk DA, Harner CD, Fu FH, Irrgang JJ.(2009). Prediction of patient-reported outcome after single-bundle ACL reconstruction. *Arthroscopy,* 25, No.5 (May), pp 457–463.

Krych AJ, Jackson JD, Hoskin TL, Dahm DL. (2008). A meta-analysis of patellar tendon autograft versus patellar tendon allograft in anterior cruciate ligament reconstruction. *Arthroscopy,* 24, No. 3 (March), pp 292-298

Lee MC, Seong SC, Lee S, Chang CB, Park YK, Kim CH. (2007). Vertical femoral tunnel placement results in rotational knee laxity after anterior cruciate ligament reconstruction. *Arthroscopy,* 23, pp 771-778.

Lewis PB, Parameswaran AD, Rue JPH, Bach BR Jr. (2008). Systematic review of single-bundle anterior cruciate ligament reconstruction outcomes: a baseline assessment for consideration of double-bundle techniques. *Am J Sports Med,* 36, No.10 (October), pp 2028-2036

L'Insalata JC, Klatt B, Fu FH, Harner CD. (1997). Tunnel expansion following anterior cruciate ligament reconstruction: a comparison of hamstring and patellar tendon autografts. *Knee Surg Sports Traumatol Arthrosc.,* 5, No.4, pp234-238.

Loh JC. Fukuda Y, Tsuda E. Steadman RJ. Fu FH. Woo SL-Y. Knee stability and graft function following anterior cruciale ligament reconstruction: Comparison between 11 o'clock and 10 o'clock femoral tunnel placement: 2002 Richard O'Connor Award paper. *Arihroscopy.* 2003:19:297-304.

Lubowitz JH (2009) Anteromedial portal technique for the anterior cruciate ligament femoral socket: pitfalls and solutions. *Arthroscopy* 25:95–101

Maletis GB, Cameron SL, Tengan JJ, Burchette RJ. (2007). A prospective randomized study of anterior cruciate ligament reconstruction: A comparison of patellar tendon and quadruple-strand semitendinosus/gracilis tendons fixed with bioabsorbable interference screws. *Am J Sports Med,* 35, pp 384-394.

Markolf KL. Hame S. Hunter DM. et al. (2002). Effects of femoral tunnel placement on knee laxity and forces in an anterior cruciate ligament graft. *J Orthop Res,* 20, pp 1016-1024.

Markolf KL, Park S, Jackson SR, McAllister DR. (2009). Anteriorposterior and rotatory stability of single and double-bundle anterior cruciate ligament reconstructions. *J Bone Joint Surg Am,* 91, pp 107-118.

Meredick RB, Vance KJ, Appleby D, Lubowitz JH. (2008). Outcome of single-bundle versus double-bundle reconstruction of the anterior cruciate ligament: A meta-analysis. *Am J. Sports Med,* 36; 1414-1421

Miller MD, Gerdeman AC, Miller CD, Hart JM, Gaskin CM, Golish SR, Clancy WG Jr.(2010). The effects of extra-articular starting point and transtibial femoral drilling on the intra-articular aperture of the tibial tunnel in ACL reconstruction. *Am J Sports Med,* 38, No. 4, pp 707-712

Mochizuki T. Muneta T. Nagase T. Shirasawa S. Akita Kl, Sekiya I. Cadaveric knee observation study for describing anatomic femoral tunnel placement for two-bundle anterior cruciate ligament reconstruction. *Arthroscopy.* 2006:22:356-361,

Morgan CD, Kaiman VR. Graw DM.(1995). Definitive landmarks for reproducible tibial tunnel placement in anterior cruciate ligament reconstruction. *Arthroscopy,* 11, pp 275-288.

Muneta T. Yamamoto H, lshibashi T. Asahina S. Murakami S, Furuya K. (1995). The effects of tibial tunnel placement and roofplasty on reconstructed anterior cruciate ligament. *Arthroscopy,* 1, pp 57-62.

Muneta T, Sekiya I, Yagishita K, et al. (1999). Two-bundle reconstruction of the anterior cruciate ligament using semitendinosus tendon with Endobuttons: Operative technique and preliminary results. *Arthroscopy,* 15, pp 618-624.

Muneta T, Koga H, Mochizuki T, et al. (2007). A prospective randomized study of 4-strand semitendinosus tendon anterior cruciate ligament reconstruction comparing single-bundle and double-bundle techniques. *Arthroscopy,* 23, pp 618-628.

Musahl V, Plakseychuk A, VanScyoc A, et al. (2005). Varying femoral tunnels between the anatomical footprint and isometric positions: Effect on kinematics of the anterior cruciate ligament-reconstructed knee. *Am J Sports Med,* 33, pp 712-718.

Nishimoto K, Kuroda R, Mizuno K, Hoshino Y, Nagamune K, Kubo S, Yagi M, Yamaguchi M, Yoshiya S, Kurosaka M (2009) Analysis of the graft bending angle at the femoral tunnel aperture in anatomic double bundle anterior cruciate ligament reconstruction: a comparison of the transtibial and the far anteromedial portal technique. *Knee Surg Sports Traumatol Arthrosc,* 17, pp270–276

Pandarinath R, Ciccotti M, DeLuca PF, Frederick RW. (2011). Current trends inACL reconstruction among professional team physicians. *Proceedings of the AAOS 2011 Annual Meeting,* 12, paper 324

Park SJ, Jung YB, Jung HJ, Jung HJ, Shin HK, Kim E, Song KS, Kim GS, Cheon HY, Kim S. (2010). Outcome of arthroscopic single-bundle versus double-bundle reconstruction of the anterior cruciate ligament: a preliminary 2-year prospective study. *Arthroscopy.* 26, No.5 (May), pp 630-636.

Paulos LE, Cherf J, Rosenberg TD, Beck CL. (1991). Anterior cruciate ligament reconstruction with autografts. *Clin Sports Med,* 10, No. 3 (July), pp 469-85.

Petersen W, Zantop T.(2007) Anatomy of the anterior cruciate ligament with regard to its two bundles. *Clin Orthop Relat Res,* 454, pp 35–47.

Pinczewski LA, Salmon LJ, Jackson WF, von Bormann RB, Haslam PG, Tashiro S. (2008). Radiological landmarks for placement of the tunnels in single-bundle reconstruction of the anterior cruciate ligament. *J Bone Joint Surg Br.,* 90, No.2 (February), pp :172-179.

Prodromos C, Joyce B, Shi K. (2007). A meta-analysis of stability of autografts compared to allografts after anterior cruciate ligament reconstruction. *Knee Surg Sports Traumatol Arthrosc*, 15, pp 851–856

Purnell ML, Larson AI, Clancy W. (2008).Anterior cruciate ligament insertions on the tibia and femur and their relationships to critical bony landmarks using high-resolution volume-rendering computed tomography. *Am J Sports Med*,36, pp 2083-2090.

Ristanis S. Giakas G. Papageorgiou CD. Moraiti T. Stergiou N, Georgoulis AD. (2003).The effects of anterior cruciate ligament reconstruction on tibial rotation during pivoting after descending stairs. *Knee Surg Sports Traumatol Arthrosc*, 11, pp 360-365.

Romano VM. Graf BK. Keenc JS. Lange RH. (1993). Anterior cruciate ligament reconstruction: The effect of tibial tunnel placement on range of motion. *Am J Sports Med*, 21, pp 415-418.

Rosenberg TD, Deffner KT. (1997). ACL reconstruction: semitendinosus tendon is the graft of choice. *Orthopedics*. 29, No.5 (May); pp396, 398.

Rosenberg T, Brown G. (1997). Anterior cruciate liagement reconstruction with a quadrupled semitendinosus autograft. *Sports Med Arthrosc Rev*, 1, pp243-258

Rue JP. Ghodadra N. Bach BR Jr. (2008). Femoral tunnel placement in single-bundle anterior cruciate ligament reconstruction: A cadaveric study relating transtibial lateralized femoral tunnel position to the anteromedial and posterolateral femoral origins of the anterior cruciate ligament. *Am J Sports Med*, 36 pp 73-79.

Rue JP, Ghodadra N, Lewis PB, Bach BR Jr. (2008). Femoral and tibial tunnel position using a transtibial drilled anterior cruciate ligament reconstruction technique. *J Knee Surg*, 21, pp 246-249.

Rue JPH, Ghodadra N, Bach, BR Jr. (2008). Femoral tunnel placement in single-bundle anterior cruciate ligament reconstruction: A cadaveric study relating transtibial femoral tunnel position to the anteromedial and posterolateral bundle femoral origins of the anterior cruciate ligament. *Am J Sports Med* 36, No.1 (January), pp 73-79.

Saharsrabudhe A, Christel P, Anne F, Appleby D, Basdekis G. (2010) Postoperative evaluation of tibial footprint and tunnels characteristics after anatomic double-bundle anterior cruciate ligament reconstruction with anatomic aimers. *Knee Surg Sports Traumatol Arthrosc*. 18, No.11 (November), pp 1599-1606.

Sbihi A, Franceschi JP, Christel P, Colombet P, Djian P, Bellier G. (2004). Comparaison biomécanique de la reconstruction du ligament croisé antérieur par greffe de tendons de la patte d'oie à un ou deux faisceaux. Une étude cadavérique. *Rev Chir Orthop*, 90, pp 643-650.

Serrano-Fernandez JM, Espejo-Baena A, Martin-Castilla B, De La Torre-Solis F, Mariscal-Lara J, Merino-Ruiz ML. (2010).Augmentation technique for partial ACL ruptures using semitendinosus tendon in the over-the-top position. *Knee Surg Sports Traumatol Arthrosc*, 18, No.9 (September), pp1214-1218

Shelton WR, Fagan BC. (2011). Autografts commonly used on anterior cruciate ligament reconstruction. *J Am Acad Othop Surg*,19, No.5 (May), pp 259-264.

Siebold R, Dehler C, Ellert T. (2008). Prospective randomized comparison of double-bundle versus single-bundle anterior cruciate ligament reconstruction. *Arthroscopy*, 24, No.2 (February), pp 137-45

Sommer C, Friederich NF, Muller W. (2000). Improperly placed anterior cruciate ligament grafts: correlation between radiological parameters and clinical results. *Knee Surg Sports Traumatol Arthrosc,* 8, pp 207–213

Stäubli HU, Rauschning W. (1994). Tibial attachment area of the anterior cruciate ligament in the extended knee position. Anatomy and cryosections in vivo comple in vivo. mented by magnetic resonance arthrography. *Knee Surg Sports Traumatol Arthrosc,* 2, pp 138-146.

Scopp JM. Jasper LE, Belkoff SM, Moorman CT IIL. (2004). The effect of oblique femoral tunnel placement on rotational constraint of the knee reconstructed using patellar tendon autografts. *Arthroscopy,* 20, pp 294-299.

Shino K, Nakata K, Nakamura N, Toritsuka Y, Horibe S, Nakagawa S, Suzuki T.(2008). Rectangular tunnel double-bundle anterior cruciate ligament reconstruction with bone-patellar tendon-bone graft to mimic natural fiber arrangement. *Arthroscopy,* 24, No.10 (October), pp 1178-1183.

Silva A, Sampaio R, Pinto E. (2010). Placement of femoral tunnel between the AM and PL bundles using a transtibial technique in single-bundle ACL reconstruction. *Knee Surg Sports Traumatol Arthrosc,* 18, No.12 (December), pp 1245–1251.

Sohn DH, Garrett WE Jr. (2009). Transitioning to anatomic anterior cruciate ligament graft placement. *J Knee Surg,* 22, No.2 (April), pp155-160

Steiner M. (2009). Anatomic single-bundle ACL reconstruction. *Sports Med Arthrosc,* 17, No.4 (December), pp:247-251.

Streich NA, Friedrich K, Gotterbarm T, Schmitt H. (2008). Reconstruction of the ACL with a semitendinosus tendon graft: a prospective randomized single-blinded comparison of double-bundle versus single-bundle technique in male athletes. *Knee Surg Sports Traumatol Arthrosc,* 16, No.3 (March), pp 232-238

Song EK, Oh LS, Gill TJ, Li G, Gadikota HR, Seon JK. (2009). Prospective comparative study of anterior cruciate ligament reconstruction using the double-bundle and single-bundle techniques. *Am J Sports Med,* 37, pp 1705–1711.

Takahashi M, Doi M, Abe M, Suzuki D, Nagano A (2006) Anatomical study of the femoral and tibial insertions of the anteromedial and posterolateral bundles of human anterior cruciate ligament. *Am J Sports Med,* 34, pp787–792

van Eck C, Lesniak bP, Schreiber VM, Fu F. (2010). Anatomic single- and double-bundle anterior cruciate ligament reconstruction flowchart. *Arthroscopy,* 26, No.2 (February), pp 258-268.

van Eck C, Working Z, Fu F. (2011). Current concepts in anatomic single- and double-bundle anterior cruciate ligament reconstruction.*Phys Sportsmed.* 39, No.2 (May), pp 140-148.

Wilson TC, Kantaras A, Atay A, Johnson DL. (2004). Tunnel enlargement after anterior cruciate Ligament surgery. *Am J Sports Med,* 32, No.2, pp 543-549.

Yagi M, Wong EK, Kanamori A, Debski RE, Fu FH, Woo SL. (2002). Biomechanical analysis of an anatomic anterior cruciate ligament reconstruction. *Am J Sports Med,* 30, pp 660–666.

Yagi M, Kuroda R, Nagamune K, Yoshiya S, Kurosaka M. (2007). Double bundle ACL reconstruction can improve rotational stability. *Clin Orthop Relat Res,* 454, pp100-107.

Yamamoto Y, Hsu WH, Woo SL, Van Scyoc AH, Takakura Y, Debski RE. (2004). Knee stability and graft function after anterior cruciate ligament reconstruction: A comparison of a lateral and an anatomical femoral tunnel placement. *Am J Sports Med*, 32, pp 1825-1832.

Yasuda K. Kondo E. Ichiyama H. et al. (2004).Anatomic reconstruction of the anteromedial and posterolateral bundles of the anterior cruciate ligament using hamstring tendon grafts. *Arthroscopy*. 20, pp 1015-1025.

Yasuda K, Kondo E, Ichiyama H, Tanabe Y, Tohyama H. (2006). Clinical evaluation of anatomic double-bundle anterior cruciate ligament reconstruction procedure using hamstring tendon grafts: comparisons among 3 different procedures. *Arthroscopy*. 22, pp 240-251.

Yunes M, Richmond JC, Engels EA, Pinczewski LA (2001) Patellar versus hamstring tendons in anterior cruciate ligament reconstruction: a meta-analysis. *Arthroscopy*, 17, pp248–257.

Zaffagnini S, Bruni D, Martelli S, Imakiire N, Marcacci M, Russo A (2008) Double-bundle ACL reconstruction: influence of femoral tunnel orientation in knee laxity analysed with a navigationnsystem—an in vitro biomechanical study. *BMC Musculoskelet Disord*, 9, pp 25-

Zantop T, Petersen W, Sekiya JK, Musahl V, Fu FH (2006) Anterior cruciate ligament anatomy and function relating to anatomical reconstruction. *Knee Surg Sports Traumatol Arthrosc*, 14, pp982–992

Zantop T, Herbort M, Raschke MJ, Fu FH, Petersen W (2007) The role of the anteromedial and posterolateral bundles of the anterior cruciate ligament in anterior tibial translation and internal rotation. *Am J Sports Med*, 35, pp 223–227.

Zantop T, Haase AK, Fu FH, Petersen W. (2008). Potential risk of cartilage damage in double bundle ACL reconstruction: impact of knee flexion angle and portal location on the femoral PL bundle tunnel. *Arch Orthop Trauma Surg*, 128, pp 509-513.

Zantop T, Diermann N, Schumacher T, Schanz S, Fu FH, Petersen W. (2008). Anatomical and nonanatomical double-bundle anterior cruciate ligament reconstruction: importance of femoral tunnel location on knee kinematics. *Am J Sports Med*, 36, pp 678–685.

10

The Role of Arthroscopy in Mini-Invasive Treatment of Tibial Plateau Fractures

Şt. Cristea, A. Prundeanu,
Fl. Groseanu and D. Gârtonea
Clinic of Orthopaedic and Trauma Surgery,
St. Pantelimon Hospital
Romania

1. Introduction

The treatment of tibial plateau fractures represents a challenge in current activity of an orthopedic surgeon, because these kind of fractures have an intraarticular trajectory. It is important in this kind of fractures to have a good mobility after treatment (Mills & Nork SE, 2002). Instead of the standard treatment with one or two plates and screws, one should try to use the reduction of the fracture's fragment with Kirschner wires under Rx control and fix the fragments with K wires, screws and external fixation (Marsh et al., 1995; Morandi & Pearse, 1996). Open reduction and internal fixation has a significant complication rate and this has encouraged interest in percutaneous techniques, most of which associate arthroscopy and fluoroscopy. Arthroscopy is useful to provide a good view of the articular surface and allows assessment of associated intra-articular lesions.
The objectives of this treatment are to obtain a good articular congruity, axial alignment, joint stability and functional motion.

2. Method

Minim invasive treatment and arthroscopic postreduction control are performed based on the Schatzker's classification, (Buchko & Johnson, 1996; Cristea et al., 2010; Kenneth A.E.& Kenneth J. K., 2006).

3. Diagnostic

The clinical diagnostic is sustained by the following clinical signs:
- swelling of the knee;
- hemarthrosis;
- pain;
- varus or valgus tibial deviation;
- impossible weight bearing;
- restriction for active movements of the knee joint.

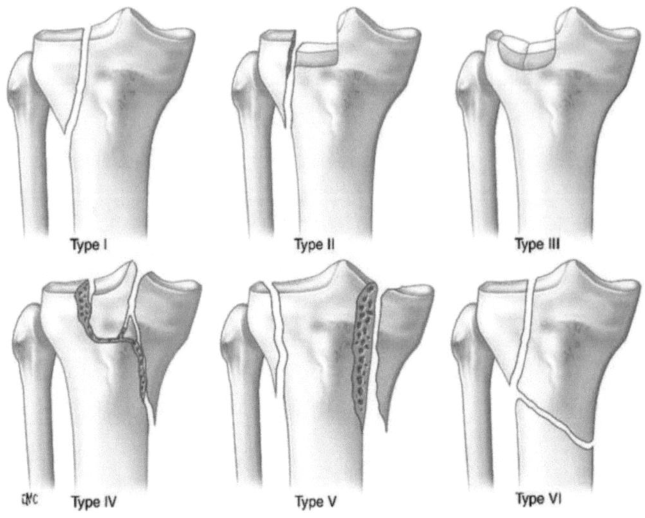

Fig. 1. Schatzker's Classification

3.1 Radiological diagnostic

Different kinds of Xray exposures are used :

- antero-posterior;
- lateral;
- oblique internal or external;
- in tension-evaluate the reduction (ligamentotaxis)

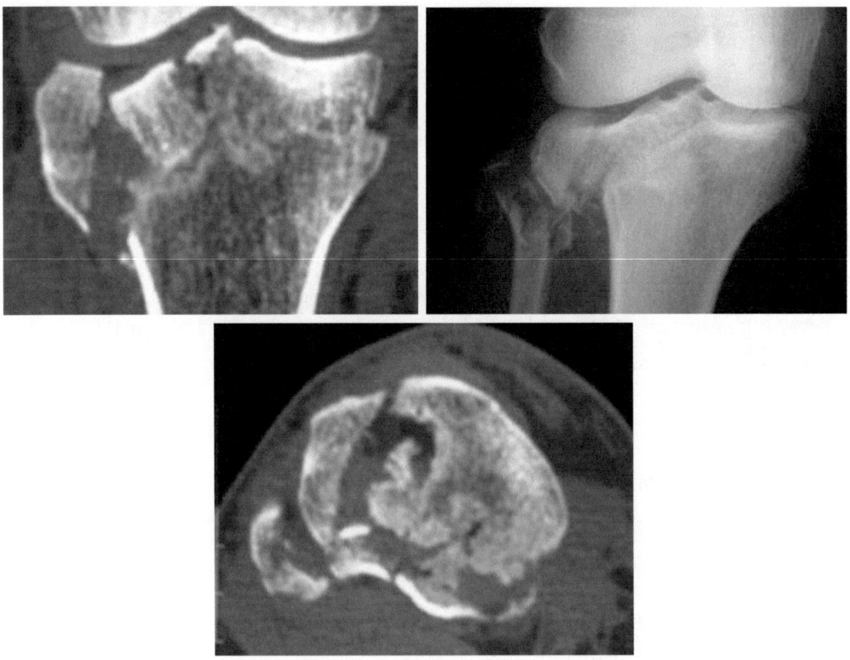

Fig. 2. Schatzker's V - CT and X Ray aspects

3.2 CT diagnostic

Using the reconstruction in sagital and coronal plane of the images more information about the type and localization of the fracture is obtained (Rafii et al., 1987). CT exam is mandatory for the surgical treatment planning in type IV, V and VI Schatzer. By all experience of using CT and Xray exams, after several different cases, the surgeon will understand the fracture aspect only by Xray exams.

4. Surgical treatment

Most surgeons use different kind of plates with screws with open reduction of the fracture:

- ''L'' plate;
- LC DCP plate;
- two plates;
- plate and external fixation.

The minimal invasive surgical treatment of these kind of fractures should be done under fluoroscopic and arthroscopic control.

This technique is particularly adapted to each Schatzker type, inspite of others (Casteleyn & Handelberg, 2001) considering a limited role of arthroscopy only in relative simple split, depression and split-depression fracures.

The patient is under spinal anesthesia, then the fragments of the fracture are identified using Xray control. The reduction of the fracture is then atempted by flexion, extension, traction (ligamentotaxis) (Sirkin et al., 2000).

Standard arthroscopic portals can be used, joint irrigation is mandatory with a low pressure gravity feed, and a tourniquet is always necessary to reduce bleeding. Some arthrocopic surgical experience is necessary. The scope must be left for a few seconds in the same position in order to flush the blood and visualise the lessions. Prolonged operation time may lead to increased fluid effusion with compartimental syndrome or deep venous thrombosis.

The technique will be described particularly adapted to each Schatzker type.

In case of fractures with pure cleavage, split fractures, K wires are inserted rectangularly on the fracture's line, subchondral, under Xray and arthroscopic guidance. Eventually compression forces are applied by putting cannulated cancellous screws in paralel planes.

In case of fractures with depression, a K wire is inserted in the depressed bone fragment. Then this bone fragment is lifted under Xray and arthroscopic control and then another K wire is inserted through these reduced bone fragments, subchondral. Eventually compression forces are applied by putting cancellous screws in paralel planes.

In case of combinated fractures, cleavage and depression a K wire is inserted through the fracture's cleavage directly in the depressed bone fragment, and this depressed bone fragment is lifted using strong forces till the K wire is bend, under Xray and arthroscopic control. Then another K wire is inserted through these reduced bone fragments, perpendiculary to the cleavage fracture, then compression forces are applied by putting paralel cancellous screws. After the alignment of the articular surface is obtained these fragments are fixed with cancellous screws or another K wire. In case of cominuted fractures, first the depression is reduced and then the cleavage. The forces applied on the K wire for the alignment of the fracture are very strong (Cristea et al., 2010).

In case of Schatzker type V-VI external fixation is used after obtaining the alignment of the articular surface (Cristea et al., 2010).

Indirect reduction techniques have the advantage of minimal soft tissue striping and fragment devitalization (Kenneth A.E.& Kenneth J. K., 2006). For badly comminuted fractures an external fixator is used such as femoral - tibial distractor, eventually articulated. Closed methods are prefered in order to elevate depressed fragments, which can be carried out under fluoroscopic or arthroscopic guidance (Buchko & Johnson, 1996; Cristea et al., 2010). Bone tamps are placed under image and the depressed segments are elevated. Accuracy of reduction may be checked with the aid of the arthroscope. In type IV-VI because there are significant forces, lag screws alone are not sufficient to stabilize these fractures and external fixation is used.

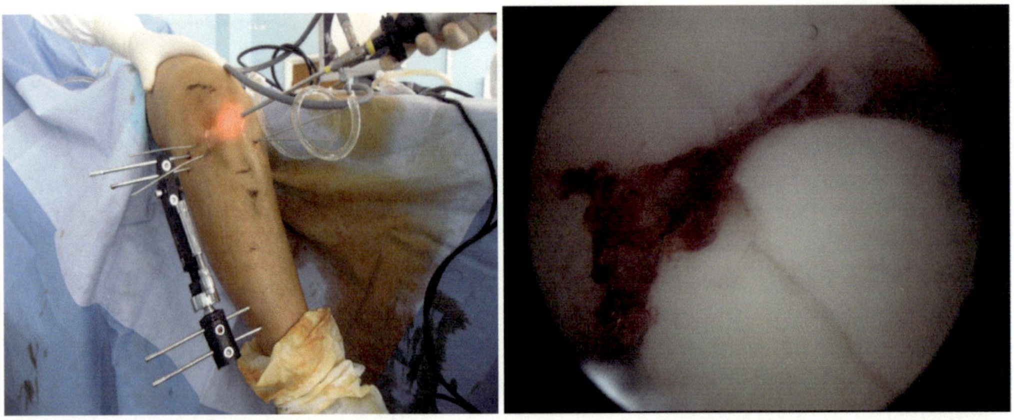

Fig. 3. External fixator and minim invasive reduction under X ray and arthroscopic control - intraoperative aspects

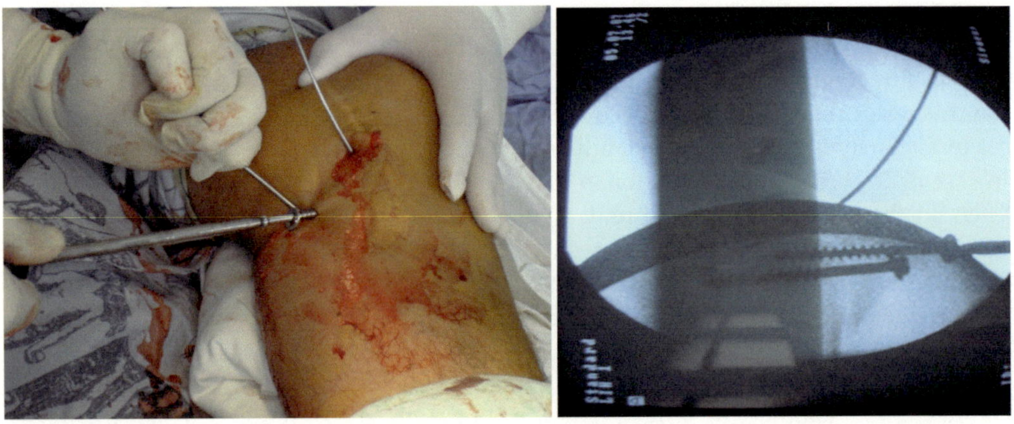

Fig. 4. Minim invasive reduction under X ray and arthroscopic control - intraoperative aspects

4.1 Asociated meniscal and ligamentous lesions

Diagnosis and immediate treatment of associated meniscal lesions by partial meniscectomy and debridement can be performed during initial arthroscopy. These may account for a lower incidence of degenerative changes in arthroscopically treated fractures cases. The collateral ligaments sprains do not require surgical treatment. They can be futher protected during mobilisation with an articulated cast-brace or a rehabilitation brace when the joint immobilisation is not necessary. The ACL lesions are reevaluated after the fracture healing and late reconstruction could be necessary.

Various lessions of soft tissue are associated with tibial plateau fractures. These are usually neglected by most traumatic surgeons. All the meniscus lessions type, capsular disruption, intraarticular haematomas, osteochondral small fragments, ACL various lessions or collateral ligaments are associated with tibial plateau fractures.

Based on the OR findings, in our opinion, the following classification of soft tissue lessions should be added to each type of Schatzker fractures:

- A1-without lesions of the meniscus or ACL
- A2-with tears of the meniscus – repaired by excision and debridement
- B1-lesions of the meniscus - which must be sutured
- B2-fracture of the tibial plateau spine - which must be repared in emergency
- C1- with desinsertion of ACL from femoral insertion - which should be repared in emergency

  C2-with ireparable rupture of ACL , which can be repared later in another surgical session.

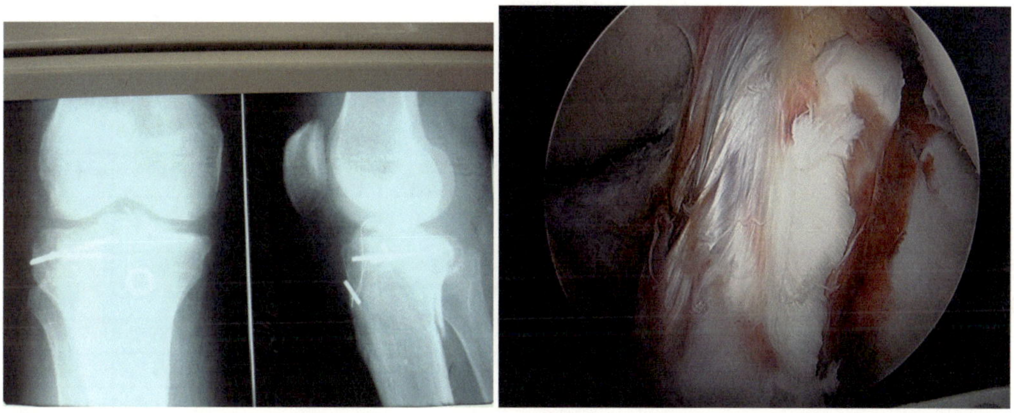

Fig. 5. Minim invasive reduction of complex fracture which includes the spinal plateau. X ray and Arthroscopic control – after reduction

4.2 Author's experience and statistical analysis

Between 2006-2010 we had 398 tibial plateau fractures and for 262 we used surgical treatment. Of those 68% were external plateau fractures; 18% were internal plateau fractures and 14% were bilateral plateau fractures. We saw a great discrepancy between radiology and CT. On the Xray and CT we follow and appreciate the deplacement degree, fracture's type and indication of treatment (Tscherne & Lobenhoffer, 1993).

We obtained very good results in 80% of cases, but also we have one case with infection after a month which neccessitate extraction of the screws and wires; in 15% of cases we obtained a mobility of the knee around 95-105 degree of fexion; in 4% of cases we were not able to restore the entire surface of the tibial plateau.

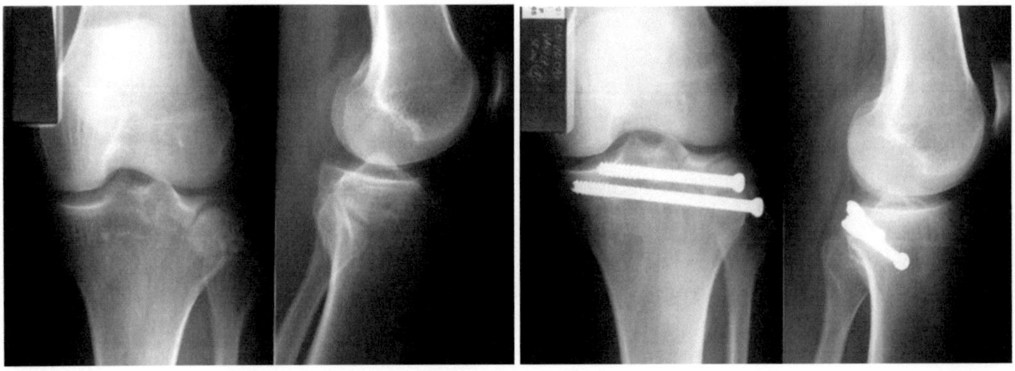

Fig. 6. X ray Pre and postoperative aspects

The statistical analysis was obtained with the use of SASTM computer software, version 9.1.3, Cary U.S. To compare the subgroups on the basis of quantitative variables, a Student test was used. For the qualitative variables, a Pearson's Khi^2 was used or a Fisher's exact test if the theoretical numbers were too low.. The degree of significance chosen for the overall risk of the first case was fixed at 5 % in both situations.

In our study several international systems of evaluation were used (KOOS scores, IKS, Lysholm, Tegner and Rasmussen) thus permiting a comparison with a larger number of literature series. In general our functional results were satisfying and comparable to other series.

In table 1 and 2 we compare our results with other international studies in literature.

	Scheerlin C.K., 1998	Cassard, 1999	Rossi,2008	Siegler, 2009	Our series, 2010
Number of patients	52	44	57	28	262
Number of follow-up patients	38	44	46	21	184
Average age	47	46	48	43	51
Average follow-up (months)	62	69	60	59,5	60
Associated lessions (%)	53,8	–	39	32,1	63
Meniscal lesions (%)	–	–	28	7,1	53
ACL Lessions (%)	–	–	11	3,6	10
Postoperative complications (%)	15,4	–	3,5	0	4,9
IKS average	–	92	93,2	85,2	93
IKS functional average	–	96	94, 8	91	95
Clinical Rasmussen average	–	–	28,2	25,5	9
Radiological Rasmussen average	–	–	–	25,5	9
Arthrosis Xray (%)	28,9	20	8,6	47,6	25
Malalignment (%)	15,8	–	8,7	32,1	4,9

ACL : anterior cruciate ligament ; IKS : International Knee Society.

Table 1. Mean results of tibial plateau fractures.

	Bobic, 1993	Cassard, 1999	Mazoue, 1999	Gill, 2001	Kieffer, 2001	Roerdink, 2001	Asik 2002	Pogliacomi, 2005	Levy, 2008	Kayali, 2008	Siegler 2009	Our series, 2010
Number of patients	31	26	17	25	29	30	48	19	16	21	28	262
Average age	44,4	42,3	43,6	45,2	47,4	72	39	36	44,8	41	43	51
Average follow-up (months)		32,7	14,6	24	25,1	36	36	12	41	38	59,5	60
Meniscal lesions (%)	23	30,8	29,4	36	13,8	40	47,9	22,2	56,2	42,8	7,1	53
ACL Lessions (%)	13	11,5	5,9	32	10,3	6,6	6,2	11,1	6,2	0	3,6	10
Postoperative complications (%)	6,4	7,7	17,6	0	6,9	3,3	4,2	–	0	0	0	4,9
IKS average	–	94,1	–	–	–	–	–	–	–	–	85,2	93
IKS functional average	–	94,7	–	–	–	–	–	–	–	–	91	95
Lysholm average	–	–	80,9	–	–	–	–	–	–	–	86	92
Clinical Rasmussen average	–	–	–	27,5	–	–	–	–	29,25	–	25,5	9
Radiological Rasmussen average	–	–	–	–	–	–	–	–	16,87	–	8	9
Arthrosis Xray (%)	–	26,3	21,4	–	12,9	–	63	27,8	12,5	24	47,6	25
Malalignment (%)	–	10,5	–	–	6,9	–	–	–	12,5	–	32,1	4,9

Table 2. Short term results of the tibial plateau fractures

ACL : anterior cruciate ligament ; IKS : International Knee Society.
We reduced the infection rate by:

- reduced time of surgery;
- minimal dissection;
- extraperiosteal dissection;
- minimal size of implants;
- antibiotics.

We use anticoagulant therapy for thrombembolism profilaxy. There were no DVT or pulmonary embolism (PE) complications in our series. There was no compartmental syndrome in our series due to low pressure during joint irrigation in arthroscopy, no pump was used.

5. Postoperative care

5.1 Deep venous thrombosis (DVT) prevention

As tibial plateau fractures are associated with considerable soft tissue trauma and sometimes with prolonged operation times using a tourniquet, DVT is not a rare complication (Williams et al., 1995).
The use of one of the low-molecular-weight heparins is advisable. One should prolong their use for more than 3 weeks until the complete mobilisation of the knee and the pacient. Foot and calf mechanical compression devices can also be used with success. Compressive antithromboembolic stockings are always mandatory.

5.2 Mobilisation

Once a satisfactory fracture reduction and stabilisation have been obtained, the immediate mobilisation is done. The soft tissue and skin coverage lesions are limited. Immediate continuous passive motion (CPM) can be beneficial for the restoration of the articular homeostasis and the remodelling of the small articular fragments. When the external fixator locks the knee, a stable construct to early mobilisation of the pacient is mandatory. In generaly at 3-6 weeks the articular mobility is achieved, depending of the fracture type and stability of the fixation.

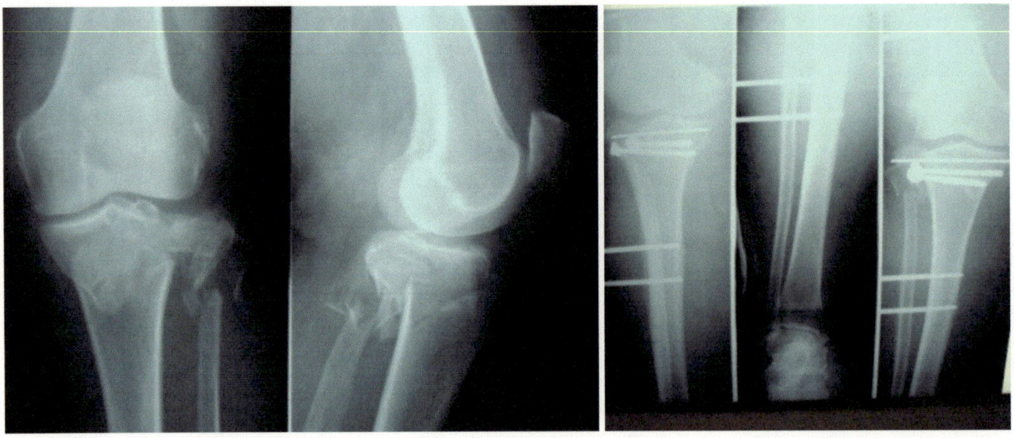

Fig. 7. X ray Pre and postoperative aspects

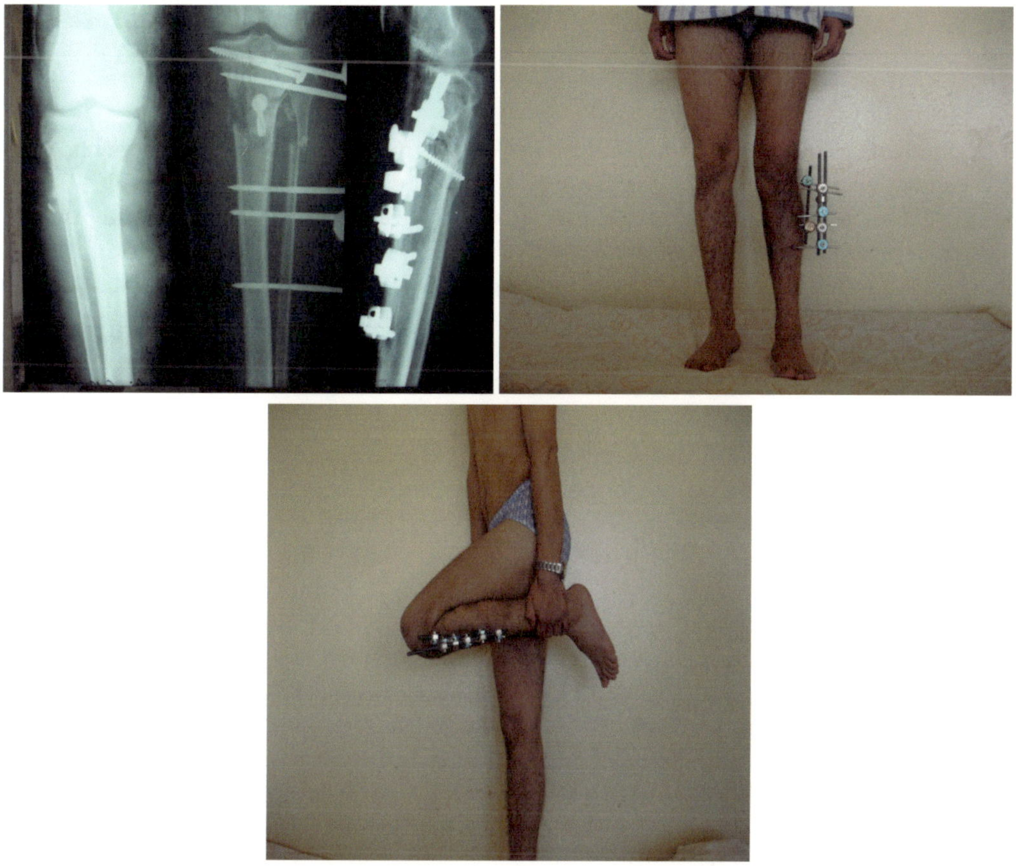

Fig. 8. X ray Pre and postoperative aspects

5.3 Weight-bearing

In general, walking with crutches with minimal load bearing is possible after a few days. In simple fractures, or stable construct fixation full bearing is allowed at 10-12 weeks. The articulated cast braces or rehabilitation braces can be usefull in early rehabilitation. Secondary, progressive impaction of the depressed zone can occur due to weight bearing, even 4 to 5 months postoperatively, especially in obese patients or those with ostheoporotic bone.

6. Complications

The risk of infection is reduced due to: shortened time of surgery, minimal dissection, extraperiosteal dissection, minimal size of implants, antibiotics. The implants ablation and antibiotics resolve that rare complication, while in classical open surgery the rate of infections and stiffness is 10 %.

Posttraumatic arthritis in 4a patient with bicondylar fracture could be a good indication for total knee replacement. In only 4% of cases the restore of the entire surface of the tibial plateau was not achieved. The varum deviation was finally observed in 3% of patients, with maximum value of 5^0.

7. Conclusion

This kind of articular fractures requires perfect alignment of fracture's fragments. It is difficult to treat these fracture especially type V and type VI Schatzker.

Beside the standard treatment with one or two plates and screws, one could use the reduction of the fracture's fragment with K wire under Xray and arthroscopic control, and then fix the fragments with K wire and screws. First of all it is important to establish the fracture's type. Schatzker classification is commonly used for their identification. The preoperative planning is necessary and also the X-ray and CT scan. For this technique different kind of material is used: K wire, screws, external fixation, fluoroscope, and arthroscopy.

The role of arthroscopy in these fractures is twofold: 1. To confirm the quality of a good reduction, 2. To accurately asses and treat the associated lesions of the soft tissue - menisci, cruciate ligaments, capsular disruption.

This minimal invasive technique is useful for the treatment of this kind of fractures and in most cases has good outcome.

Good results are obtained by using this method (Cristea et al., 2010) in the surgical treatment of tibial plateau fractures. This technique is adapted to resolve all tibial fractures type, not only Schatzker I - III, like some authors (Siegler et al., 2011).

The advantages of this method are: minimal blood lost, small infection rate, good mobilization of the knee without pain, cheaper implants, reproductibility of the technique, it can be made in emergency, cost - efficient.

A single dose of antibiotics is admninistrated during surgery and anticoagulant for thrombembolism prophylaxis is done.

8. References

Asik M, Cetik O, Talu U, Sozen YV. Arthroscopy-assisted operative management of tibial plateau fractures. Knee Surg Sports Traumatol Arthrosc 2002;10:364—70.

Bobic V., O'Dwyer K. J. Tibial plateau fractures: the arthroscopic option Knee surg, sports Traumatol, Arthrosopy (1993) 1: 239-242

Buchko GM, Johnson DH: Arthroscopy assisted operative management of tibial plateau fractures, Clin Orthop 332:29, 1996;

Cassard X, Beaufils P, Blin JL, Hardy P. Osteosynthesis under athroscopic control of separated tibial plateau fractures. 26 case reports. Rev Chir Orthop 1999;85: 257—66.

Casteleyn P.P., Handelberg F.: Fractures of the upper part of the tibia , Surgical Techniques in Orthopaedics and Traumatology, Elsevier, 55-510-A-10, 2001

Cristea St., Prundeanu A., Groseanu F., Atasiei T.: Minimal invasiv treatment of tibial plateau fractures Seventh SICOT/SIROT Annual International Conference on 31 August - 3 September 2010 in Gothenburg, Sweden poster 23768; 2010

Cristea Şt., Prundeanu A., Groseanu F., Predescu V., Gârtonea D., Păpălici A., Olaru R.: Le rôle de l'arthroscopie dans le traitement percutané des fractures du plateau tibial Revue de Chirurgie Orthopédique Ms. Ref. No.: OTSR-RCO-D-11-00169 / 2011

Gill TJ, Moezzi DM, Oates KM, Sterett WI. Arthroscopic reduction and internal fixation of tibial plateau fractures in skiing. Clin Orthop Relat Res 2001;383:243–9.

Kayali C, Oztürk H, Altay T, Reisoglu A, Agus H. Arthroscopically assisted percutaneous osteosynthesis of lateral tibial plateau fractures. Can J Surg 2008;51:378–82.

Kenneth A.Egol and Kenneth J. Koval: Fractures in Adults Rockwood and Green's sixth edition Lippincott 2006 : vol 2 pag 1999 - 2029; 2006

Kiefer H, Zivaljevic N, Imbriglia JE Arthroscopic reduction and internal fixation (ARIF) of lateral tibial plateau fractures. Knee Surg Sports Traumatol Arthrosc. 2001 May;9(3):167-72.

Levy BA, Herrera DA, Macdonald P, Cole PA. The medial approach for arthroscopic-assisted fixation of lateral tibial plateau fractures: patient selection and mid- to long-term results. J Orthop Trauma 2008;22:201–5.

Marsh JL, Smith ST, Do TT: External fixation and limioted internal fixation for complex fractures of tibial plateau, J Bone Joint Surg 77A:661,1995;

Mazoue CG, Guanche CA, Vrahas MS. Arthroscopic management of tibial plateau fractures: an unselected series. Am J Orthop 1999;28:508–15.

Mills WJ, Nork SE: Open reduction and internal fixation of high-energy tibial plateau fractures, Orthop Clin North Am 33:177,2002;

Morandi M, Pearse MF: Management of complex tibial plateau fractures with Ilizarov external fixator, Tech Orthop 11:125, 1996;

Pogliacomi F., Verdano M. A., Frattini M., Costantino C., Vaienti E., Soncini G.: Combined arthroscopic and radioscopic management of tibial plateau fractures: report of 18 clinical cases ACTA BIOMED 2005; 76; 107-114

Prundeanu A., Groseanu Fl., Gavrila M., Cristea St.: Treatment of tibial plateau fractures with minimal incision Archives of The Balkan Medical Union ISSN 0041 - 6940 VOL. VOL. 44, NO. 3, PP. 186-190, 2009

Rafii M, Lamont JG, Firooznia H: Tibial plateau fractures: CT evaluation and classification, Crit Rev Diagn Imaging 27:91,1987;

Roerdink WH, Oskam J, Vierhout PA. Arthroscopically assisted osteosynthesis of tibial plateau fractures in patients older than 55 years. Arthroscopy 2001;17:826–31.

Rossi R, Bonasia BE, Blonna D, Assom M, Castoldi F. Prospective follow-up of a simple arthroscopic-assisted technique for lateral tibial plateau fractures: results at 5 years. Knee 2008;15: 378–83.

Scheerlinck T, Ng CS, Handelberg F, Casteleyn PP. Medium-term results of percutaneous, arthroscopically-assisted osteosynthesis of fractures of the tibial plateau. J Bone Joint Surg Br 1998;80:959–64.

Siegler J., Galissier B., Marcheix P.S., Charissoux J.J., Mabit C., Arnaud J.P. : Osteosynthese percutanee sous arthroscopie des fractures des plateaux tibiaux : evaluation a moyen terme des resultats, Revue de chirurgie orthopedique et traumatologique , Vol.97, Nr 1, Fevr. 2011

Sirkin MS, Bono CM, Reilly MC, Behrens FF: Percutaneous methods of tibial plateau fixation, Clin Orthop 375:60, 2000;

Tscherne H, Lobenhoffer P: Tibial plateau fractures: management and expected results, Clin Orthop 292:87,1993

Williams S., Hulstyn M., Fadale P., Lindy P., Ehrlich M., Coran J., Dorfman G. : Incidence of deep vein thrombosis after arthroscopic knee surgery, a prospective study, Arthroscopy, 1995, 11:701-705, 1995

11

Arthroscopy Following Total Knee Replacement

Vaibhav Bagaria[1], Jami Ilyas[2], Bhawan Paunipagar[3], Darshna Rasalkar[4] and Rohit Lal[5]
[1]Columbia Asia Hospital and ORIGYN Clinic, Ghaziabad,
[2]Royal Perth Hospital, Perth,
[3]Department of Diagnostic Radiology and Organ Imaging Prince of Wales Hospital and Child Cancer Centre,
[4]Kokilaben Dhirubhai Ambani Hospital, Mumbai,
[5]ORIGYN Clinic, INDIRAPURAM, Ghaziabad,
[1,4,5]India
[2]Australia
[3]Hong Kong

1. Introduction

Total Knee replacement although an extremely successful procedure is occasionally complicated by conditions such as pain of unknown etiology, clunk and stiffness. Diagnosing and managing the patients with pain and dysfunction following joint replacement is difficult and can be challenging. The underlying cause could be impinging soft tissue under the patella with the clunk syndrome, impinging hypertrophic synovitis elsewhere in the knee, impinging PCL stump, prosthesis loosening and wear, arthrofibrosis and subclinical infections.

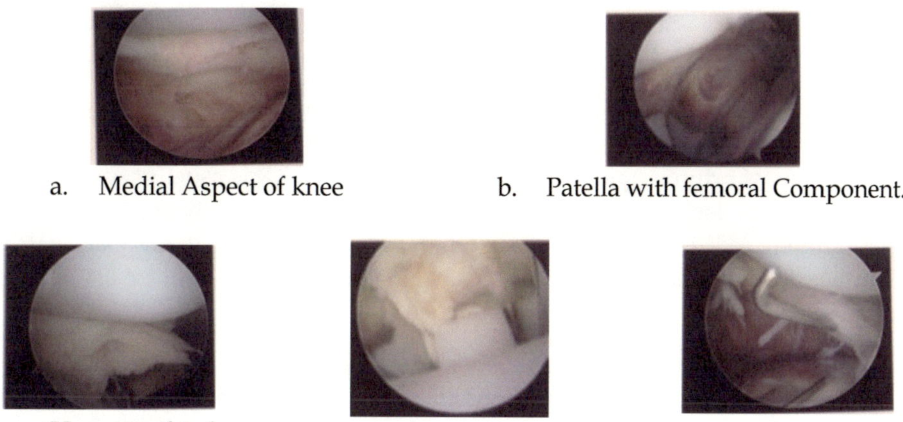

a. Medial Aspect of knee
b. Patella with femoral Component.
c. Hypertrophied Synovium
d. Poly Insert with Cam
e. Suprapatellar pouch

Fig. 1a. Normal Arthroscopic appearance after TKR

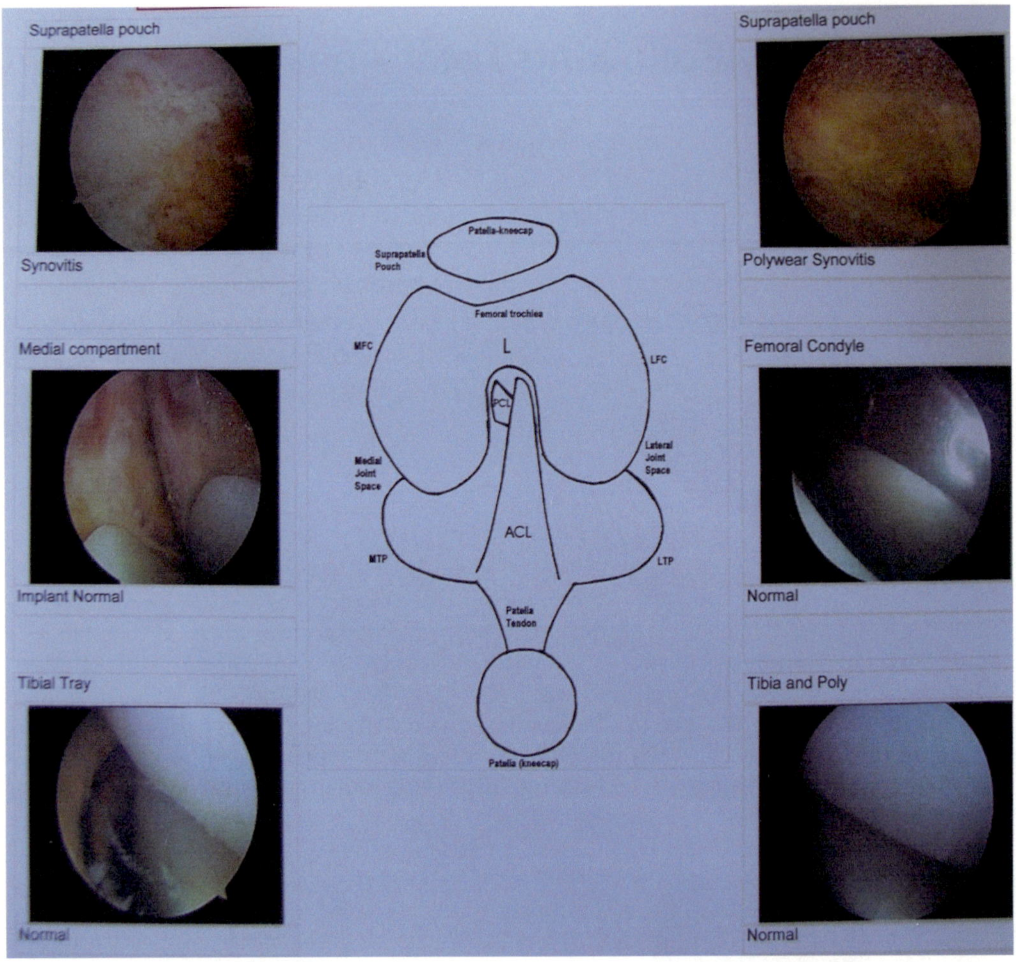

Fig. 1b. Sequence of arthroscopic examination of Knee post TKR is usually same as normal Knee - Patellofemoral joint, Medial compartment, Intercondylar notch, lateral compartment. Extra precaution needs to be taken while handling scope so as not to damage or scratch the metal surface. It could also be technically challenging in tight knees and due to scarring around knee.

Many of the problems can be diagnosed after clinical examination, radiography, bone scan and aspiration. Most of the remaining conditions can be resolved (except infection) using arthroscopic techniques. The chapter describes the indications and surgical techniques for arthroscopy following the knee replacement, along with a description of the various conditions that can be encountered. Arthroscopic images of arthroscopy after knee replacement are also included for teaching purposes.

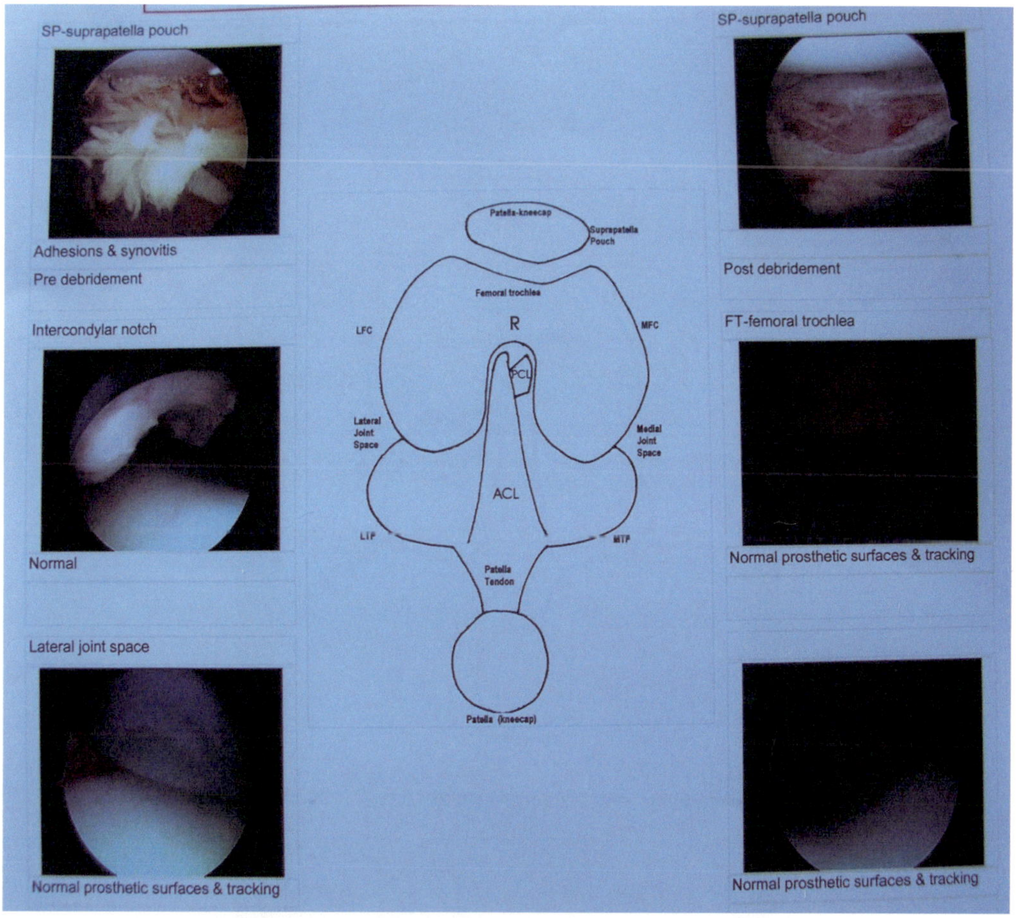

Fig. 2. Ceramic Knee - Arthroscopic appearance

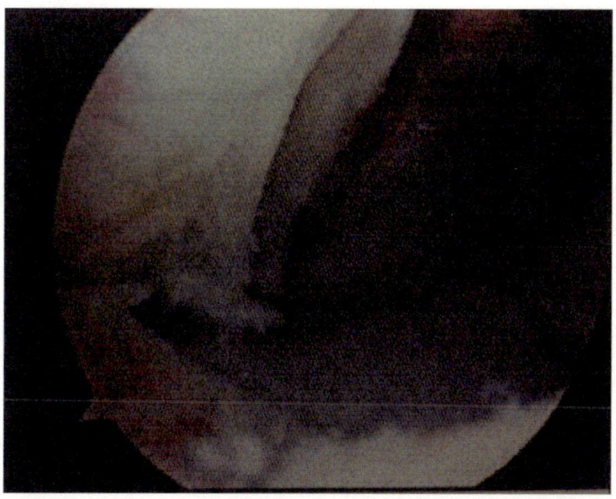

Fig. 3. Unicompartmental Knee Replacement - Arthroscopy Appearance.

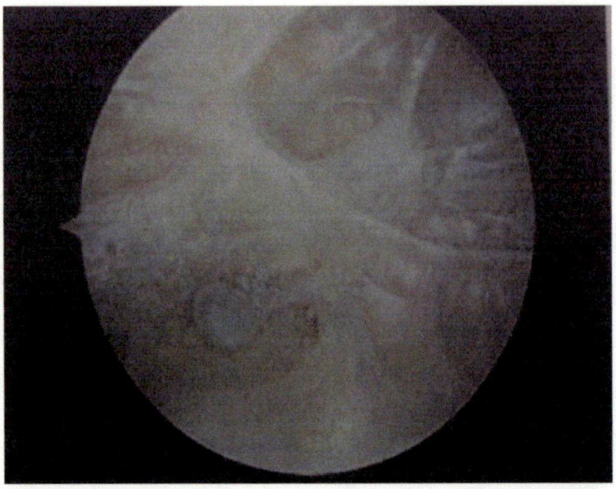

Fig. 4.1. Painful TKR without any clinically identifiable cause. O Arthroscopy synovium showed signs of metallosis.

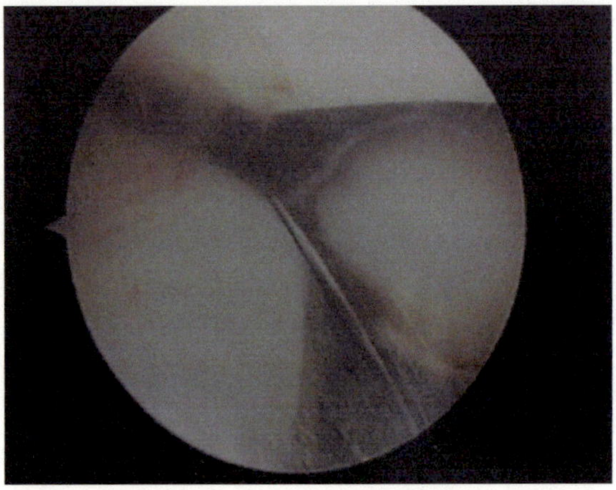

Fig. 4.2. Note the scratches on the metal surface of the same knee.

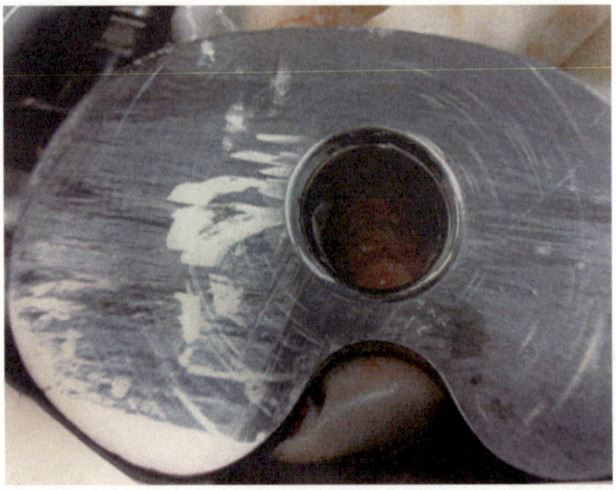

Fig. 4.3. Same knee implant at the time of revision. The knee was a part of global recall. Note the scratches on the tibial base plates

2. Arthrofibrosis

The incidence of arthrofibrosis or stiffness following TKR varies considerably and has been cited to be between 1 and 11%. Arthrofibrosis or knee stiffness is clinically defined as an inadequate range of movement that results in functional limitations affecting activities of daily living. The cutoff range of motion (ROM) for which stiffness requires surgical treatment is defined as having a flexion contracture of 15 degrees or flexion of less than 75 degrees. This decreased range of movement can severely affect the patient's ability to perform tasks of daily living such as walking, climbing stairs, or getting up from a seated position. Biomechanical studies and gait analysis have shown that patients required 67 degrees of knee flexion during the swing phase of gait, 83 degrees of flexion to climb stairs, 90- 100 degrees of flexion to descend stairs, and 93 degrees of flexion to stand from a seated position

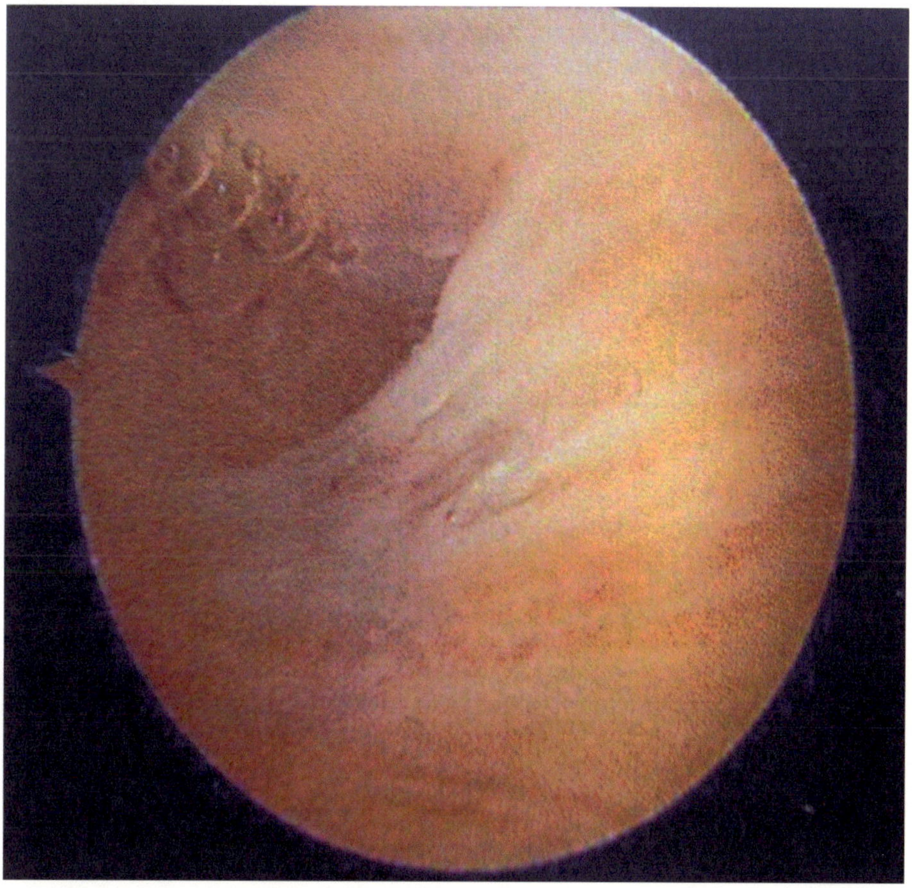

Fig. 5. Adhesion in suprapatellar pouch.

2.1

Arthrofibrosis may be secondary to numerous factors, including limited preoperative range of motion, faulty surgical technique, incorrect sizing, inappropriate implant placement, or inadequate postoperative rehabilitation and limiting motion until wound healing occurs. It could be also due to a biological predilection as some patients may be predisposed to extensive scar tissue formation as a response to the tissue trauma itself, which occurs during total knee replacement.

2.2

Managing stiff knee involve a thorough clinical exam to rule out any extrinsic contributing factor, ruling out infection and revisiting the surgical notes to identify any surgery related causes. One of the important aspects is identifying or excluding low grade infections. Initial step in managing these cases is a step by step incremental rehabilitation program. If this fails, a closed manipulation may be the next step. Recalcitrant cases may require arthroscopic or open arthrolysis. Arthroscopic management allows minimally invasive access to focal lesions (e.g. nodules, loose bodies) and is helpful in addressing cases of severe diffuse arthrofibrosis refractory to closed methods as well as in avoiding potential catastrophic complications associated with manipulation alone. Arthroscopic treatment of painful knee arthroplasty provides reliable expectations for improvement in function, decrease in pain, and improvement in knee scores.

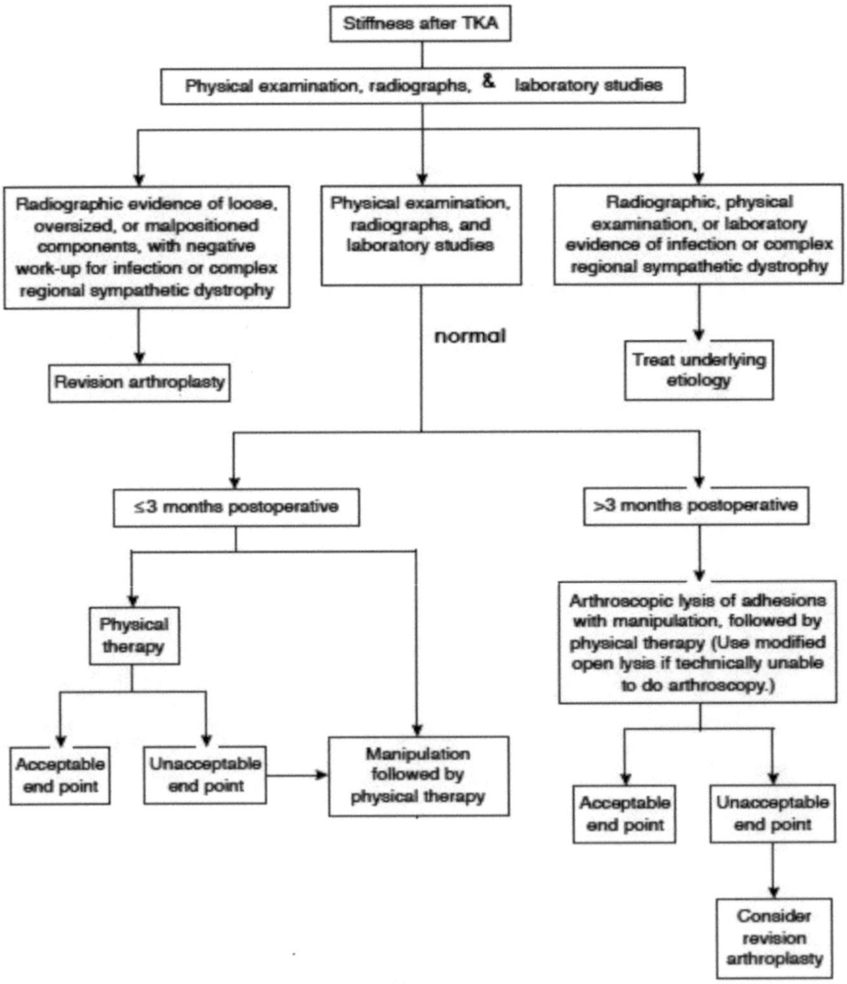

Flowchart for management of Arthrofibrosis after TKR

2.3

Performing arthroscopy for arthrofibrosis however may be a technically demanding. Insertion of the arthroscope into a markedly stiff knee with an arthro-fibrotic patello-femoral compartment can be challenging and one posing potential risk of damaging the prosthesis. Arthroscopic debridement of adhesions in combination with manipulation has been shown to substantially improve knee range of movement in patients with postoperative arthrofibrosis resulting from surgical procedures other than TKA. However, arthroscopic lysis of adhesions after TKA has not been as successful as lysis after procedures other than TKA. Bocell et al observed that only two of seven patients maintained pain-free improvements in range of movement after arthroscopic debridement of arthrofibrosis and manipulation after TKA. Campbell observed an increase in flexion of only 11° and an increase in extension of only 5.5° in eight patients 1 year after arthroscopy. Others have reported more marked improvements in range of movement. After arthroscopic debridement and manipulation, Diduch et al reported a 26° improvement in mean flexion in eight patients, and Scranton observed a 31° gain in mean range of movement; however, neither study examined the effect of arthroscopy on flexion contractures. Bae et al reported a mean improvement of 42° in the total arc of motion at 1-year follow-up in 13 knees; the improvement in flexion contractures was less clear. Patients with flexion limitations who receive a PCL-retaining total knee component may benefit from arthroscopic release of the PCL. Williams et. al observed an increase in mean flexion of 30° and an improvement in mean knee extension from 4° to 1.5° at 20-month follow-up in 10 knees after arthroscopic PCL release. When adhesions are more extensive, electro-cautery, arthroscopic scissors, and large-radius shavers can be used to debride the supra-patellar pouch and the medial and lateral gutters.

Study	Number of Patients (Knees)	Technique	Time from TKA to Secondary Surgery (Months)	Total Gain in Range of Motion (Degrees)	Time to Follow-up (Months)
Williams et al	9 (10)	PCL release	29	30°	20
Campbell	8 (8)	Lysis	11.6	16.5°	12
Diduch et al	8 (8)	Lysis	7.4	26°	20
Bae et al	11 (13)	Lysis	20	42°	12
Sprague et al	1 (1)	Lysis	12	23°	3
Scranton et al	7 (7)	Lysis	N/A	31°	12
Scranton et al	4 (4)	Modified Open	N/A	62°	12
Nicholls & Dorr	12 (13)	Revision	N/A	33°	N/A
Ries & Badalamente	5 (6)	Revision	20	50°	33
Babis et al	7 (7)	Open Lysis with Tib. Insert Exchange	12	28°	50

2.4
Loss of knee flexion often indicates involvement of the supra-patellar pouch, patello-femoral joint or anterior interval. Involvement of the intercondylar notch can affect both flexion and extension. Extension loss can result from intra-articular nodules and arthrofibrosis of the posterior capsule.

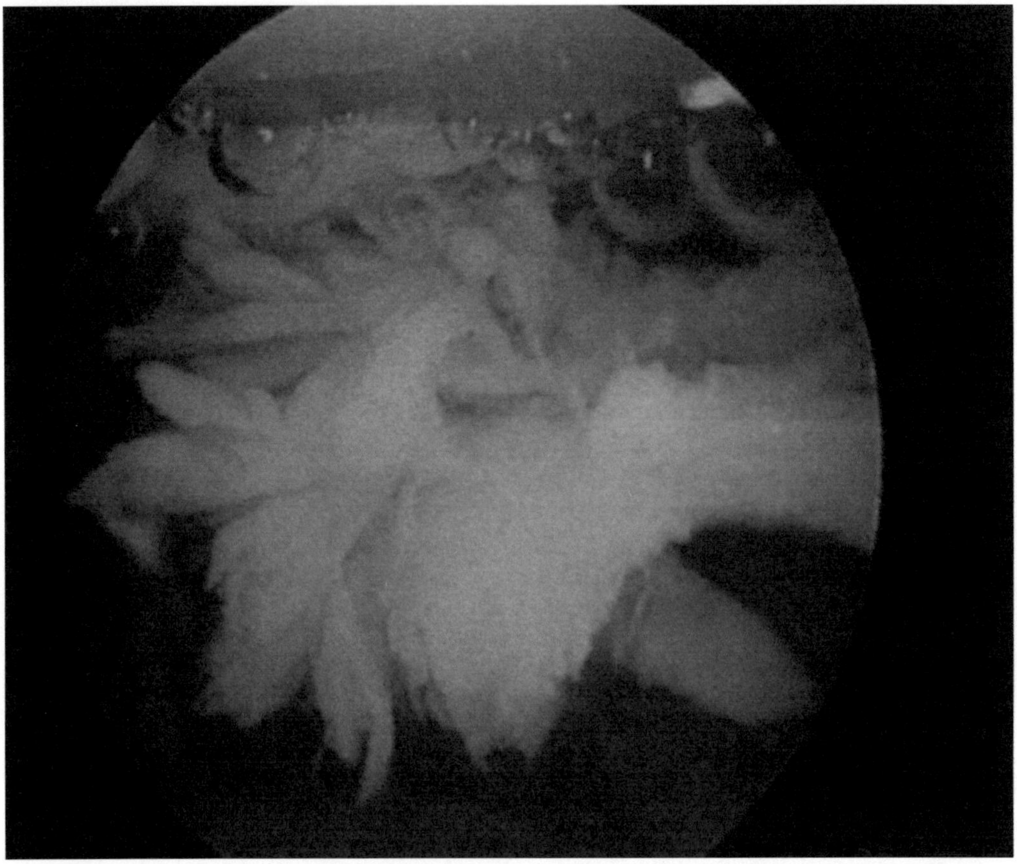

Fig. 6. Suprapatellar pouch with adhesion and synovitis

Kim et al (Ref) described a systematic approach when performing arthroscopic debridement of an arthrofibrotic knee. The use of regional anesthesia can effectively manage perioperative pain and facilitate postoperative rehabilitation (Ref: Millet). Prior to portal placement; capsular distention is achieved by saline injection into the supra-patellar pouch. Arthroscopy of prosthetic knees is initially approached through the conventional anterior-medial and anterior-lateral portals. If necessary, additional superolateral or superomedial portals can be utilized. Extreme care must be exercised when trocars and other instruments are inserted or manipulated in the joint, so as not to scratch the metallic surfaces or the polyethylene. Raab et al noted in an in vitro study, that a stainless steel cannulae could produce surface alterations in the femoral component with loads as small as 8 Newton. The supra-patellar pouch is reestablished first, followed by the medial and lateral gutters. The anterior interval is identified by releasing the infra-patellar fat pad from the anterior tibia, allowing for reestablishment of the pretibial recess. Medial and/or lateral retinacular release may be required in the patient with reduced patellar mobility or a tight patello-femoral joint. Once in the intercondylar notch, the surgeon must evaluate notch stenosis. If present, a notchplasty is performed. Scar tissue, bony nodules, and loose bodies are removed. Depending on the severity of the scarring, release or excision is performed. Once complete, the knee should be ranged and motion reassessed. Persistent loss of extension usually indicates posterior capsular involvement. Care needs to be taken, as decreased joint space by intra-articular adhesions bands and hypertrophied synovium, iatrogenic damage to the prosthesis and polyethylene during arthroscopy may be the major disadvantage of arthroscopy following total knee replacement.

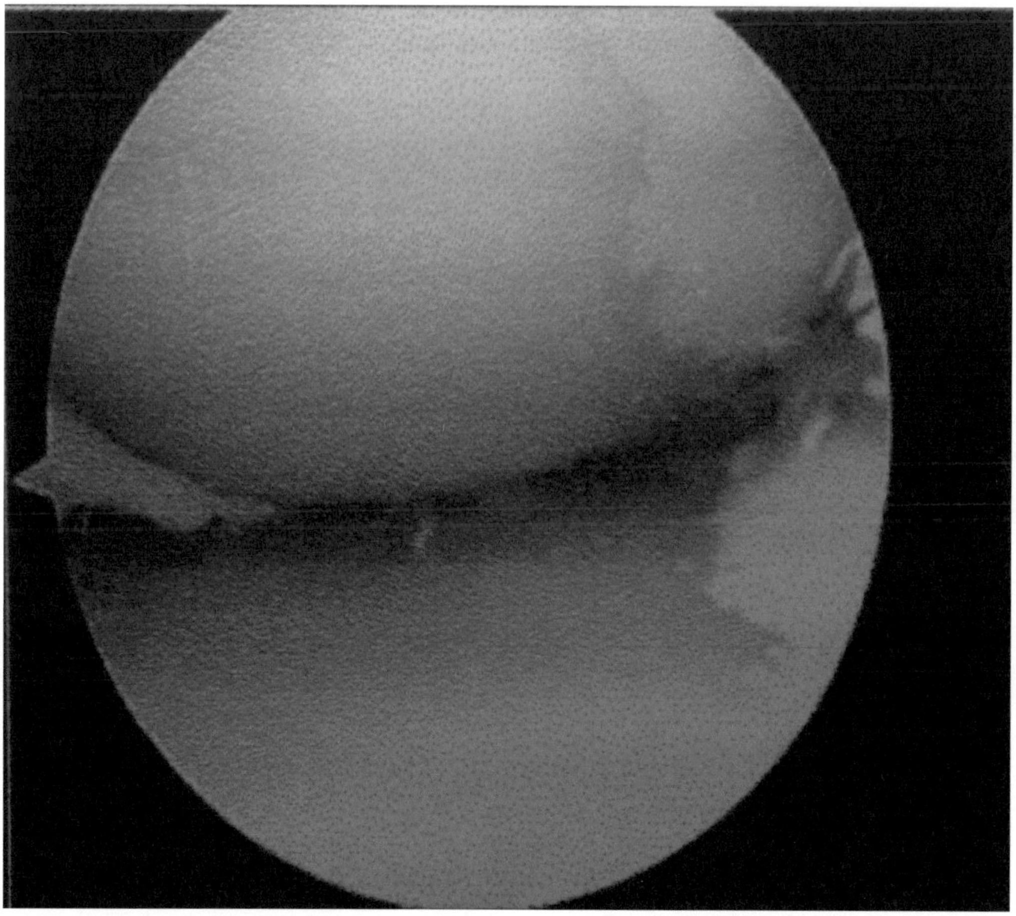

Fig. 7. Scar Tissue within joint space.

3. Patella clunk syndrome

This condition was first described by Insall in 1982 who termed it as "peripatellar nodule" caused by peripatellar soft-tissue impingement against the anterior margin of the intercondylar box of the femoral component". The term "patellar clunk syndrome" however was coined by Hozack in 1989 who described the pathology as a prominent fibrous nodule at the junction of the proximal patellar pole and the quadriceps tendon which wedged into the inter-condylar notch during flexion and dislodged during extension, generating the symptoms. Thorpe and Bocell described a syndrome of similar presentation in 1990. The symptoms they described were "painful and usually visible popping, catching, or locking in the patello-femoral articulation as the knee was brought from flexion to extension." They used the term "tethered patella syndrome" to describe this condition. Condition described by Insall, Hozack, and Thorpe is within the spectrum of the same disease entity. It was caused by peripatellar fibrous hyperplasia, especially prominent in the suprapatellar region and the lateral parapatellar gutter. It was actually a spectrum of disease, which ranged from painful crepitation to full-blown patellar clunk syndrome.

3.1

The exact cause of patellar clunk syndrome had not been identified. Most authors believed that it was multi-factorial. The design of prosthesis, extent of surgical trauma, change in joint line, patellar height, patellar thickness, and abnormal patellar tracking has been proposed as possible causes. The presence of unilateral patellar clunk syndrome in a patient with bilateral TKA of the same prosthesis provided a good model in examining this complex situation as some of the variables were controlled (i.e. same patient, same disease, and same prosthesis). The presence of excessive peri-patellar fibrosis is a prerequisite of this syndrome.

3.2

Patellofemoral synovial hyperplasia is a less well-described syndrome, characterized by a more diffuse proliferation of tissue proximal to the patella. Symptoms include pain and crepitus, most prominent during active knee extension from a 90° flexed position during stair climbing or rising from a chair. Knee range of motion (ROM) tends not to be affected and the lack of a discrete "clunk" is also criterion for this diagnosis.

3.3

Typically the syndrome appears 4 - 6 month after knee replacement surgery but the cases have been reported almost up to 4 years after surgical intervention. Posterior stabilized Knees are the ones that are commonly affected possibly due to nature of its design. The cases have been reported in cases where patella have been resurfaced and also in the cases where patella has not been resurfaced. The diagnosis is a clinical one, and the impressive clunking and jumping of the involved patella can often be seen or heard across the examining room. The fibrous nodule tends to lodge into the femoral component inter-condylar notch during flexion and displaces with an audible and often painful clunk at approximately 30° to 45° from full extension. The diagnosis can be reached based on the history and clinical examination although some surgeons may use a Doppler ultrasound to confirm the diagnosis.

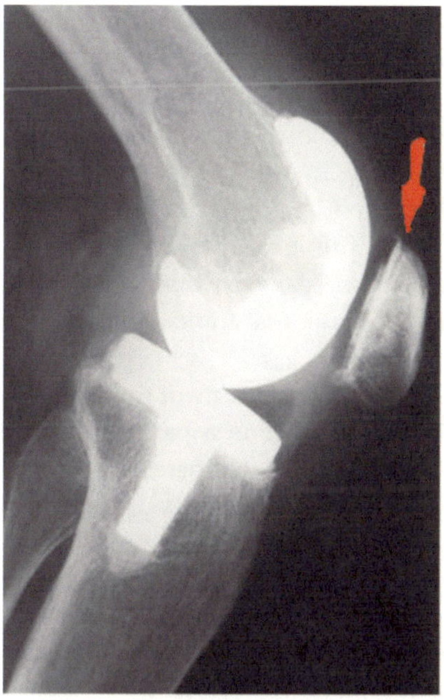

Fig. 8. Arrow denoting a narrow hair thin lucent line at the superior pole of patella. Also note that patella at the lower pole is thicker than the upper pole

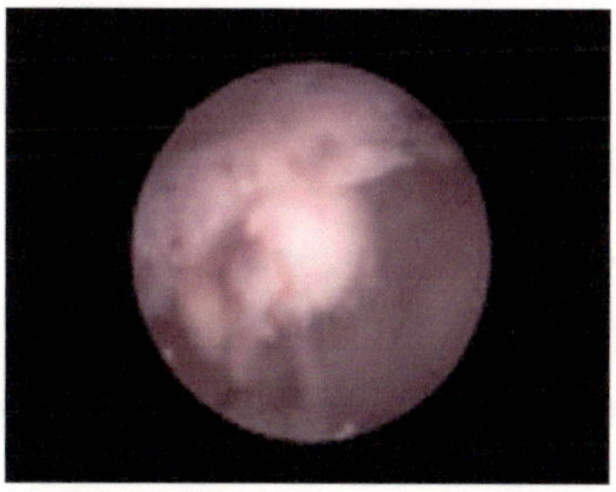

Fig. 9. Arthroscopic image of the nodule at the superior pole of the patella.

3.4 Causes of patellar clunk syndrome

1. Poor Patellar Tracking.
2. Peripatellar Fibrosis
3. Implant Design Related Issues
4. Implant malpositioning.
5. Quadriceps Impingement secondary to superior placement of patellar button.
6. Inadequate synovial tissue debridement at superior pole of patella during primary procedure.

3.5

Before 1990s, post-TKR patellar clunk syndromes were managed by open arthrotomy and excision of the offending fibrous nodule and adhesion. Although it has been effective in treating the symptoms of "clunk" and had successful results without recurrence, there are morbidities associated with this approach such as wound complication and delay in regaining range of motion. The requirement of postoperative analgesics for pain control is higher, and the length of hospitalization is often prolonged.

Advantages of using arthroscopy in treating patellar clunk syndrome included clear visualization of the pathology and few associated complications. The recovery period required for patients to regain full range of motion and normal activity is shorter. However, the synovitis itself could easily be removed with a motorized shaver. On the technical side, the supra-patellar joint space and the medial and lateral gutters are often contracted.

Arthroscopic debridement is an accepted treatment option for both patellar clunk syndrome and synovial hyperplasia; however, there is a paucity of functional outcome data in the literature, especially with respect to synovial hyperplasia.

Adhesions around the knee are usually debribed, first to make room for instrument insertion and then for the subsequent debridement of the dense fibrous nodules. Instrument insertion into the suprapatellar space and parapatellar gutters could therefore avoid causing iatrogenic damage to the surface of the prosthesis. The fibrous nodules are normally tough. Punch forceps and scissors are needed to shred them before the motorized shaver could debride them effectively. Care must be taken to avoid damaging the prosthesis components, as the potential risk of increasing the rate of wear of the prosthesis is theoretically possible.

Takahashi et al. classified the soft tissue impingement under patella after total knee arthroplasty into 3 categories [19]: Patella Clunk Syndrome

Type I	Fibrous firm nodule just proximal to the patella button without the other fibrous tissues causing the impingement
Type II	Impinging hypertrophic synovitis, generalized hypertrophic synovitis without fibrous nodule
Type III	Combination of a fibrous nodule proximal to the patella button and generalized hypertrophic synovitis

Arthroscopic Classification (Thorpe & Bocell): Tethered Patella Syndrome

Type I	Transverse fibrous band at the junction between the patella and quadriceps tendon
Type II	Longitudinal band in the lateral parapatellar gutter
Type III	Band in the infrapatellar region

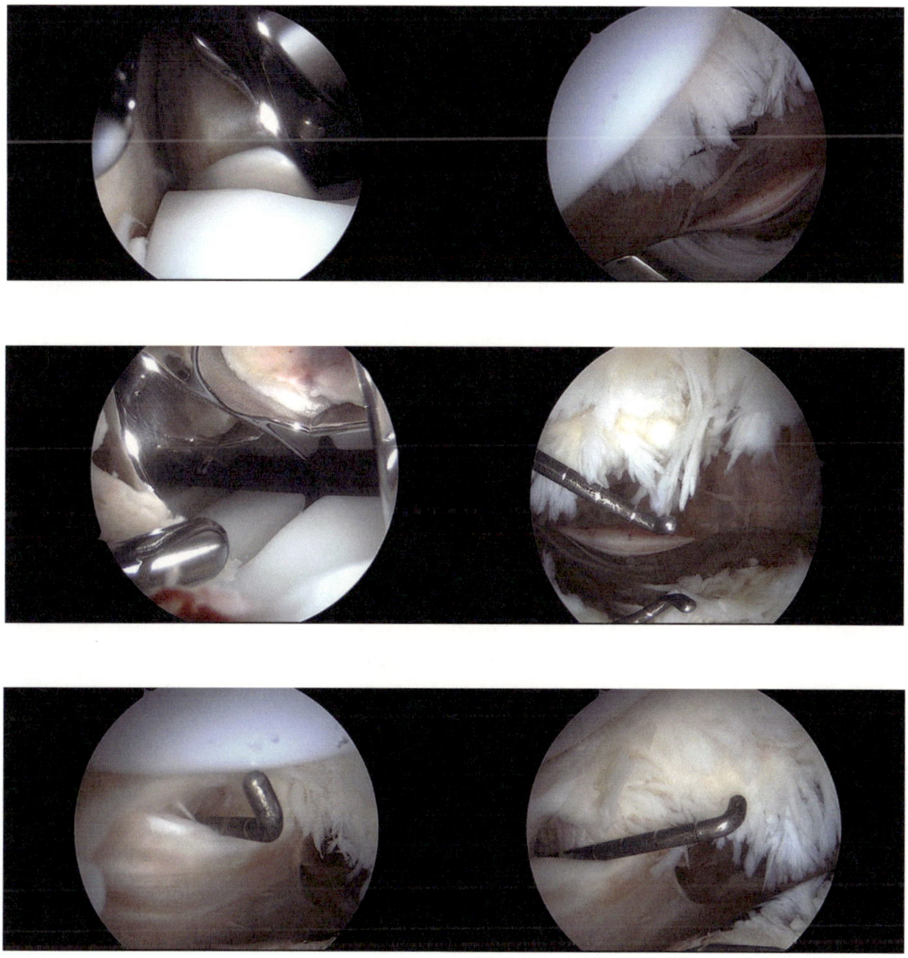

Fig. 10. Arthroscopic sequence of resection of the nodule.

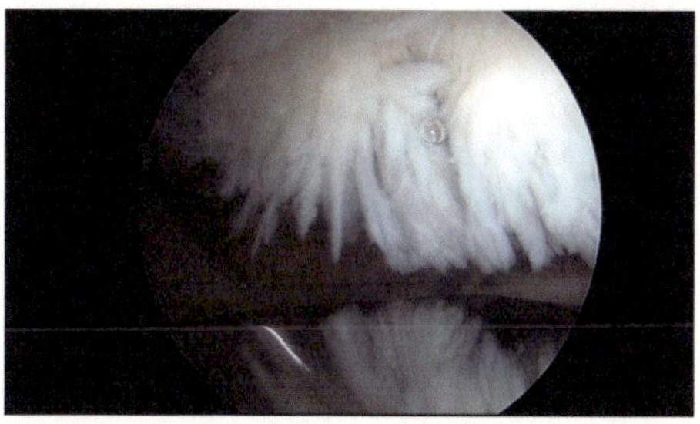

Fig. 11. Appearance after resection of the nodule

4. Posterior cruciate ligament stump impingement

Despite the clinical experience, most patients with symptomatic TKA complain about anterior knee pain, there is small number of patients with posterior knee pain. Although a rare scenario it can be painful and debilitating for the patients with total knee replacements. There is limited evidence in the literature regarding this particular impingement, probably because of difficulty in diagnosing the pathology. Diduch has reported only 4 cases of PCL stump impingement in his study on cruciate substituting knees. The posterior cruciate ligament stump may be quite prominent in the case of posterior cruciate sacrificing (PS) knees and are prone for impingement and interference with cam mechanism. Rarely, PCL impingement as a whole can also be seen after total knee replacement using cruciate retaining prosthesis, especially if the debridement around the notch and PCL is inadequate.

4.1 Pathogenesis

Generally in a routine total knee replacement using cruciate sacrificing prosthesis, removing the PCL makes it easier to balance the collateral ligaments. Since the evolution of high flexion mobile bearing posterior cruciate ligament substituting knee designs, it is necessary to completely resect the PCL. Any residual stump of the PCL may impinge in the cam/spine mechanism causing pain and limited motion. Keeping in mind, resection of the PCL may influence the height of the flexion and extension gaps. It has been postulated, that most likely, it is the postero-medial bundle of PCL stump, which is the main culprit. However, there have been only few reported cases of PCL impingement after cruciate retaining total knee replacements.

4.2 Clinical features

The patients usually come with severe posterior knee pain while flexing of the knee over 70° to 90°, which increases posterior translation of the tibia. This is seen when the PCL stump from the intercondylar notch gets entrapped in the medial tibio-femoral joint, resulting in severe posterior pain. This residual stump can get incarcerated and interfere with cam mechanism of the knee preventing any further flexion.

4.3 Investigations

It is very hard to diagnose PCL stump impingement clinically as the symptoms are not usually typical. Special scans like MRI and CT scans are also of limited value due to their scatter and artifacts associated with metallic implants. However, arthroscopy has an important role in this with regards to both diagnostic and therapeutic significance. If an arthroscopy is performed in these patients, it is recommended a complete inspection of the joint including the posterior compartments as is done in non-TKA patients with posterior knee pain.

4.4 Treatment

Non-operative treatments involve measures for pain relief and frequent visits to the physical therapists. These measures are effective only in few cases, since patients continue to be in a vicious cycle of increasing pain and reduced range of movement. As we know it is usually confirmed only on arthroscopy, it can certainly be treated at the same time. Diduch, in his study, claims 75% success of pain relief after arthroscopic debridement of impinged PCL stump in total knee replacement patients.

4.5 Arthroscopy technique

Literature suggests that on few occasions' additional portals to assist adequate visualization of the posterior compartments and also to avoid iatrogenic damage to prosthetic component in a struggle to see at the back of total knee replacement is required. Although Diduch describes adequate view with standard anterior portals, there are suggestions of posteromedial and posterolateral portals in addition to the standard anterior ones (Landsiedl). Before attempting to see into posterior compartment, it is advised to release or resect any adhesions, which enables complete inspection of the anterior compartment of the knee joint, including soft tissue impingements, evaluation of the inlays and tracking of the patella.

It is recommended, through the standard anteromedial portal, a wide semicircular notchplasty should be performed (diameter of about 8 to 10 mm) in the posterior superolateral region of the notch just above the posterior condyle of the femoral component, to allow entrance of the arthroscope into the posterolateral compartment from the anteromedial portal. Due to the semicircular shape of the notchplasty, the arthroscope and the resecting instruments are mobile and otherwise inaccessible areas can be inspected and treated. A 1.2-mm can be inserted through posterolateral portal into the joint under arthroscopic control. A posterolateral portal is established with a stab incision. After blunt preparation down to the capsule, a working cannula is inserted using a sharp trocar for penetration parallel to the cannula to avoid slipping along the posterolateral capsule, frequently happens with blunt trocars. This usually provides an adequate view of the posterolateral compartment. Impingement of degenerated tissue in flexion can be seen much better from this portal than from the trans-fossa approach. Similarly, posteromedial portal can be established to work your way around the PCL stump. After resection of the PCL stump and its posterior synovial sheath, the posteromedial compartment can be inspected completely using the anteromedial or posterolateral portals.

4.6 Technical challenges

Technical problems lay in mirror images with problems in orientation, and the possibility of damaging the components by manipulation of the optic sheet or motorized instruments. The key points are the exact location of the portals and a smooth introduction of the trocar. For orientation, the use of a probe is mandatory to distinguish between reality and mirror image. The use of additional portals helps to avoid damaging the prosthesis components, especially by using motorized shavers and visualizing the tracing behavior of the patella. Alterations to the surface of cobalt-chromium femoral components can occur during arthroscopy with stainless-steel cannulae. Damage and degradation of the articulating surfaces of a total knee replacement have been associated with release of wear debris. There is a correlation between surface roughness of cobalt-chromium femoral components and polyethylene wear of the tibial component. In addition, studies have shown extensive foreign-body giant-cell reactions to polyethylene particles and synovial membrane reactions to loose cobalt chromium particles. To avoid this Raab recommends the use of plastic cannulae instead of metallic ones.

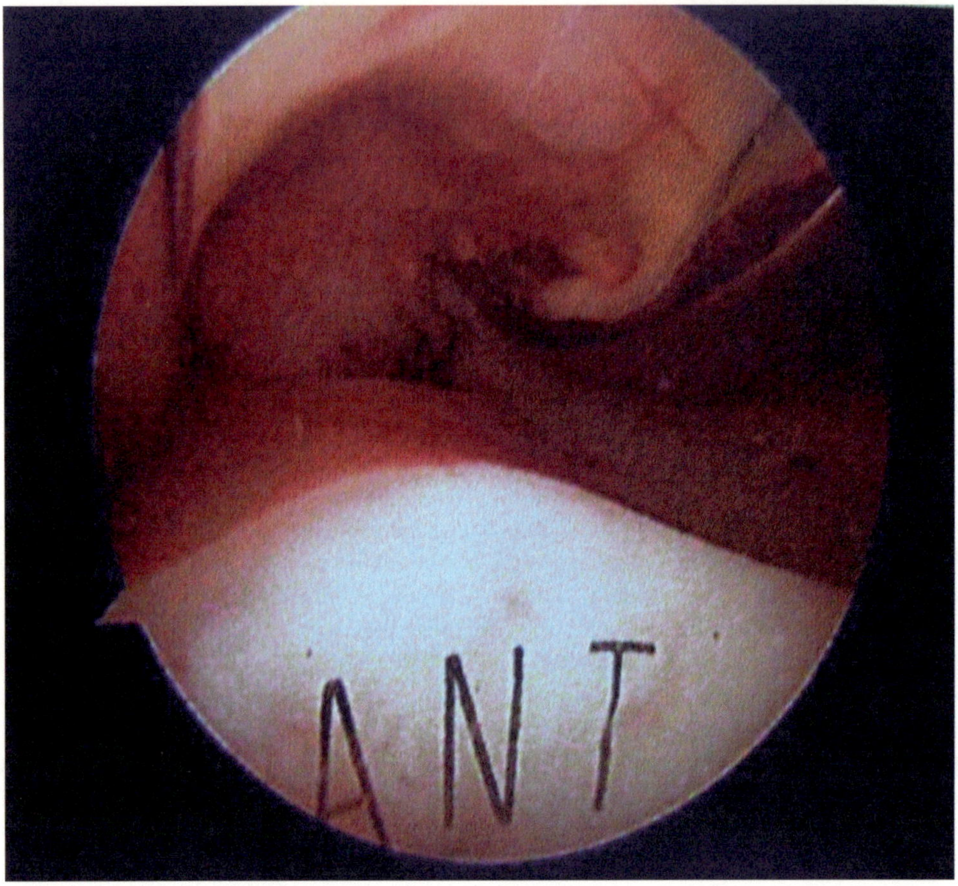

Fig. 12. PCL impingement seen during arthroscopic examination of PCL retaining prosthesis.

5. References

[1] Daumer KM, Khan AU, Steinbeck MJ. Chlorination of pyridinium compounds. Possible role of hypochlorite, N-chloramines, and chlorine in the oxidation of pyridinoline cross-links of articular cartilage collagen type II during acute inflammation. J Biol Chem. 2000; 275:34681-92

[2] Xavier S, Piek E, Fujii M, Javelaud D, Mauviel A, Flanders KC, Samuni AM, Felici A, Reiss M, Yarkoni S, Sowers A, Mitchell JB, Roberts AB, Russo A. Amelioration of radiation-induced fibrosis: inhibition of transforming growth factor-beta signaling by halofuginone. J Biol Chem. 2004; 279:15167-76.

[3] Diamond JR, Ricardo SD, Klahr S. Mechanisms of interstitial fibrosis in obstructive nephropathy. Semin Nephrol. 1998; 18:594-602
[4] Poli G, Parola M. Oxidative damage and fibrogenesis. Free Radic Biol Med. 1997; 22:287-305
[5] Swindle EJ, Hunt JA, Coleman JW. A comparison of reactive oxygen species generation by rat peritoneal macrophages and mast cells using the highly sensitive real-time chemiluminescent probe pholasin: inhibition of antigen-induced mast cell degranulation by macrophage-derived hydrogen peroxide. J Immunol. 2002; 169:5866-73.
[6] Baran CP, Zeigler MM, Tridandapani S, Marsh CB. The role of ROS and RNS in regulating life and death of blood monocytes. Curr Pharm Des. 2004; 10:855-66.
[7] Jackson RW. The role of arthroscopy in the management of the arthritic knee. Clin Orthop. 1974;101:28–35.
[8] Sprague N, O'Connor RL, Fox JM. Arthroscopic treatment of postoperative knee fibroarthrosis. Clin Orthop. 1982; 166:165–172.
[9] Jens G. Boldt, Urs K. Munzinger, Arthrofibrosis Associated with Total Knee Arthroplasty: Gray-Scale and Power Doppler Sonographic Findings AJR 2004;182:337–340
[10] Giovagnorio F, Martinoli C, Coari G. Power Doppler ultrasonography in knee arthritis: a pilot study. Rheumatol Int 2001; 20:101–104
[11] Scranton PE Jr: Management of knee pain and stiffness after total knee arthroplasty. J Arthroplasty 2001; 16:428-435
[12] Brassard MF, Scuderi GR: Complications of total knee arthroplasty, in Insall JN, Scott WN (eds): Surgery of the Knee, ed 3. New York, NY: Churchill Livingstone, 2001, pp 1814-1816
[13] Fox JL, Poss R: The role of manipulation following total knee replacement. J Bone Joint Surg Am 1981; 63:357-362
[14] Shoji H, Solomonow M, Yoshino S, D'Ambrosia R, Dabezies E: Factors affecting postoperative flexion in total knee arthroplasty. Orthopedics 1990; 13: 643-649
[15] Sprague NF III, O'Connor RL, Fox JM: Arthroscopic treatment of postoperative knee fibroarthrosis. Clin Orthop 1982; 166:165-172.
[16] Sprague NF III: Motion-limiting arthrofibrosis of the knee: The role of arthroscopic management. Clin Sports Med 1987; 6:537-549.
[17] Bocell JR, Thorpe CD, Tullos HS: Arthroscopic treatment of symptomatic total knee arthroplasty. Clin Orthop 1991; 271:125-134.
[18] Campbell ED Jr: Arthroscopy in total knee replacements. Arthroscopy 1987; 3: 31-35
[19] Diduch DR, Scuderi GR, Scott WN, Insall JN, Kelly MA: The efficacy of arthroscopy following total knee replacement. Arthroscopy 1997; 13:166-171.
[20] Bae DK, Lee HK, Cho JH: Arthroscopy of symptomatic total knee replacements. Arthroscopy 1995; 11:664-671
[21] Williams RJ III, Westrich GH, Siegel J, Windsor RE: Arthroscopic release of the posterior cruciate ligament for stiff total knee arthroplasty. Clin Orthop 1996; 331:185-191

[22] Kim DH, Gill TJ, Millett PJ: Arthroscopic treatment of the arthrofibrotic knee. *Arthroscopy* 2004;20(suppl 2): 187-194.

[23] Millett PJ, Williams RJ III, Wickiewicz TL: Open debridement and soft tissue release as a salvage procedure for the severely arthrofibrotic knee. *Am J Sports Med* 1999;27:552-561

[24] Beight JL, Yao B, Hozack WJ, et al: The patellar clunk syndrome after posterior stabilized total knee arthroplasty. CORR 299:139, 1994

[25] Hozack WJ, Rothman RH, Booth RE, et al: The patellar clunk syndrome: a complication of posterior stabilized total knee arthroplasty. CORR 241:203, 1989

[26] Diduch DR, Scudeii GR, Scott WN, et al: The efficacy of arthroscopy following total knee replacement. Arthroscopy 13:166, 1997

[27] Insall JN, Lachiewicz F, Burstein AH: The posterior stabilized condylar design. Two to four year clinical experience. J Bone Joint Surg A 64A: 1317, 1982

[28] Thorpe CD, Bocell JR, Tullos HS: Intra-articular fibrous bands patellar complications after total knee replacement. J Bone Joint Surg A 72A:811, 1990

[29] Bocell JR, Thorpe CD, Tullos HS: Arthroscopic treatment of symptomative total knee arthroplasty. CORR 271:125, 1991

[30] Lintner DM, Bocell JR, Tullos HS: Arthroscopic treatment of intraarticular fibrous band after total knee arthroplasty. A follow-up note. CORR 309:230, 1994

[31] Figgie HE, Goldberg VM, Heiple KG, et al: The Influence of tibial-patellofemoral location on function of the knee in patients with the posterior stabilized condylar knee prosthesis. J Bone Joint Surg A 68A:1030, 1986

[32] Insall JN, Salvati E: Patella position in the normal knee joint. Radiology 101:101, 1971

[33] Okamoto T, Fukani H, Atsui K, Fukunishi S, Koezuka A, Maruo S (2002) Sonographic appearance of fibrous nodules in patellar clunk syndrome: a case report. J Orthop Sci 7:590–593

[34] Scott RD, Volatile TB (1986) 12 years experience with posterior cruciate retaining total knee arthroplasty. Clin Orthop 205: 100–107

[35] Sculco TP, Martucci EA (2001) Knee arthroplasty, chapter 6. Patellofemoral joint. Springer, Berlin Heidelberg New York

[36] Shoji H, Shimozaki E (1996) Patellar clunk syndrome in total knee arthroplasty without patella resurfacing. J Arthroplasty 11:198–201

[37] Vertullo CJ, Easley ME, Scott N, Insall JN (2001) Mobile bearings in primary knee arthroplasty. J Am Acad Orthop Surg 9: 335–364 602

[38] Callaghan JJ, Insall JN, Greenwald AS (2000) Mobile-bearing knee replacement: concepts and results. J Bone Joint Surg Am 82:1020–1041

[39] Pollock DC, Ammeen DJ, Engh GA. Synovial entrapment: a complication of posterior-stabilized total knee arthroplasty. J Bone Joint Surg 2002; 84A:2174.

[40] Takahashi M, Miyamoto S, Nagano A. Arthroscopic treatment of soft-tissue impingement under the patella after total knee arthroplasty. Arthroscopy 2002; 18:E20.

[41] Brassard MF, Insall JN, Scuderi GR. Complications of total knee arthroplasty. In: Insall JN, Scott WN, editors. Surgery of the Knee. 4th ed. New York: Churchill Livingstone; 2006. p. 1752–3.

[42] Ip D, Wu WC, Tsang WL. Comparison of two total knee prosthesis on the incidence of patella clunk syndrome. Int Orthop 2002;26:48–51.
[43] Anderson MJ, Becker DL, Kieckbusch T. Patellofemoral complications after posterior-stabilized total knee arthroplasty: a comparison of 2 different implant designs. J Arthroplasty 2002; 17:422–6.
[44] Lucas TS, DeLuca PF, Nazarian DG, et al. Arthroscopic treatment of patellar clunk. Clin Orthop 1999; 367:226.
[45] Clarke HD, Fuchs R, Scuderi GR, et al. The influence of femoral component design in the elimination of patellar clunk in posterior-stabilized total knee arthroplasty. J Arthroplasty 2006; 21:167.
[46] Lonner J, Jasko J, Bezwada H, et al. Incidence of patellar clunk with a modern posterior-stabilized knee design. Am J Orthop 2007; 36: 550.
[47] Maloney WJ, Schmidt R, Sculco TP. Femoral component design and patellar clunk syndrome. Clin Orthop 2003; 410: 199.
[48] Yau WP, Wong JWK, Chiu KY, Ng TP, Tang WM. Patellar clunk syndrome after posterior stabilized total knee arthroplasty. J Arthroplasty 2003; 18: 1023–8.
[49] Larson CM, Lachiewicz PF. Patellofemoral complications with the Insall Burstein II posterior-stabilized total knee arthroplasty. J Arthroplasty 1999; 14: 288–92.
[50] Sringari T, Maheswaran SS. Patellar clunk syndrome in patellofemoral arthroplasty—a case report. Knee 2005; 12: 456–7.
[51] Vernace JV, Rothman RH, Booth RE. Arthroscopic management of the patellar clunk syndrome following posterior stabilized total knee arthroplasty. J Arthroplasty 1989;4:179–82
[52] Ranawat AS, Ranawat CS, Slamin JE, Slamin JE, Dennis DA. Patellar crepitation in the P.F.C. sigma total knee system. Orthopedics 2006; 29: S68–70.
[53] Diduch. D, Giles. R. The efficacy of arthroscopy following total knee replacement. Arthroscopy: The Journal of Arthroscopic and Related Surgery, Vol 13, No 2 (April), 1997
[54] Franz Landsiedl, M.D., Nicolas Aigner. A New Arthroscopic Technique for Revision of the Posterior Compartment in Symptomatic Total Knee Arthroplasty; Arthroscopy: The Journal of Arthroscopic and Related Surgery, Vol 21, No 4 (April), 2005
[55] Dowson D, Taheri S, Wallbridge N. The role of counterface imperfections in the wear of polyethylene. Wear. 1987; 119:277.
[56] Hood RW, Wright TM, Burstein AH. Retrieval analysis of total knee prostheses: a method and its application to 48 total condylar prostheses. J Biomed Mater Res. 1983;17:829-42.
[57] Levesque M, Livingston BJ, Jones WM, Spector M. Scratches on condyles in normal functioning total knee arthroplasty. Trans Orthop Res Soc. 1998;23:247.
[58] Howie DW, Vernon-Roberts B. The synovial response to intraarticular cobaltchrome wear particles. Clin Orthop. 1988; 232:244-54.
[59] Mintz L, Tsao AK, McCrae CR, Stulberg SD, Wright T. The arthroscopic evaluation and characteristics of severe polyethylene wear in total knee arthroplasty. Clin Orthop. 1991; 273:215-22.

[60] Damage to Cobalt-Chromium Surfaces During Arthroscopy of Total Knee Replacements, Raab, G, Christopher, J, The Journal of Bones and Joint Surgery, Vol 83-A · Number 1 · January 2001

12

Arthroscopic Soft Tissue Releases of the Knee

Michael R. Chen and Jason L. Dragoo
Stanford University Department of Orthopaedic Surgery, USA

1. Introduction

Intra-articular fibrosis, which includes a family of disorders such as anterior interval scarring, posterior capsular contracture, a tight lateral retinaculum, as well as arthrofibrosis, may lead to alterations in joint biomechanics and can result in pain. 1, 2, 3 Specific releases for each region of fibrosis, along with characteristic physical examination findings, have been described. Familiarity with the diagnosis and arthroscopic treatment of these disorders may lead to improved treatment outcomes in this patient population.

2. Anterior interval release

2.1 History and physical examination

The anterior interval has been defined as the space between the infrapatellar fat pad and patellar tendon anteriorly, and the anterior border of the tibia and transverse meniscal ligament posteriorly.1 Trauma or previous surgery may cause hemorrhage or inflammation of the fat pad (Hoffa's Syndrome), which may be followed by fibrosis. If fibrosis occurs between the fat pad and transverse ligament or anterior tibia, it will lead to dysfunction of the anterior knee structures, such as decreased excursion of the patellar tendon and result in stretching of the surrounding synovial tissue, which may lead to pain or even loss of knee extension. 1 Fibrosis within the anterior interval can exist on a spectrum of severity. Paulos et al. described infrapatellar contracture syndrome, a severe form of anterior interval scarring, with fibrosis of the fat pad and severe limitations in range of motion. 5

Patients with anterior interval scarring complain of anterior knee pain, and frequently describe a sense of fullness within the knee, especially with extension. Physical examination may demonstrate a small flexion contracture, decreased proximal excursion of the patella, as well as a positive Hoffa's test 1. Hoffa's test is performed by placing the thumb at the margin of the infrapatellar fat pad and patellar tendon medially and laterally with the knee flexed at 30° (Figure 1). Pressure is applied with the thumb, and the knee is fully extended. Increased pain in the fat pad with knee extension indicates a positive result. Patients may also have pain in the fat pad with forceful hyperextension of the knee. The patellar tendon and patella should also be carefully examined to ensure they are not also causes of the anterior knee pain.

Scarring in the fat pad can be visualized on standard T1- and T2-weighted magnetic resonance imaging (MRI). Low T1- and T2- signal identified on sagittal images coursing from the posterior portion of the fat pad to the anterior surface of the tibia and/or transverse meniscal ligament indicates anterior interval scarring.

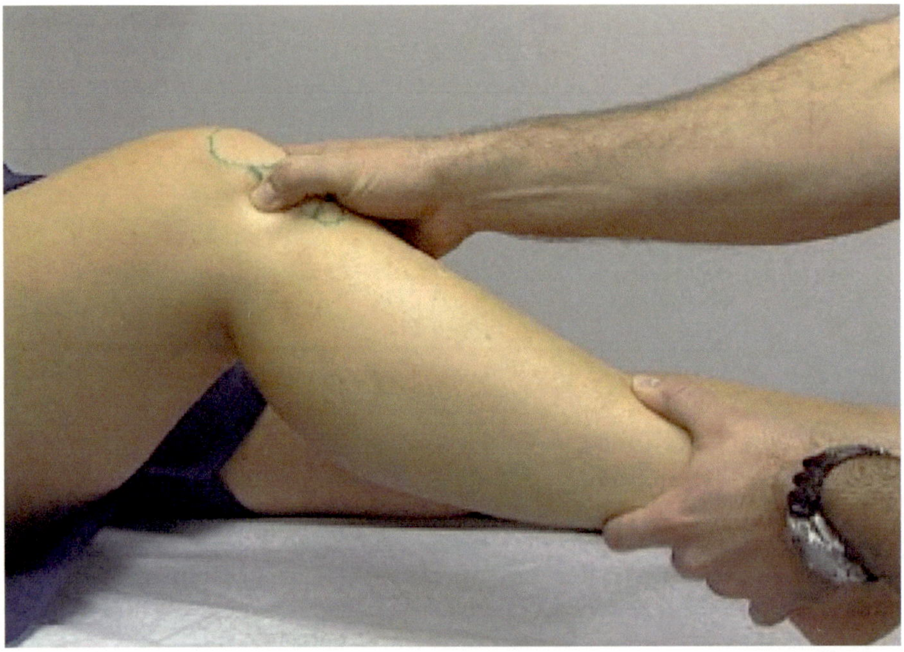

Figure 1A

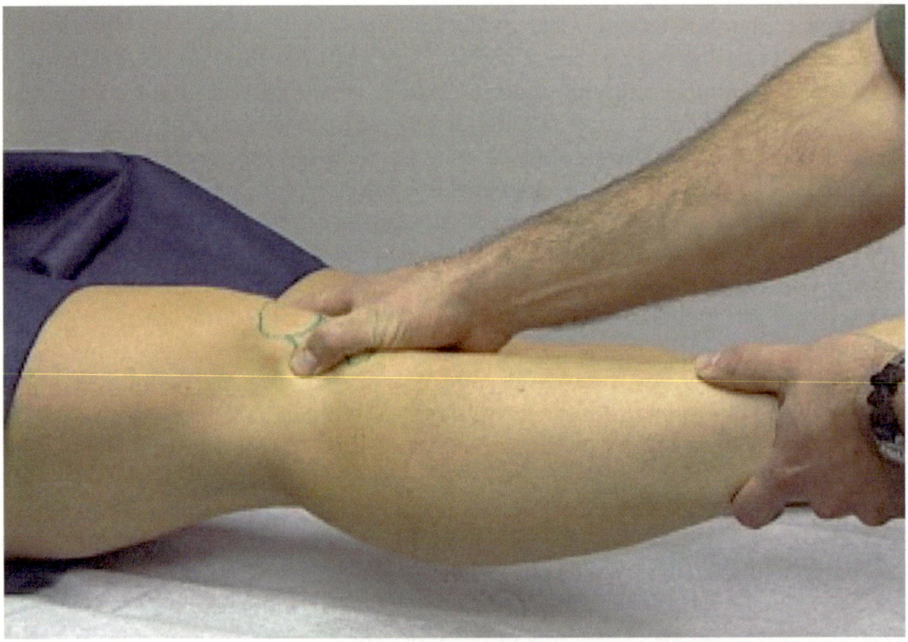

Figure 1B

Fig. 1. Demonstration of Hoffa's test. A, The thumb is placed at the margin of the infrapatellar fat pad and the patellar tendon with the knee in 30° of flexion. B, Pressure is applied with the thumb and the knee and then brought into full extension. Increased pain in the fat pad indicates a positive result.

2.2 Anterior interval release

Arthroscopic treatment of anterior interval scarring begins with establishment of a modified anterolateral viewing portal. The portal is established slightly more lateral and proximal to the standard placement to allow easier visualization of the anterior interval structures (Figure 2). Viewing of anterior interval scarring with the 30º arthroscope will demonstrate decreased opening of the interval with extension as well as fibrosis of the infrapatellar fat pad.

Fibrosis can be released with use of a 70º electrothermal probe via a modified anteromedial portal (Figure 2). Systematic release begins anterior to the transverse ligament, starting just anterior to the anterior horn of the medial meniscus, and proceeding laterally and anterior to the anterior horn of the lateral meniscus (Figure 3). The release is continued until the anterior tibial cortex in encountered or until normal fat pad tissue is seen. Adequate release is confirmed by visualization of interval widening with knee extension and closing with flexion. Care is taken to avoid disrupting the anterior meniscal attachments or the transverse meniscal ligament. Meticulous hemostasis is obtained to prevent postoperative bleeding and recurrent scarring 1.

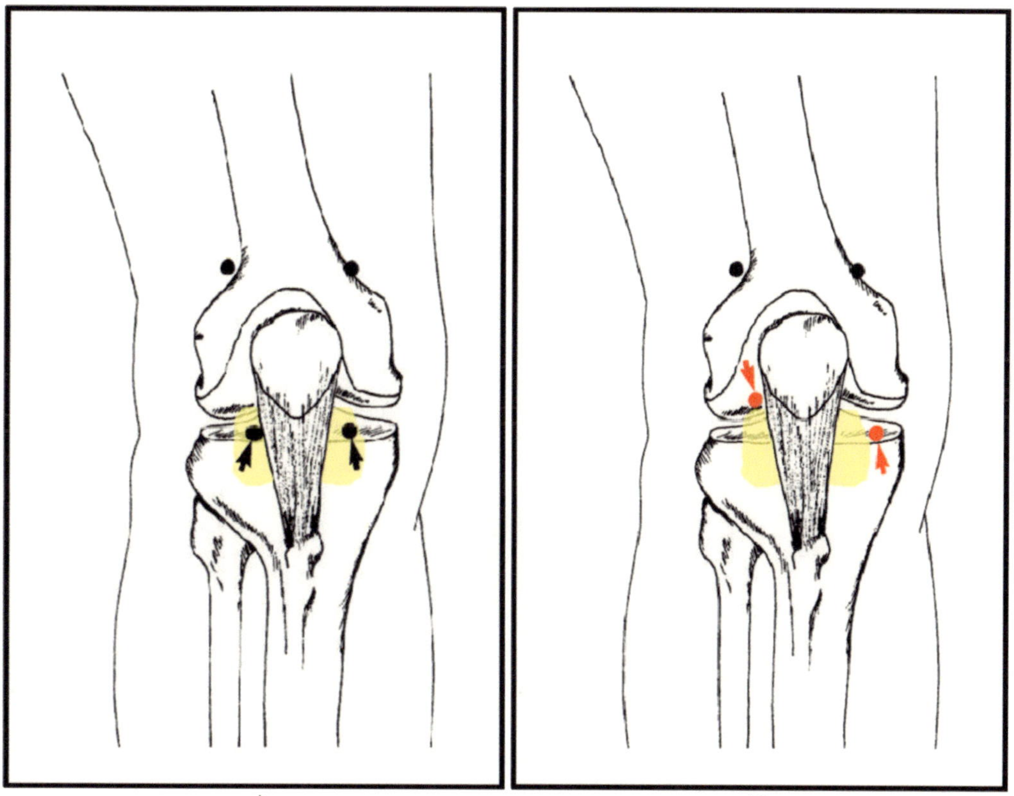

A B

Fig. 2. Modified arthroscopic portals for anterior interval release. A, Standard arthroscopic portals. B, The modified anterolateral portal established slightly more lateral and proximal to the standard placement to allow easier visualization of the anterior interval and the modified anteromedial portal established more medial to allow instrumentation of the anterior interval.

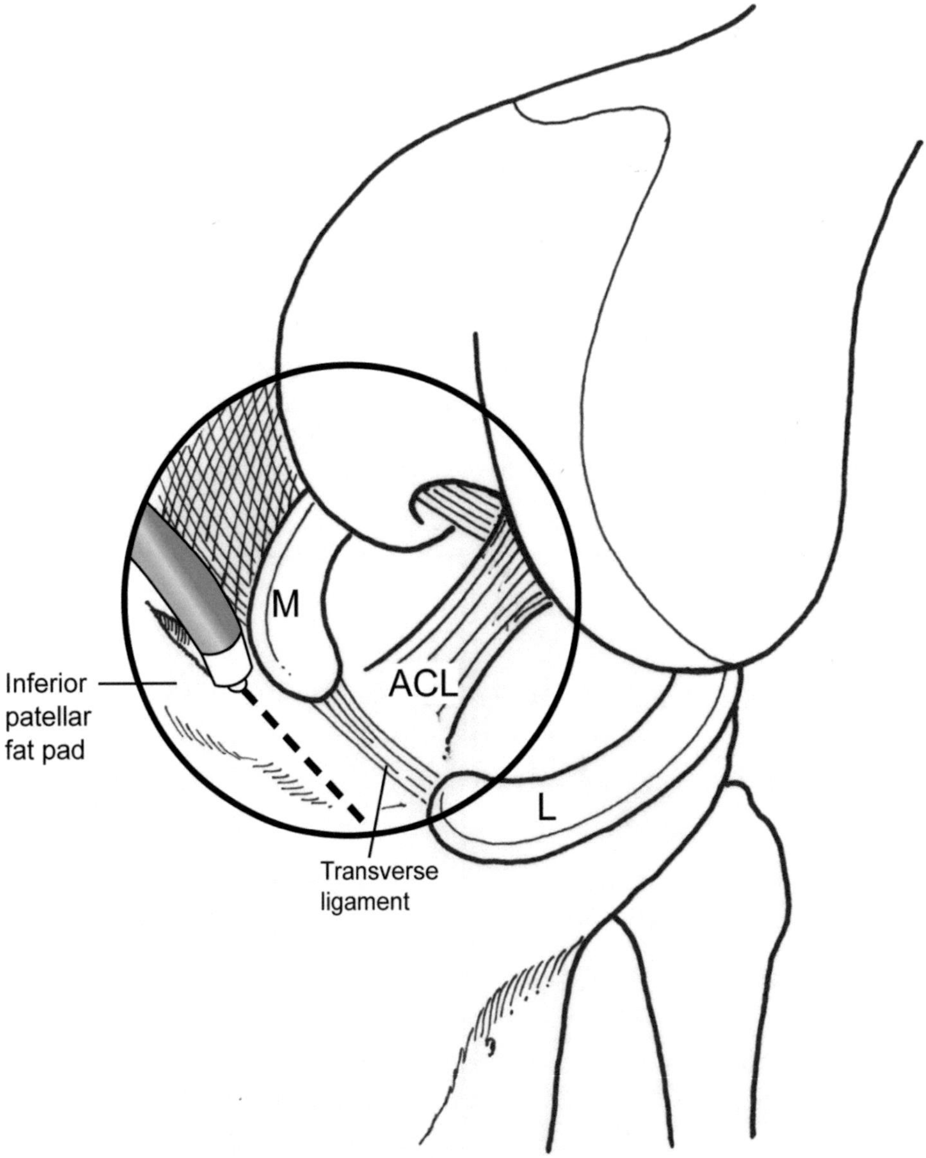

Fig. 3. Location of anterior interval release. The release is made anterior to the transverse meniscal ligament and proceeds anterior to the anterior horn of the medial and lateral meniscus.

Postoperatively, the goal is to prevent scar reformation, while preserving joint mobility. Initially, rehabilitation is focused on establishing full range of motion and patellar and patellar tendon mobility. Patients are limited to touch-down weight bearing for 2 weeks to limit inflammation and to maximize interval excursion. 4 Patients are also usually prescribed anti-inflammatory medications for 4 to 6 weeks following surgery. After 6 weeks, the goal is the return functional strength followed by sports specific exercise and gradual return to sport.

2.3 Results

Steadman et al 1 described the results of isolated anterior interval release in twenty-five consecutive patients. Patients failed a minimum of six months of physical therapy and non-steroidal anti-inflammatory medications. Following arthroscopic release, the average Lysholm score significantly improved from 59 preoperatively to 81 postoperatively, while the average International Knee Documentation Committee (IKDC) score improved from 49 to 70. Four patients had failed results, requiring a second surgical release. Ogilvie-Harris and Giddens described arthroscopic resection of the infrapatellar fat pad in patients with Hoffa's syndrome. 6 Patients had significant improvement in symptoms and function after surgery at an average follow-up of 76 months.

Conversely, patients with severe scarring, or infrapatellar contracture syndrome, had symptoms of patellofemoral arthritis and tibiofemoral arthritis and could not return to pre-injury sport or work despite improvements in range of motion after arthroscopic and open treatment. 5

3. Posterior capsular release

3.1 History and physical examination

Flexion contractures are one of the main factors that adversely affect patient outcome and knee function following surgery. 5, 7, 8 A 5° loss of extension can cause a noticeable limp during ambulation and patellofemoral irritability, and a loss of 10° is poorly tolerated. 3 Deficits greater than 20° result in a significant leg-length discrepancy. 8 Contracture of the posterior capsule is the primary cause of extension loss, however anterior interval scarring, patellar entrapment, anterior cruciate ligament (ACL) graft malposition and hamstring tightness can also contribute. 5, 7, 8, 9

Patients with an extension deficit should be systematically evaluated for the multiple potential causes of a flexion contracture. A thorough history of any trauma or surgical procedures should be obtained. Knee range of motion should be carefully measured and the quality of the endpoint should be recorded. Flexion contractures exhibiting a firm endpoint tend to involve the posterior capsule, while a spongier endpoint typically indicates involvement of the patellofemoral mechanism or anterior interval.

MRI is the imaging modality of choice. Thickening or scarring of the posterior capsule, indicated by low T1 and T2 signal, may sometimes be observed.

3.2 Posterior capsular release

Surgical intervention is indicated in a patient with a 10-15 degree flexion contracture with an unyielding endpoint that has failed non-operative management, 10 however even smaller degrees of contracture may not be tolerated in the elite athletic population. Both open 9,10,11 and arthroscopic posterior capsular releases 12,13 have been described, however arthroscopic releases are more technically demanding.

The patient is positioned for standard arthroscopy, however the contralateral leg is placed in a well-leg holder and the foot of the bed is dropped. Care should be taken to place the tourniquet high on the thigh to allow adequate draping for the creation of a posteromedial and/or posterolateral portal (Figure 4). An arthroscopic pump is generally recommended to maintain a constant intra-articular pressure and ensure distension of the posterior capsule. Anterolateral and anteromedial arthroscopic portals are created near the edge of the patellar tendon to allow instrumentation to be used in the posterior compartment.

The posteromedial compartment is visualized with a 30° arthroscope via the anterolateral portal by placing it between the medial femoral condyle and posterior cruciate ligament (PCL). 12 Often, a blunt arthroscopic obturator must first be used to break through scar tissue or adhesions, prior to inserting the arthroscope. 12 A spinal needle is placed under direct visualization from the posteromedial skin through the posteromedial capsule to localize the posteromedial arthroscopic portal (Figure 4). The portal is then created by making a small incision and advancing an arthroscopic cannula through the incision into the posteromedial compartment under direct visualization. Similarly, the arthroscope may be placed between the ACL and lateral femoral condyle to visualize the posterolateral compartment. A posterolateral portal can be created in a similar manner; however care must be taken to avoid the peroneal nerve, which lies on the posteromedial border of the biceps tendon. Incision must be anterior to the biceps and blunt dissection must be performed during portal placement.

Two methods of arthroscopic capsular release have been described. Laprade et al. 12 described an isolated posteromedial release for flexion contractures. Separation of the posteromedial capsule from the posteromedial structures, including the medial gastrocnemius tendon and muscle, using a blunt arthroscopic obturator or a small periosteal elevator was recommended. An arthroscopic basket punch and shaver, with the shaver blade facing anteriorly, are then used to release the posteromedial capsule. The procedure

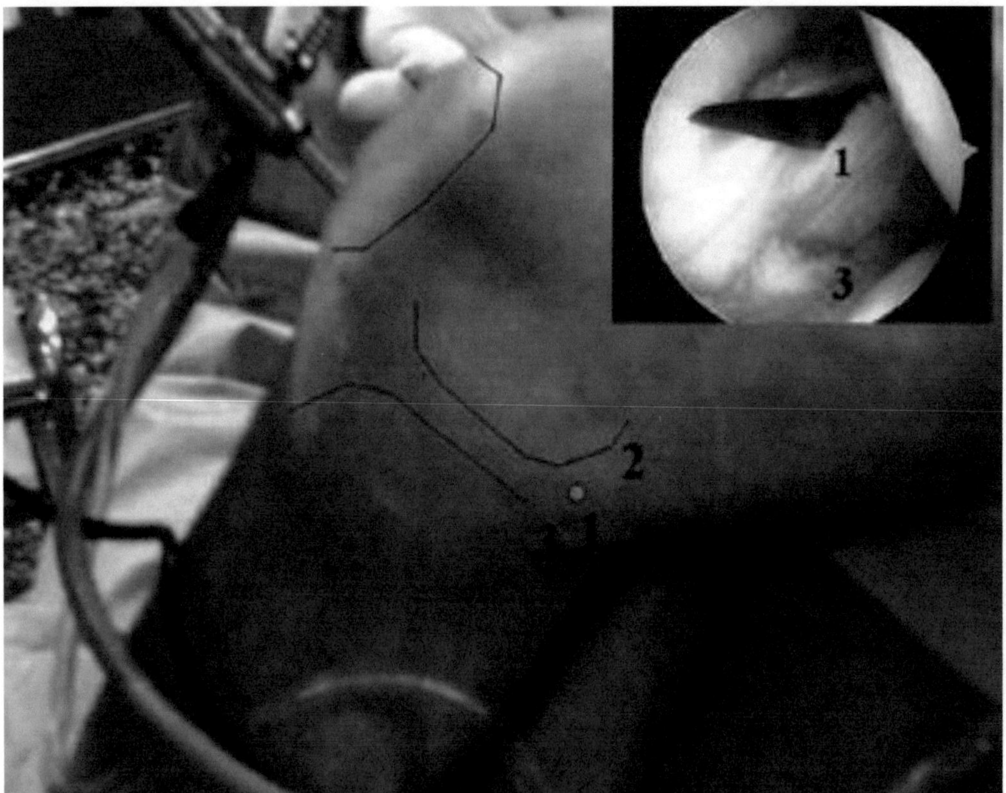

Figure 4A

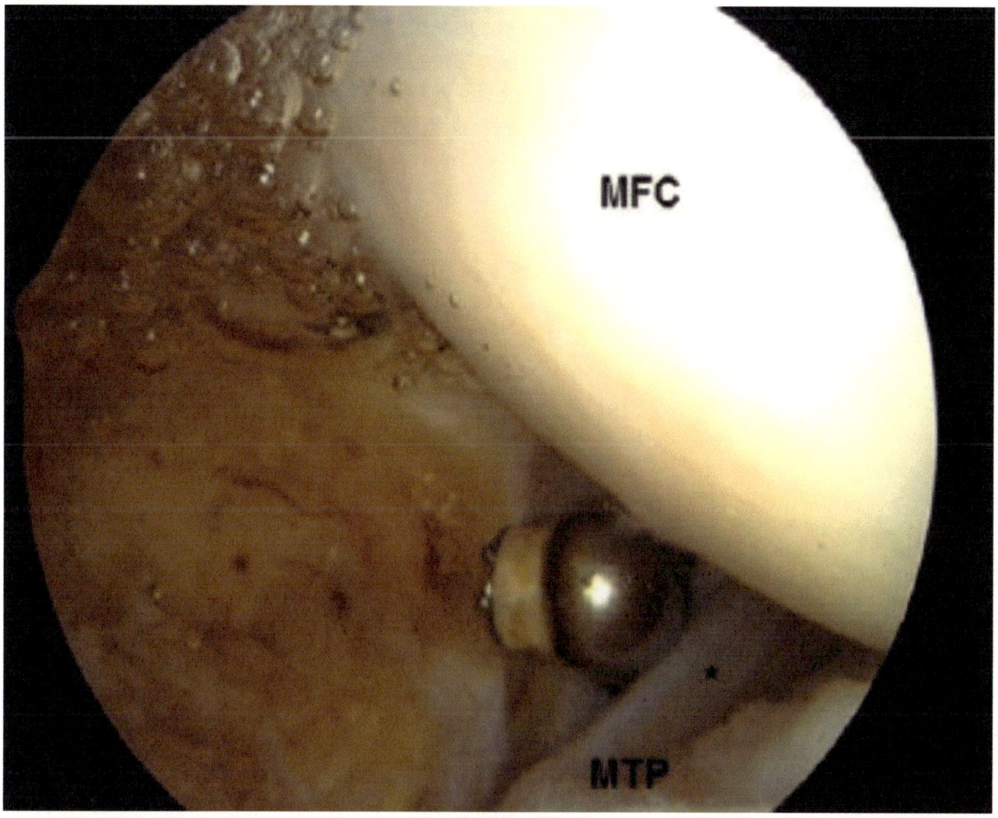

Figure 4B

Fig. 4. Posteromedial arthroscopic portal. A, The entry site (1) is between the posterior medial femoral condyle (2) and posterior medial tibial plateau (3) and created under direct visualization. B, View from the posterolateral portal toward the posteromedial aspect of the knee during capsular release. MFC: medial femoral condyle. MTP: medial tibial plateau.

starts medially and proceeds laterally to the midline, in line with the PCL at the mid-capsular level. The gastrocnemius muscle and tendon become visible as the capsule is released.

Mariani 13 described posteromedial and posterolateral arthroscopic capsular releases. The arthroscope may be placed in either posteromedial or posterolateral portals to visualize the contralateral compartment. Often there is a posterior septum that must first be released. A blunt trocar may be used to perforate the septum and then expanded with a shaver or radiofrequency probe. Posterior adhesions are removed until the femoral condyles become visible. A punch or radiofrequency probe is then directed toward the superior capsular attachments at the condyle. The capsule is then progressively released. The tendon of the gastrocnemius is then recognized and can also be released to allow for a greater posterior release.

Postoperatively, patients may be admitted to the hospital for pain management and initial physical therapy. An indwelling epidural catheter is often beneficial, in addition to oral and intravenous analgesics. Early, aggressive physical therapy is begun on the first postoperative day. A continuous passive motion machine is used and is alternated in cycles with extension splinting. Patients are advanced to weight bearing as tolerated and weaned from crutches when they are able to ambulate pain free. Patients are also placed on deep venous thrombosis prophylaxis for two weeks. At discharge, patients continue with outpatient physical therapy and nighttime extension splinting for at least 6 weeks.

3.3 Results

Laprade et al 12 reported the results of isolated arthroscopic posteromedial release in 15 patients with an average follow-up of 24 months. Preoperative knee extension averaged 15° and significantly improved to 0.7° at the final follow-up.

Mariani 13 reported the results of arthroscopic posterior capsular release in 18 patients. Extension deficits averaged 34° preoperatively and improved to 3° at final one year follow-up. Patients with more severe pre-operative flexion contractures need more aggressive releases of *both* the posteromedial and posterolateral capsule and possibly partial release of the gastrocnemius tendon if the results are not adequate.

4. Lateral retinacular release

4.1 History and physical examination

The patellofemoral joint is an intrinsically unstable articulation, stabilized dynamically by the vastus medialis obliqus (VMO) and statically by the medial patellofemoral ligament and lateral retinaculum. 14, 15, 16 Imbalance may arise because of weakness in the VMO or tightness from the lateral retinaculum. Axial alignment and bony morphology of the patellofemoral joint may also contribute to this imbalance.

Evaluation of anterior knee pain begins with a history of aggravating factors such as inclined ambulation, squatting, prolonged sitting, or going up and down stairs. If present, patellar instability needs to be identified, as this can affect surgical decision making.

Physical examination begins with inspection of patellar glide, or excursion, which should be examined in all directions. 17 The VMO can be inspected for atrophy or weakness, and the medial and lateral patellar facets should be palpated for tenderness. Patellar tilt should be carefully assessed. 17 The inability to elevate the lateral aspect of the patella to neutral with the knee in full extension and the patella centered in the trochlea indicates a tight lateral retinaculum and possible over-constraint of the patellar mechanism (Figure 5). A patellar apprehension test should also be performed to evaluate for instability at 30° of flexion.

Radiographic evaluation consists of standard weight bearing AP and lateral radiographs of the knee, as well as an axial view of the patellofemoral joint in 30° or 45° of flexion. Patellar tilt and subluxation, as well as trochlear and patellar bony morphology can be evaluated on the axial view. MRIs are not routinely indicated for isolated patellofemoral pathology unless the articular surface warrants evaluation or there is history of patellar instability.

Initial, non-operative treatment generally begins with physical therapy. Specific therapy is aimed at strengthening of the hip external rotators and abductors, VMO and core musculature, as well as patellar mobilization. Patellar taping using the McConnell method may also be beneficial. 18 Surgical intervention is only indicated after failure of non-operative management.

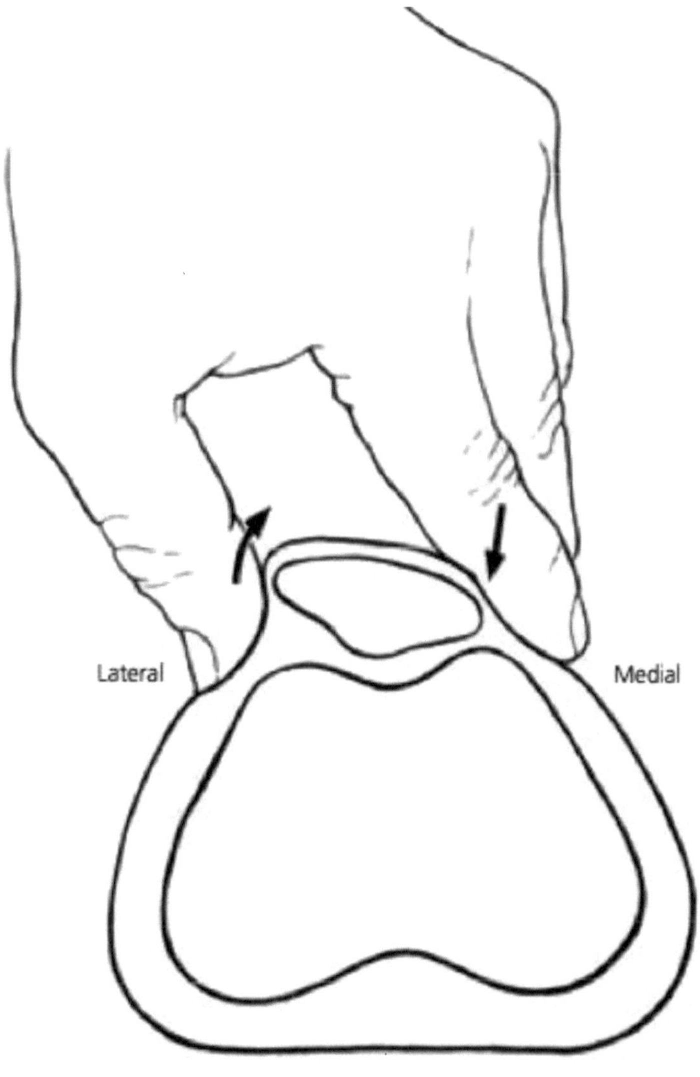

Fig. 5. Patellar tilt test. The patella is centralized in the femoral trochlea with the knee in full extension. The medial and lateral aspect of the patella is stabilized and the lateral aspect is elevated. Inability to elevate the lateral aspect of the patellar to neutral indicates a tight lateral retinaculum.

4.2 Lateral release

Lateral release is indicated in patients who have failed physical therapy and have increased lateral facet pressure demonstrated either radiographically or clinically with a tight lateral retinaculum on tilt testing. 2,18,19 Isolated lateral release is contraindicated for patellar instability. 19,20,21

A tight lateral retinaculum is confirmed on patellar tilt testing once the patient is under anesthesia. 20 Patellar tilt and areas of chondromalacia are also visually assessed and documented arthroscopically.

Modern lateral releases are generally performed using an arthroscopic electrothermal probe to aid in hemostasis, since hemarthrosis is the most common complication of this procedure. 23 The anterolateral portal is often used as the working portal and the anteromedial portal as the viewing portal. Placement of the electrothermal probe through a superior portal is possible, but usually unnecessary. The lateral release is performed approximately 1cm posterior to the lateral border of the patella to avoid devascularization. A complete release begins at the level of the proximal pole of the patella and is continued distally to the level of the distal pole. Modified releases begin distal to the vastus lateralis insertion on the patella and are continued distally only far enough to achieve a neutral tilt test. The release is performed in layers to prevent over-release.
Complications of lateral releases are common, especially with excessive release, which continues beyond the fat and muscle layers or disrupts the vastus lateralis tendon insertion. Over-release can result in wound complications or medial patellar instability. Hemarthrosis is the most common complication; therefore meticulous hemostasis is required due to the proximity of the geniculate arteries. 23
Weight-bearing is generally limited for several days to decrease the incidence of hemorrhage and inflammation. Bracing after lateral release is not routinely used. Patellar mobilization is begun immediately after surgery in physical therapy, followed by quadriceps strengthening.

4.3 Results

Several studies have demonstrated 60-90% satisfactory results with arthroscopic lateral release for patellofemoral pain with maltracking and without instability. 22,23,24,25 Increasing amounts of chondromalacia and instability were associated with less favorable results in these studies. When arthroscopic lateral release has been performed for indications other than lateral patellar compression, the results have been poor. 19,20,21,22,25,27,28

5. Lysis of adhesions

5.1 History and physical examination

Arthrofibrosis is the development of intra-articular scarring and adhesions due to trauma, previous surgery, prolonged immobilization and infection. In general, arthrofibrosis of the anterior structures of the knee cause of loss of flexion, while scarring of the posterior structures can cause loss of extension. Scarring and adhesions lead to loss of capsular compliance and pain. 29
Physical examination of the patella typically exhibits decreased excursion in all directions. Tenderness in the region of the supra-patellar pouch and/or infrapatellar fat pad is common, along with loss of range of motion.
If arthrofibrosis is recognized early, non-operative measures such as physical therapy modalities, range of motion exercises and anti-inflammatory medications may successfully improve motion. Manipulation under anesthesia has been a commonly performed procedure, however it is falling out of favor due to complications such hemarthrosis, which can predispose to further scar tissue formation, distal femur fractures and patellar tendon rupture. Arthroscopic lysis of adhesions avoids these complications and allows for controlled, focused treatment.

5.2 Arthroscopic lysis of adhesions

A systematic evaluation as described by Kim, et al. allows for assessment and treatment of intra-articular sources of motion loss. 30 Capsular distension before arthroscopy is useful, as it re-establishes effective joint space, allows easier and safer insertion of instruments, enhances visualization, and may disrupt intra-articular adhesions. 31 Injection of sterile saline should be performed slowly to allow for capsular stretching and to avoid rupture of the capsule, preventing extravasation of fluid during arthroscopy. 29,31

Intra-articular volume capacity can be assessed by injecting the knee with 60cc's of sterile saline. 29,31 After injection, the 18 gauge needle is disconnected from the syringe. If the saline drips out of the needle, the capsule is under little tension and the intra-articular volume is considered normal (Figure 6B). If, however, the saline is expressed from the joint in a stream (Figure 6A), the capsule is under significant pressure indicating insufficient volume. The knee should then be evaluated for stuctures known to reduce interarticular volume. 29

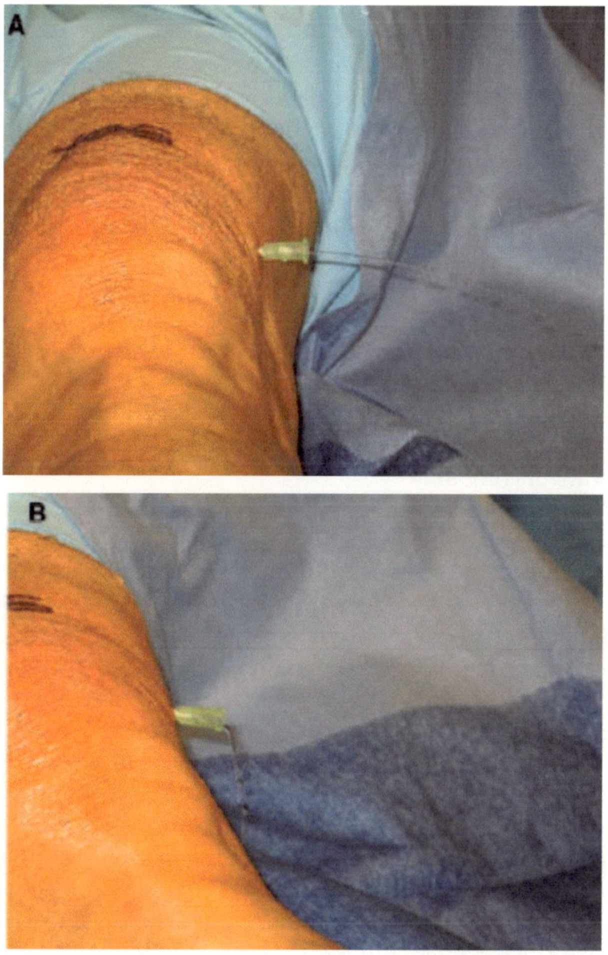

Fig. 6. Assessment of intra-articular volume. The preoperative knee is injected with 60mL of sterile saline. A, Rapid outflow suggests insufficient intra-articular volume. B, Slow egress (drip) indicates normal volume.

Using an electrothermal probe, adhesions are lysed and scarring is released to re-establish the suprapatellar pouch. Adhesions between the capsule and the femoral condyles are often observed and require release. The anterior interval is then re-established as necessary. 1 The medial and lateral patellar retinaculum are partially released if they are scarred, which improves patellofemoral mobility and capsular compliance. The intercondylar notch is then assessed for cyclops lesions.

After completing all anterior releases, the knee is then taken through a range of motion. If a persistent extension deficit remains, then the posterior compartment is assessed and released as previously described.

Postoperatively, an indwelling epidural catheter can help provide adequate pain management, which allows for immediate intensive physical therapy. Patients are placed in a continuous passive motion (CPM) machine immediately, and patellar mobilization and range of motion exercises are emphasized.

5.3 Results

Numerous authors have reported significant improvements of range of motion after lysis of adhesions from 35º to 68º. 32,33,34,35 The most common adverse outcome of this procedure is the inability to restore complete range of motion. 32,33,35 Several authors have also noted marked post-operative tenderness in the region of the infrapatellar fat pad, which resolved with non-operative measures. 32,33 Hematoma is rare with modern techniques using radiofrequency ablation and meticulous hemostasis during the procedure.

6. Plica excision

6.1 History and physical examination

Plicae are remnants of synovial membranes, which divide the embryologic knee into compartments. Plicae are traditionally described based on their anatomic location as suprapatellar, infrapatellar, and medial patellar or medial shelf. Lateral plicae have also been described, but are uncommon.

The suprapatellar plica is seen as a complete or partial synovial membrane that lies proximal to the proximal pole of the patella in the suprapatellar pouch. Arthroscopic studies have described an incidence of some form of suprapatellar plica as high as 87%. 36 The infrapatellar plica originates in the intercondylar notch and inserts into the synovium around the infrapatellar fat pad. Posteriorly, it may be separate from the ACL or attached to it. It is commonly seen during arthroscopy, with an incidence up to 86%. 36 The medial patellar plica originates on the medial wall of the knee, passes obliquely and inferiorly, sometimes crossing the suprapatellar plica, and inserts into the synovium surrounding the infrapatellar fat pad. The true incidence of the medial plica is unknown.

The presence of a plicae does not necessarily indicate a pathologic condition. However, plicae may become symptomatic if thickened, hypertrophic, inflamed and/or fibrotic. 37 The medial plica is most commonly pathologic, resulting in snapping or abrasion against the femoral condyle.

Pathologic plicae are notoriously difficult to diagnose because of their relative rarity, and shared symptoms with other more common knee pathology. There is often a history of trauma or repetitive stress, which may convert a non-pathologic plica into a symptomatic one. Patients mostly complain of pain in the location of the plica, which is usually exacerbated by activity, specifically kneeling or crouching. The incidence of swelling, clicking, or catching varies widely. Provocative meniscal tests and test for patellofemoral pathology are often positive, which further complicates the diagnosis. A thickened medial plica is occasionally palpable medially, just proximal to the joint line, which may be tender and felt to catch with flexion and extension. MRI can often demonstrate the presence of a plica, but not whether it is pathologic.

6.2 Plica excision

A standard diagnostic arthroscopy is always performed to ensure that other more common intra-articular pathologies are not present as the source of pain. Normal plicae appear soft and may be almost translucent at its edge and can be moved freely. In contrast, pathologic plicae often appear thickened and hypertrophic, while having the feel of a tight bowstring. Underlying chondral degeneration of the medial femoral condyle is often present with medial plica impingement.

When the diagnosis of a symptomatic plica is made, it should be resected along its entire length using an electrothermal probe. Care is taken to ensure that only the plica is resected, while protecting the surrounding structures.

The normal suprapatellar pouch extends to approximately 3-4cm proximal of the proximal pole of the patella. With the arthroscope in the suprapatellar pouch, failure to visualize the quadriceps tendon suggests the presence of a complete suprapatellar plica dividing the suprapatellar pouch. The presence of an incomplete or complete suprapatellar plica can result in a decrease of knee volume, and pain. 29 Thus, suprapatellar plicae can be resected in patients with parapatellar pain with an electrothermal probe.

6.3 Results

The majority of results of arthroscopic plica excision have described medial plica excision and mostly been limited to small retrospective reviews. Kent et al. summarized the results of arthroscopic treatment of medial plica in studies published since 1980. 38 In all the studies reviewed, patients had 66% to 98% good to excellent outcomes with plica excision. Weckstrom et al. also recently described retrospective results of military recruits with arthroscopic medial plica resection at median 6-year follow-up. 39 Functional results as determined by the Kujala and Lysholm knee scores were good to excellent in 68% of patients.

Few reports exist of pathologic infrapatellar or suprapatellar plica. Demirag et al. 40 and Boyd et al., 41 in small series described 85% to 91% good or excellent results with arthroscopic resection of symptomatic infrapatellar plica, while Bae et al. 42 reported 90% good or excellent results with excision of a complete, symptomatic suprapatellar plica.

7. Summary

A myriad of inta-articular soft tissue disorders can cause significant morbidity within the knee. Arthroscopic techniques provide minimally-invasive efficacious alternatives to open treatment. Anterior interval release is a simple procedure for treating anterior interval scarring, a fibrotic condition still commonly unrecognized as a cause of anterior knee discomfort. Posterior capsular release, although technically demanding, is effective for treating flexion contractures secondary to scarring and contracture of the posterior capsule. Isolated lateral release provides satisfactory results for patellofemoral pain with maltracking without instability. Arthroscopic lysis of adhesions allows for controlled, focused treatment of all intra-articular causes of motion loss, with decreased risk of complications. Pathologic synovial plicae are an uncommon source of knee pain, but can be easily resected if symptomatic.

8. References

[1] Steadman JR, Dragoo JL, Hines SL, Briggs KK. Arthroscopic release for symptomatic scarring of the anterior interval of the knee. *Am J Sports Med* 2008 Sep;36(9): 1763-1769.

[2] Clifton, R, Ng CY, Nutton RW. What is the role of lateral retinacular release? J Bone Joint Surg Br 2010 Jan; 92(1):1-6.

[3] Sachs RA, Daniel DM, Stone ML, Garfein RF. Patellofemoral problems after anterior cruciate ligament reconstruction. Am J Sports Med 1989; 17(6):760-765

[4] Dragoo JL, Phillips C, Schmidt JD, Scanlan SF, Blazek K, Steadman JR, Williams A. Mechanics of the anterior interval of the knee using open dynamic MRI. Clin Biomech 2010 Jun; 25(5):433-437.

[5] Paulos L, Rosenberg T, Drawbert J, Manning J, Abbott P. Infrapatellar contracture syndrome: An unrecognized cause of knee stiffness with patella entrapment and patella infera. *Am J Sports Med* 1987 July-Aug;15(4): 331-341.

[6] Ogilvie-Harris DJ, Giddens J. Hoffa's disease: Arthroscopic resection of the infrapatellar fat pad. *Arthroscopy* 1994 April;10(2): 184-7.

[7] Saito T, Takeuchi R, Yamamoto K, Yoshida T, Koshino T. Unicompartmental arthroplasty for osteoarthritis of the knee: remaining postoperative flexion contracture affecting overall results. *J Arthroplasty* 2003 Aug;18(5): 612-618.

[8] Cosgarea AJ, DeHaven KE, Lovelock JE. The surgical treatment of arthrofibrosis of the knee. *Am J Sports Med* 1994 Mar; 22(2): 184-191.

[9] Lobenhoffer H, Bosch U, Gerich T. Role of posterior capsulotomy for the treatment of extension deficits of the knee. *Knee Surg Sports Traumatol Arthrosc* 1996;4(4) 237-241.

[10] Noyes FR, Barber-Westin SD in Noyes FR, Barber-Westin SD (eds.): Noyes' Knee Disorders: Surgery, Rehabilitation, Clinical Outcomes. Saunders, 2009, pp1053-1095.

[11] Millett P, Williams R, Wickiewicz T. Open debridement and soft tissue release as a salvage procedure for the severely arthrofibrotic knee. *Am J Sports Medi 1999* Sept-Oct;27(5) 552-561.

[12] Laprade RF, Pedtke AC, Roethle ST. Arthroscopic posteromedial capsular release for knee flexion contractures. *Knee Surg Sports Traumatol Arthrosc* 2008 May;16(5) 469-475.

[13] Mariani PP. Arthroscopic release of the posterior compartments in the treatment of extension deficit of knee. *Knee Surg Sports Traumatol Arthrosc* 2010 Jun;18(6) 736-741.

[14] Conlan T, Garth WP Jr, Lemons JE. Evaluation of the medial soft-tissue restraints of the extensor mechanism of the knee. *J Bone Joint Surg Am* 1993; 75-A:682-693.

[15] Fulkerson JP, Gossling HR. Anatomy of the knee joint lateral retinaculum. *Clin Orthop* 1980;153:183-188.

[16] Merican AM, Amis AA. Anatomy of the lateral retinaculum of the knee. *J Bone Joint Surg Br* 2008; 90-B: 527-534.

[17] Post WR. Clinical evaluation of patients with patellofemoral disorders. *Arthroscopy* 1999 Nov;15(8): 841-851.

[18] Fulkerson JP. Diagnosis and treatment of patients with patellofemoral pain. *Am J Sports Med* 2002; 30(30): 447-456.
[19] Panni AS, Tartarone M, Patricola A, Paxton EW, Fithian DC. Long-term results of lateral retinacular release. *Arthroscopy* 2005;21:526-531.
[20] Colvin AC, West RV. Patellar Instability. *J Bone Joint Surg Am* 2008;90:2751-2762.
[21] Lattermann C, Toth J, Bach BR Jr. The role of lateral retinacular release in the treatment of patellar instability. *Sports Med Arthrosc* 2007;15:57-60.
[22] Grana WA, Hinkley B, Hollingsworth S. Arthroscopic evaluation and treatment of patellar malalignment. *Clin Orthop Relat Res* 1984 Jun; 186: 122-128.
[23] Ogilvie-Harris DJ, Jackson RW. The arthroscopic treatment of chondromalacia patellae. *J Bone Joint Surge Br* 1984 Nov; 66(5):660-665.
[24] Panni AS, Tartarone M, Patricola A, Paxton EW, Fithian DC. Long-term results of lateral retinacular release. *Arthroscopy* 2005 May; 21(5):526-531.
[25] Alemdaroglu KB, Cimen O, Aydogan NH, Atlihan D, Iltar D. Early results of arthroscopic lateral release in patellofemoral arthritis. *Knee* 2008 Dec;15(6):451-455.
[26] Aglietti P, Pisaneschi A, Buzzi R, Gaudenzi A, Allegra M. Arthroscopic lateral release for patellar pain or instability. *Arthroscopy* 1989; 5(3): 176-183.
[27] Aderinto J, Cobb AG. Lateral release for patellofemoral arthritis. *Arthroscopy* 2002 April; 18(4):299-403.
[28] Dainer RD, Barrack RL, Buckley SL, Alexander AH. Arthroscopic treatment of acute patellar dislocation. *Arthroscopy* 1988;4(4): 267-271.
[29] Dragoo JL, Miller MD, Vaugh ZD, Schmidt JD, Handley E. Restoration of knee volume using selected arthroscopic releases. *Am J Sports Med* 2010 Nov;28(11):2288-2293.
[30] Kim DH, Gill TJ, Millett PJ. Arthroscopic treatment of the arthrofibrotic knee. *Arthroscopy* 2004 Jul; 20 Supp 2:1870194.
[31] Millett PJ, Steadman JR. The role of capsular distension in the arthroscopic management of arthrofibrosis of the knee: A technical consideration. *Arthroscopy* 2001;17:E31.
[32] Sprague NF 3rd, O'Connor RL, Fox JM. Arthroscopic treatment of postoperative knee fibroarthrosis. *Clin Orthop Rel Res* 1982 Jun;(166): 165-172.
[33] Parisien JS. The role of arthroscopy in the treatment of postoperative fibroarthrosis of the knee joint. *Clin Orthop Relat Res* 1988 Apr;229:1850192.
[34] Vaquero J, Vidal C, Medina E, Baena J. Arthroscopic lysis in knee arthrofibrosis. *Arthroscopy* 1993;9(6):691-694.
[35] Klein W, Shah N, Gassen A. Arthroscopic management of postoperative arthrofibrosis of the knee joint: indication, technique, and results. *Arthroscopy* 1994;10(6):591-597.
[36] Kim SJ, Choe WS. Arthroscopic findings of the synovial plicae of the knee. *Arthroscopy* 1997 13(1):33-41
[37] Ewing JW. Plica: pathologic or not? *J Am Acad Orthop Surg* 1883;1(2):117-121.
[38] Kent M, Khanduja V. Synovial plicae around the knee. *Knee* 2010;17(2):97-102.
[39] Weckstrom M, Niva MH, Lamminen A, Mattila VM, Pihlajamaki HK. Arthroscopic resection of medial plica of the knee in young adults. *Knee* 2010;17(2):103-107.
[40] Demirag B, Ozturk C, Karakayali M. Symptomatic infrapatellar plica. *Knee Surg Sports Traumatol Arthrosc* 2006;14(2):156-160.
[41] Boyd CR, Eakin C, Matheson GO. Infrapatellar plica as a cause of anterior knee pain. *Clin J Sport Med* 2005;15(2):98-103.

[42] Bae DK, Nam GU, Sun SD, Kim YH. The clinical significance of the complete type of suprapatellar membrane. *Arthroscopy* 1998;14(8):830-835.

13

Extraarticular Arthroscopy of the Knee

Shinichi Maeno[1], Daijo Hashimoto[2], Toshiro Otani[3], Ko Masumoto[4], Itsuki Yuzawa[5], Kengo Harato[6] and Seiji Saito[1]

[1]*Department of Orthopedic Surgery, Shioya Hospital of International University of Health and Welfare, Tochigi,*
[2]*Department of Surgery, Josai Hospital, Tochigi,*
[3]*Keio University Faculty of Nursing and Medical Care, Tokyo,*
[4]*Masumoto Clinic, Tokyo,*
[5]*Department of Orthopedic Surgery, Terada Hospital, Tokyo,*
[6]*Department of Orthopedic Surgery, Kawasaki Municipal Kawasaki Hospital*
Japan

1. Introduction

Indication of the intraarticular arthroscopy, which was originally developed in knee surgery, has been expanded dramatically in accordance with the development of the instruments, including electric coagulator or pressure and flow-control pump. It is widely used not only in the major joints such as knee, shoulder, and hip, but also in the small joints, in hand and foot. It is also applied to outside the joint cavities, such as in the bursae (Verdonk et al., 1988; Klein, 1996; Bradley & Dillingham, 1998; Ogilvie-Harris & Gilbart, 2000), bone marrow of femur or tibia (Roberts et al., 2000,2001; Kwak et al., 2009), and around the tendon sheath (van Dijk et al., 1997, 1998; Steenstra & van Dijk, 2006; Lui, 2007). We describe herein extra-articular arthroscopy using a lifting hanger.

2. Indication

Possible indications for the extraarticular procedures around the knee are; lateral release for painful bipartite patella, excessive lateral pressure syndrome, and recurrent dislocation of the patella (Maeno et al., 2008,2010), bursectomy for prepatellar bursa, and medial patellofemoral ligament (MPFL) reconstruction. It can be expanded to any other extraarticular works around the knee.

3. Instruments

A conventional arthroscopy setup is used. Either a hanger or a coil shaped lifter is needed. The hanger is shaped in a semi-circular, similar to those used in infantile gasless laparoscopic surgery (Takasago Medical Industry, Tokyo, Japan). The coil-shaped lifter is created from an endotracheal tube stylet (Muranaka Medical Instruments, Osaka, Japan). The tip end is bent manually to form a spiral shape, creating a coil about 5 cm in diameter, with about 3 loops (Fig 1).

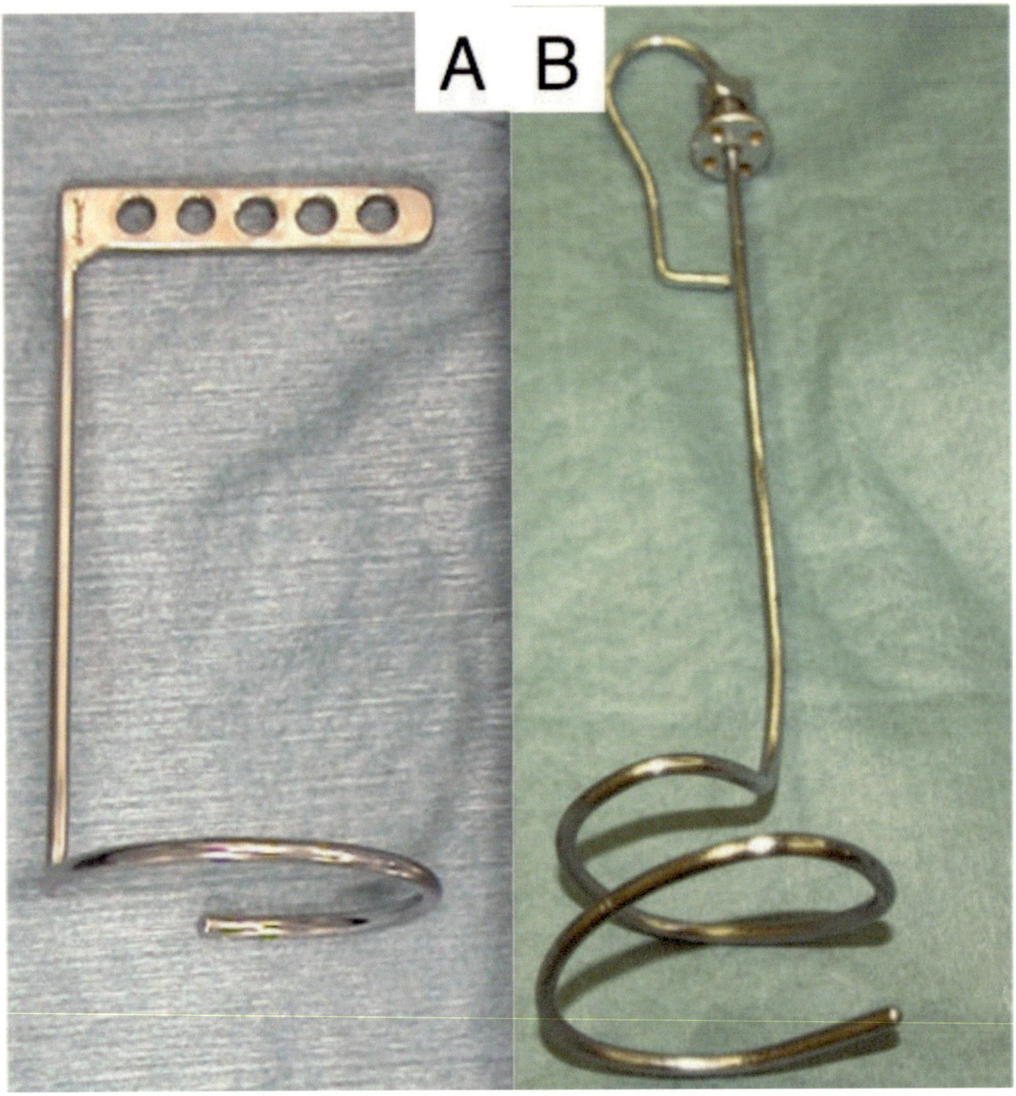

Fig. 1. A: Semi-circular hanger, B: Coil shaped lifter

4. Methods

Routine diagnostic intraarticular arthroscopy is performed from anterolateral (AL) portal. In cases of lateral release procedures, a 1 cm superolateral (SL) portal is made with care not to penetrate the joint. The subcutaneous space is then developed to establish the working space. The lifting hanger is applied. Through the superolateral portal, the ring-shaped end is inserted into the subcutaneous space, and rolled up until the end of the hanger buries under the skin (Fig.2).

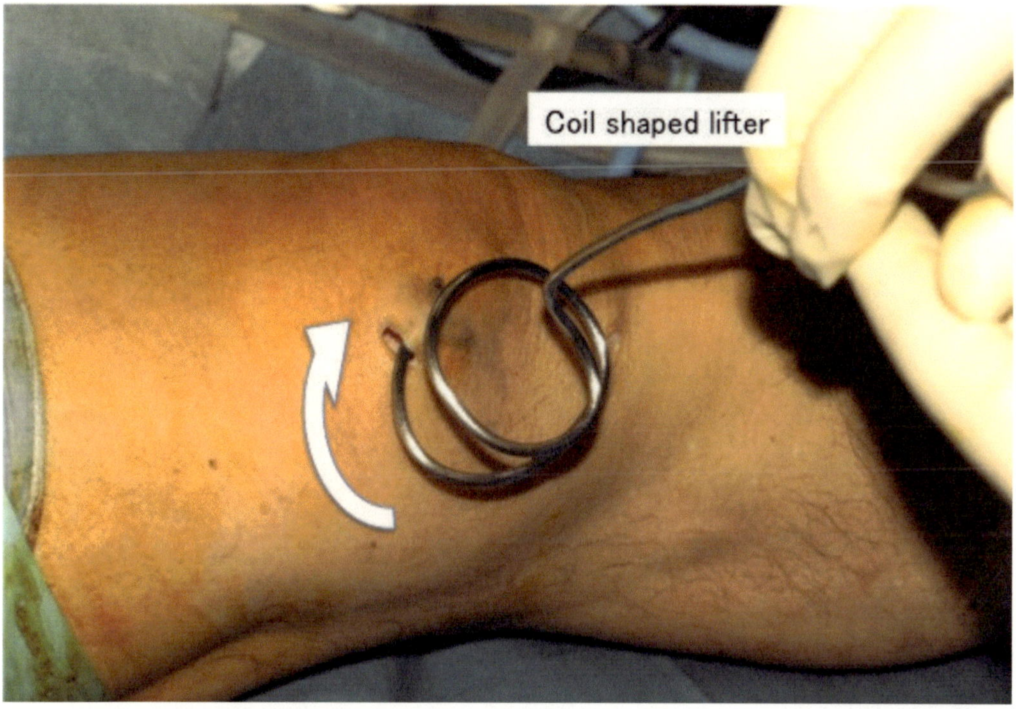

Fig. 2. Coil shaped lifter is inserted into the subcutaneous space

Once pulling the lifter, the working space is established. Care must be taken to avoid inserting the end of the hanger into the underlying muscle. Dry arthroscopy can be performed in the subcutaneous working space created by the lifter (Fig.3,4).
Lastly, the hanger is removed by turning it in the opposite direction.

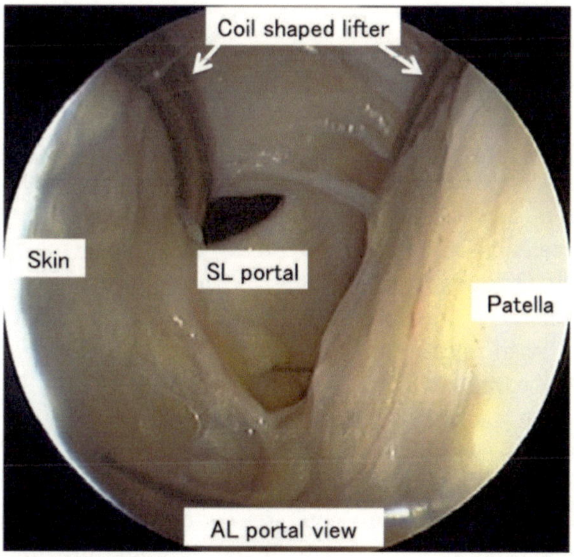

Fig. 3. Subcutaneous space created by the lifter.

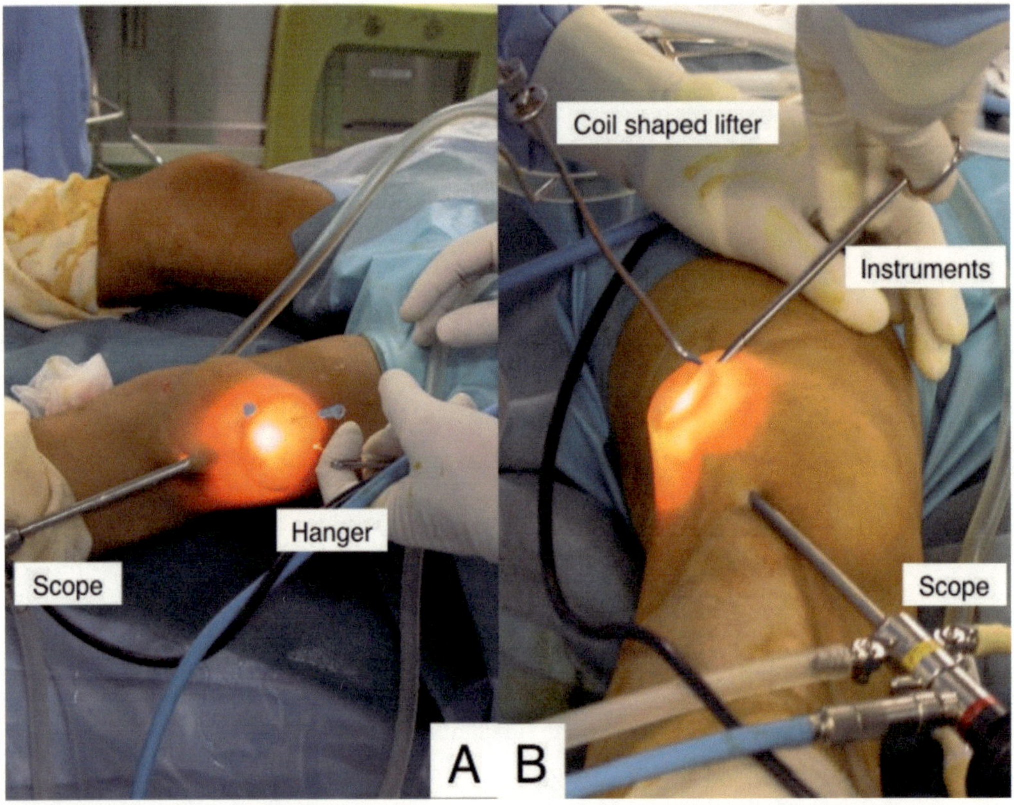

Fig. 4. Operational field during surgery. A) The hanger lifts up the skin, affording the operator a view from outside the joint. B) Likewise, coil shaped lifter is creating the space. Instruments (scissors) are introduced to the operative field. In these situations, the arthroscope is introduced from the AL portal and the hanger lifts the skin from the superolateral portal.

4.1 Lateral release

In the lateral release procedure, a subcutaneous cavity from the AL portal up to the SL portal is needed. In cases of bipartite patella, careful probing to examine instability of the fragment, the status of articular cartilage underneath the patella, and the extent of the affected area to be treated is important. Viewing the lesion from inside the joint, firstly we pierce the lesion with 23-gauge needles at the proximal and distal edges of the lesion, to ensure the extent of release. It often involves not only the lateral retinaculum but also vastus lateralis muscle. We try to release only the attachment of the vastus lateralis muscle and lateral retinaculum to the fragment.

Basically the arthroscope is in the AL viewing portal. Under a magnified arthroscopic view, careful release should be performed, including the vastus lateralis muscle and lateral retinaculum, with a No. 11 blade through the SL portal. The release should be between the needle markers with a knife and arthroscopic scissor cutters. A 1-cm portal is sufficient to introduce both the lifter and an arthroscope, or the lifter and instruments, as the portal is stretched by the lifter. Authors prefer to debride the released edge of the vastus lateralis muscle with a 4.5-mm shaver to create a gap between the muscle and fragment, which decreases the risk of the muscle scarring back down to the fragment (Fig.5).

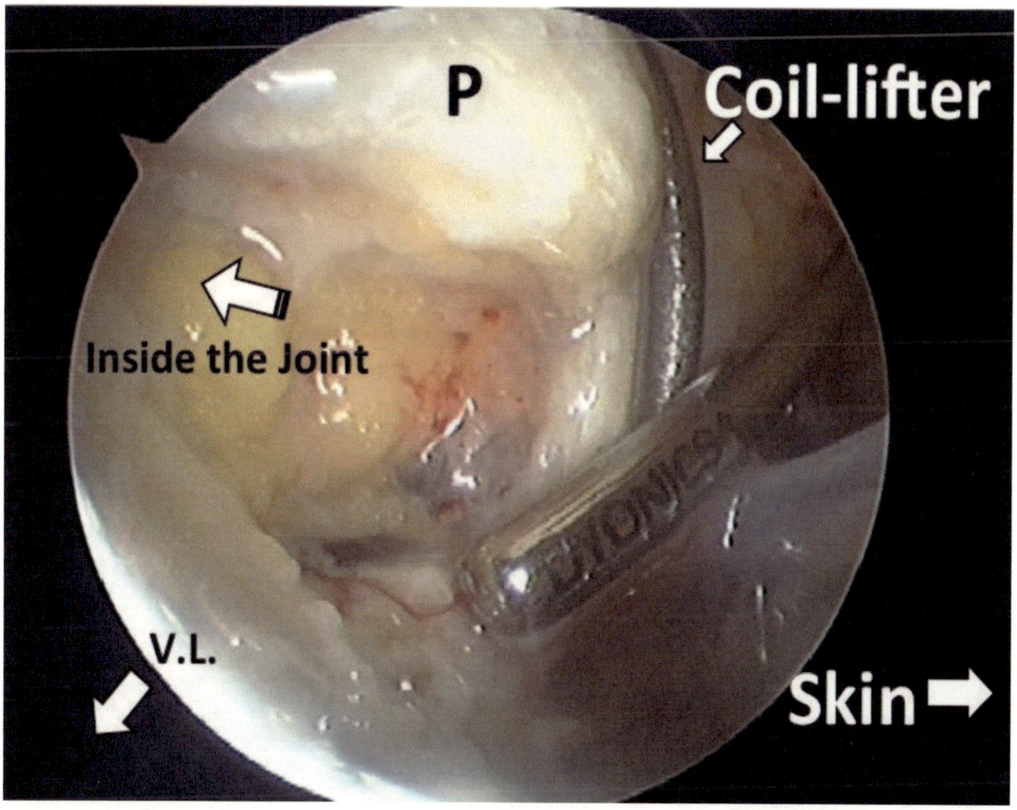

Fig. 5. SL portal view. A 4.5 mm shavor is used in order to create a gap between muscle and fragment. VL, vastus lateralis muscle; P, patella.

It should ideally be done from outside the joint with care not to penetrate the joint, so that the joint capsule can be maintained intact to help minimize the postoperative leakage of the joint fluid.

4.2 Medial patellofemoral ligament reconstruction

While numbers of MPFL reconstructions are reported, this procedure allows doing under a minimum incision. Authors' prefferred method is as follows; a 1 cm incision at the superomedial corner of the patella is made. An oblique bone tunnel through the patella is drilled with a guide pin and overdrilling method. This tunnel should be obliquely routed from the superomedial corner of the patella to the anterior center of the patella, trying to recreate the original fan-shaped attachment of the MPFL (Steensen et al., 2004). The lifting hanger is introduced into the prepatellar space, to be able to perform extraarticular dry arthroscopy. The harvested semitendinosus tendon is introduced to this space through the bone tunnel, pulled using a passing pin (Fig.6).

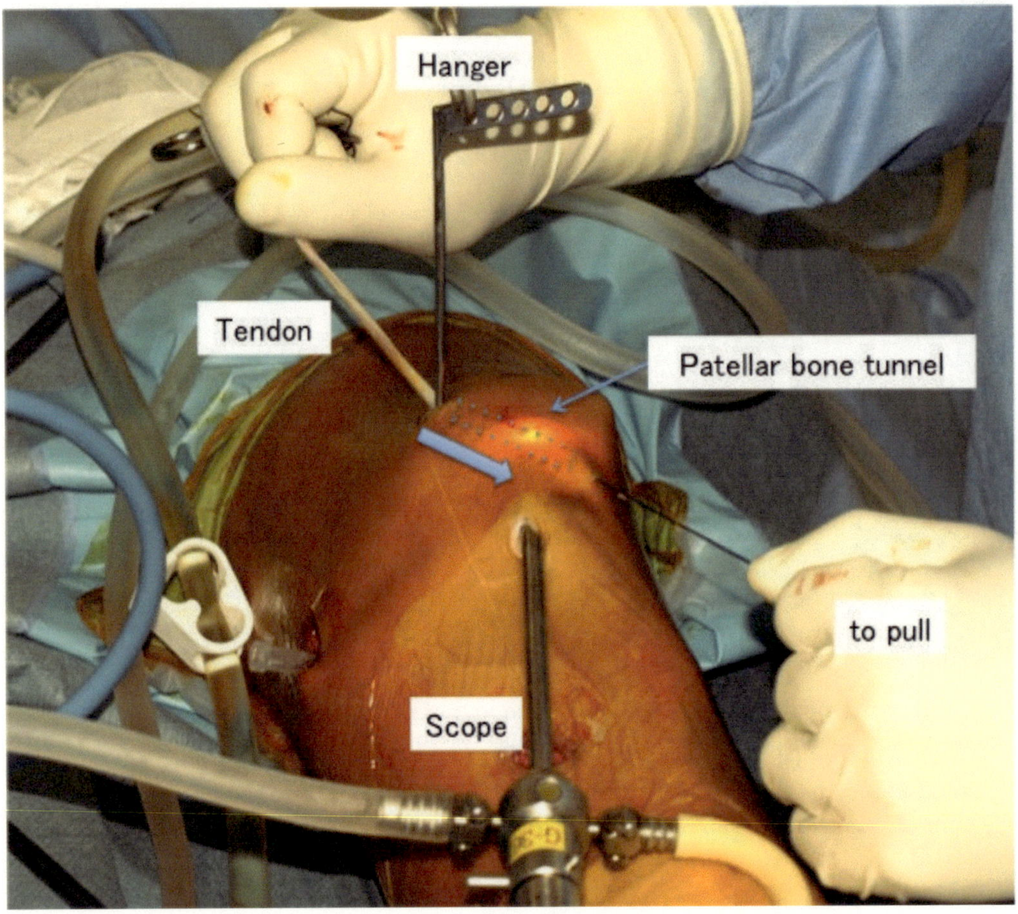

Fig. 6. Watching the drilled hole on anterior surface of the patella through the scope, absorbable sutures (No. 2 Vicryl®) connected to semitendinosus tendon is introduced by pulling through the passing pin.

The suture is caught using a grasper punch from the superomedial portal, and the tendon is drawn out to the superomedial portal, along with the existing end of the tendon (Fig.7).

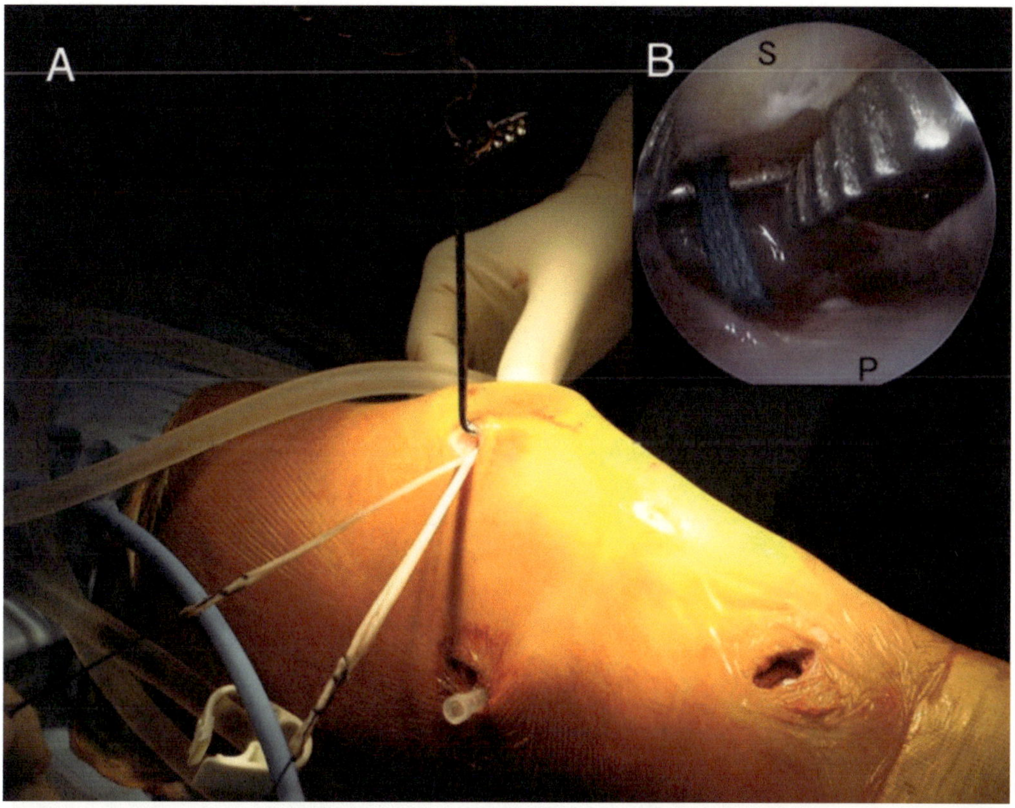

Fig. 7. A) The tendon passing through the bone tunnel is drawn out to the superomedial portal, which also exists at the other end of the tendon. B) Arthroscopic view between the patella and skin during the operation. In this situation, a hanger, an arthroscope, and forceps are introduced from the same superomedial portal. The forceps are about to grip the sutures connecting the ligament. P, patella; S, subcutaneous tissue.

Using a tendon passer, both tendon ends are lead to the femoral fixation site, which is just distal to the adductor tubercle and posterosuperior to the medial epicondyle (Nomura, 2003).
An interference screw is used to fix the ligament.

4.3 Bursectomy

Among numbers of bursae existed around the knee, the most problematic bursitis would happen in the prepatellar bursa. The incision should be at the superior and the inferior end of the bursa, with care not to cut the infrapatellar branch of the saphenous nerve. Authors prefer using dye solution prior to resection to help determine the extent of the bursal tissue, as it does not always look like typical bursa. Under dry arthroscopy in the bursa created by the lifter, bursectomy can be performed using a shavor or an electric coagulator.
Putting a drainage tube should also be considered depending on the cases.

5. Case presentation

A 10-year-old boy (football player) suffered bilateral anterior knee pain and consulted a nearby clinic in 2005, but only underwent observational studies. Radiography showed a normal patellar shape on the left, but the lateral edge of the patella seemed deficient on the right. Pain worsened to the point where he could no longer continue playing football. Bilateral bipartite patellae was diagnosed at 12 years old in 2007, and he was introduced to our hospital in October 2007.

Radiography in our hospital revealed bilateral bipartite patellae (Saupe classification, type II) (Saupe, 1943), and showed marked tenderness on the anterolateral aspect of the knees, at the site of dissociated bony fragments (Fig. 8).

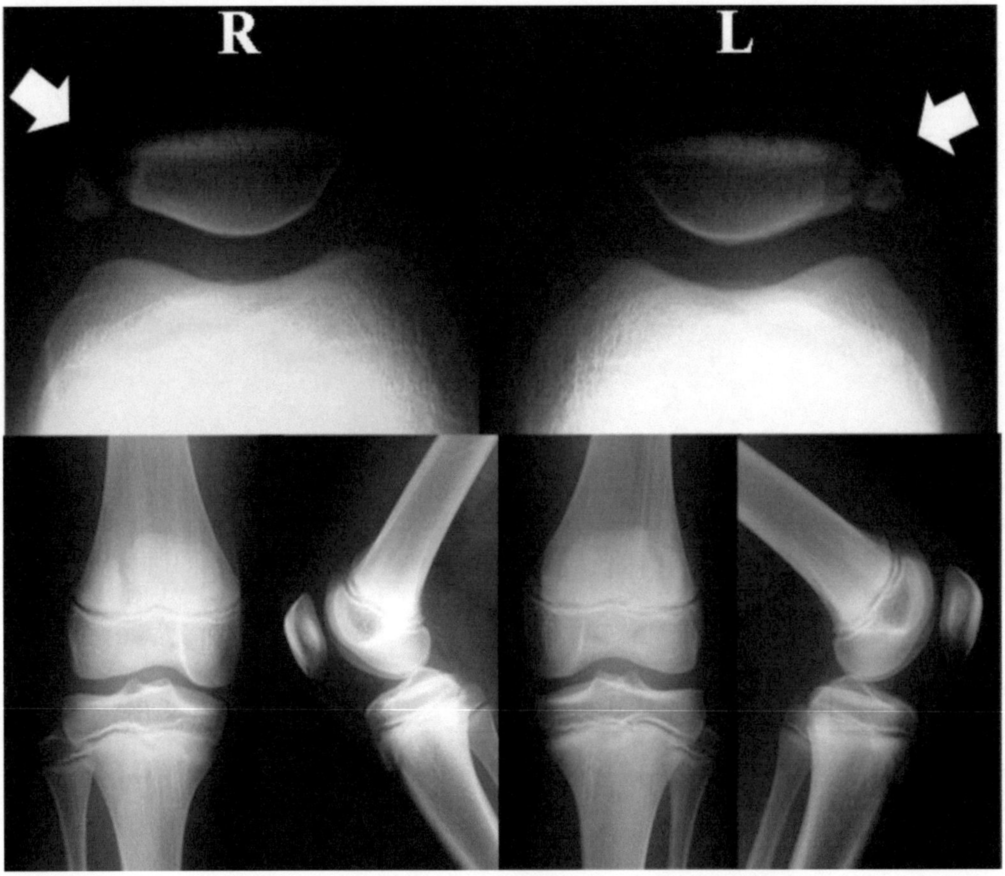

Fig. 8. Plain radiography in Case 1. Left figures show the right knee, right figures show the left knee.

Magnetic resonance imaging (MRI) showed signal hyperintensity at the dissociated fragment and fibrous connected site on T2-weighted fat-suppression images.

Lateral retinacular release accompanied by the release of vastus lateralis muscle insertion from the bony fragment were performed on both knees arthroscopically under both intra- and extra-articular views using the hanger lifting procedure in November 2007, at 13 years old. At first, conventional arthroscopy was performed to check the cartilage status. The surface of the cartilage looked almost intact on dissociated sites. We determined the range to release from the shape of the patella from inside the joint, using pierce-marks of 23-G needles for marking. The subcutaneous space was then widely developed. A semi-circular hanger was then applied through the SL access portal by placing the ring-shaped end of the hanger, with the other end of the hanger retracted by hand. Watching the patella and lateral retinaculum from outside the joint, lateral release was able to be performed. The width of release could be checked from both inside and outside the joint (Fig.9).

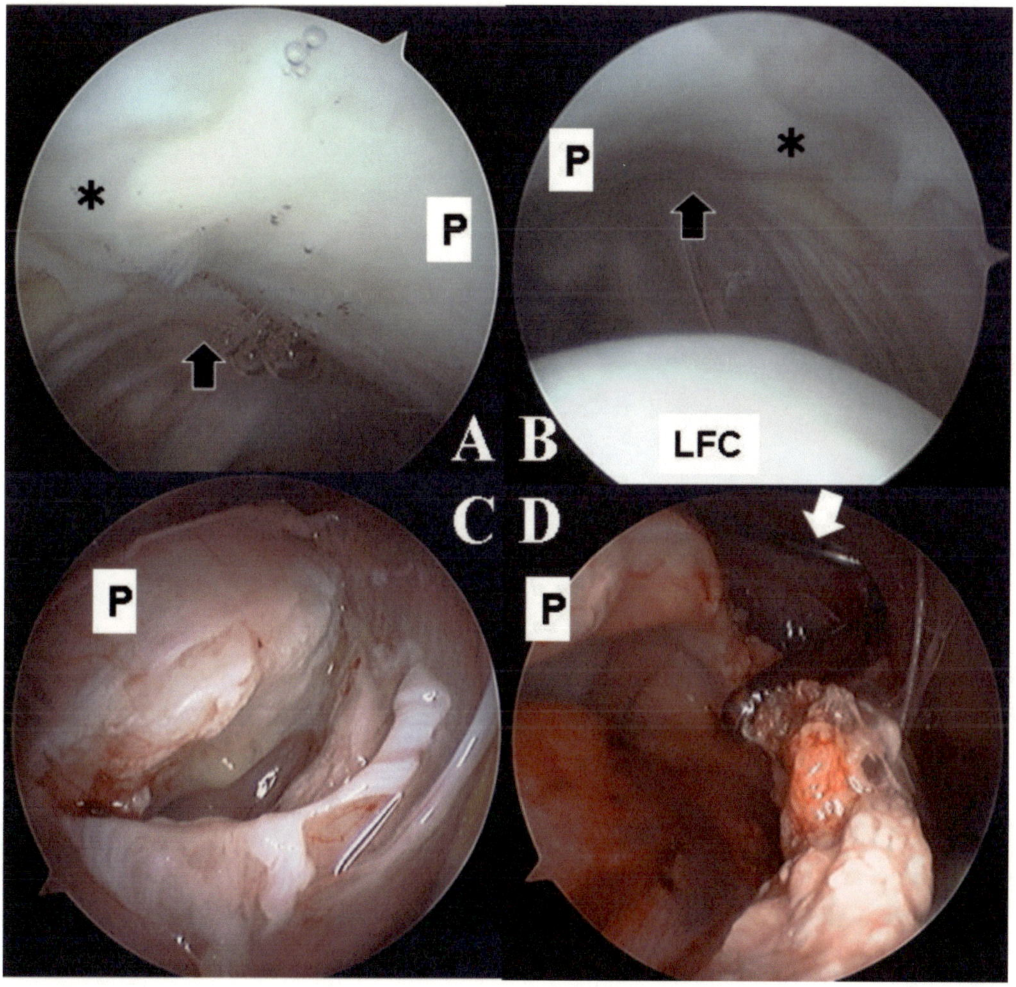

Fig. 9. Arthroscopic view from inside and outside the joint. A, C) Right knee. B, D) Left knee. A) View from inside the right knee joint, using the AL portal. Black arrow indicates the bipartite patella. No marked cartilage damage was evident. B) View from inside the left knee joint, using the AL portal. C) View from outside the right knee joint, using the SL portal. Lateral release of bipartite patella is successfully completed. The lateral femoral condyle can be seen from outside the joint. D) Lateral release performed under a view from outside the joint. A shaver is introduced from the SL portal. The camera is from the AL portal. The lifting hanger is also seen (white arrow). P, patella. *Bipartite patellae.

The patient began range-of-motion exercises from postoperative day 1, and was able to walk from postoperative day 2. Symptom resolved within 1 month, and radiography showed bone union by 2 months postoperatively in the left knee, and by 4 months in the right knee. Even the inclined bony fragment of the right knee was corrected during the course (Fig. 10).

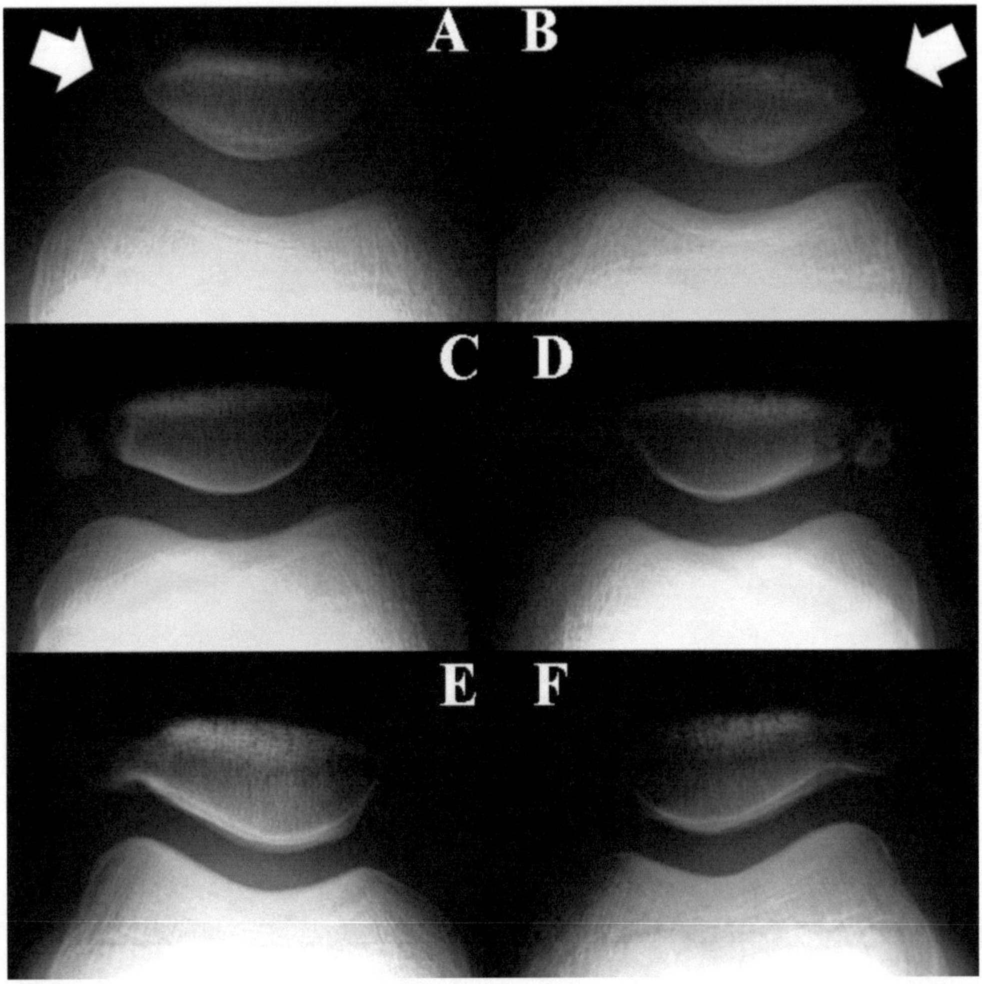

Fig. 10. Radiography of Case 1 along with time course. A, C, E) Right knee. B, D, F) Left knee. A, B) Radiography at the time of initial complaint of pain in both knees at 11 years old. The shape of the right patella seemed normal (A), but the lateral edge of the left knee seemed deficient (B). C, D) Preoperative radiography at 12 years old. Both knees displayed bipartite patella (Saupe classification, type II). E) Right knee at 4 months postoperatively. F) Left knee at 2 months postoperatively. Bone union seemed complete.

6. Discussion

Hanger lifting procedures have been developed for abdominal operations during laparoscopic surgery, to avoid the risks inherent in conventional pneumoperitoneum (Hashimoto et al., 1993, 1995, Nagai et al., 1995). The hanger we used was designed for

abdominal operations in children (Yokomori et al., 1998), but is also suitable for knee surgery because the diameter is close to that of the patella. Instead of lifting the abdominal wall, we lifted the anterior skin of the knee to achieve extra-articular arthroscopy. The most characteristic feature of this method is the provision of an extra-articular view, which seems effective for these procedures. Views can be obtained from both inside and outside the joint arthroscopically without water. Further, with regard to vastus lateralis release, the benefit of this technique is the ability to keep the joint capsule intact, which is not possible with a conventional intra-articular arthroscopic approach. In terms of MPFL reconstruction, the creation of patellar bone tunnel and tendon passage can be made under arthroscopic view.
Both intra- and extra-articular arthroscopic views seem indispensable for precise performance of those methods.
The only substantial complication is interstitial edema and subcutaneous adhesion due to developing subcutaneous space. Thus, early mobilization with compression dressing seems necessary.

7. Acknowledgement

The authors thank Drs. Yasuyuki Fukui, Makoto Nishiyama, Masayuki Ishikawa, Nobuyuki Fujita, and Soraya Nishimura, Mita Hospital, International University of Health and Welfare, for their excellent technical assistance.

8. References

Bradley DM, Dillingham MF (1998). Bursoscopy of the trochanteric bursa. *Arthroscopy*, Vol.14, No.8, pp.884-887.

Hashimoto D, Nayeem SA, Kajiwara S, Hoshino T (1993). Abdominal wall lifting with subcutaneous wiring: An experience of 50 cases of laparoscopic cholecystectomy without pneumoperitoneum. *Surg Today*, Vol.23, No.9, pp.786-790.

Klein W (1996). Endoscopy of the deep infrapatellar bursa. *Arthroscopy* Vol.12, No.1, pp. 127-131..

Kwak JH, Sim JA, Yang SH, Kim SJ, Lee BK, Ki YC (2009). The use of medulloscopy for localized intramedullary lesions: Review of 5 cases. *Arthroscopy, Vol.*25, No.12, pp.1500-1504.

Lui TH (2007). Arthroscopically assisted Z-lengthening of extensor hallucis longus tendon. *Arch Orthop Trauma Surg*, Vol.127, No.9, pp.855-857.

Maeno S, Hashimoto D, Otani T, Masumoto K, Matsumoto H (2008). Hanger-lifting procedure in knee arthroscopy. *Arthroscopy, Vol.24, No.12*, pp.1426-1429.

Maeno S, Hashimoto D, Otani T, Masumoto K, Fukui Y, Nishiyama M, Ishikawa M, Fujita N, Kanagawa H (2010). Medial patellofemoral ligament reconstruction with hanger lifting procedure, *Knee Surg Sports Traumatol Arthrosc*, Vol.18, No.2, pp.157-160.

Maeno S, Hashimoto D, Otani T, Masumoto K, Hui C (2010). The "coiling-up procedure": a novel technique for extra-articular arthroscopy. *Arthroscopy*, Vol.26, No.11, pp.1551-1555.

Nomura E, Inoue M (2003). Surgical technique and rationale for medial patellofemoral ligament reconstruction for recurrent patellar dislocation. *Arthroscopy*, Vol.19, No.5, pp.E47

Nagai H, Kondo Y, Yasuda T, Kasahara K, Kanazawa K (1993). An abdominal wall-lift method of laparoscopic cholecystectomy without peritoneal insufflation. *Surg Laparosc Endosc* Vol.3, No.3, pp.175-179.

Ogilvie-Harris DJ, Gilbart M (2000). Endoscopic bursal resection: The olecranon bursa and prepatellar bursa. *Arthroscopy* Vol.16, No.3, pp.249-253.

Roberts CS, Statton JO, Walker JA, Seligson D, Hempel D (2000). Medulloscopy of the tibia: Initial report of a new technique. *Arthroscopy* Vol.16, No.8, pp.865-868.

Roberts CS, Walker JA, Statton J, Seligson D (2001). Medulloscopy for sepsis or nonunion: Early clinical experience with the tibia and femur. *Arthroscopy* Vol.17, No.9, pp.E39.

Saupe H (1943). Primare Knochenmark seilerung der Kniescheibe. *Dtsche Z Chir* Vol. 258, pp.386.

Steensen RN, Dopirak RM, McDonald WG (2004). The anatomy and isometry of the medial patellofemoral ligament. Implications for reconstruction. *Am J Sports Med* Vol.32,pp.1509–1513

Steenstra F, van Dijk CN (2006). Achilles tendoscopy. *Foot Ankle Clin* Vol.11, No.2, pp.429-438, viii.

van Dijk CN, Kort N, Scholten PE (1997). Tendoscopy of the posterior tibial tendon. *Arthroscopy* Vol.13, No.6, pp.692-698.

van Dijk CN, Kort N (1998). Tendoscopy of the peroneal tendons. *Arthroscopy* Vol.14, No.5, pp.471-478.

Verdonk R, Van Meirhaeghe J, Van Houcke H, Verjans P, De Groof E, Van Lerbeirghe J, Claessens H (1988). Shoulder bursoscopy. *Acta Orthop Belg* Vol.54, No.2, pp.233-236.

Yokomori K, Terawaki K, Kamii Y, Obana K, Hashizume K, Hoshino T, Hashimoto D (1998). New technique applicable to pediatric laparoscopic surgery: Abdominal wall "area lifting" with subcutaneous wiring. *J Pediatr Surg* Vol.33, No.11, pp.1589-1592.

Part 5

Arthroscopy of the Foot and Ankle

14

Posterior Ankle and Hindfoot Arthroscopy

Masato Takao
Teikyo University
Japan

1. Introduction

Hindfoot pain can be caused by any part of the posterior ankle anatomy with bony and soft tissue, including os trigonum, large posterior talar process, tenosynovitis of the flexor hallucis longus tendon, osteochondral lesions of the talus, subtalar arthritis and arthrosis, prominent calcaneus posterior process and free bodies, such as synovial chondromatosis. Because these structures are deeply situated and difficult to palpate, there remain diagnostic difficulties. Posterior ankle and hindfoot arthroscopy gives excellent access to such a posterior ankle compartment[1], and it is regarded as the ideal diagnostic tool for accurate diagnosis of the hindfoot disorders. Furthermore, it is also regarded as an effective tool especially for the athletes who expect to return to their initial athletic activities with a shorter recovery time.

The arthroscopic approach to the posterior ankle was first described by Parisien and Vangsness in 1985 as a subtalar arthroscopy[2]. In 2000, van Dijk advanced an epoch-making technique, a two portal endoscopic approach, which makes it possible to obtain broad field of vision and working space[1]. Recently, posterior ankle and hindfoot arthroscopy utilizing a two portal endoscopic approach has been developed and widely used for diagnosis and treatment of hindfoot disorders. In this part, the author describes the posterior ankle and hindfoot arthroscopy utilizing a two portal endoscopic approach.

2. Basics and clinical applications

2.1 Indications

The indications of hindfoot endoscopy are posterior ankle joint pathologies including osteochondral lesions of the posterior talus, loose bodies, ossicles, posttraumatic calcification or avulsion fragment; posterior subtalar joint pathologies including osteophyte, loose bodies, osteoarthritis or intraosseous talar ganglion; periarticular pathologies including posterior ankle impingement syndrome, deltoid ligament avulsion, tenosynovitis or intratendinous ganglion of the flexor hallucis longus, tenosynovitis or partial rupture of the peroneal tendon and posterior tibial tendon, retrocalcaneal bursitis and entrapment of the tibian nerve within the tarsal tunnel[3].

2.2 Set-up and normal anatomy

2.2.1 Set-up

Hindfoot endoscopy was performed under spinal lumbar anesthesia. The patient was placed in a prone position on an operating table (Figure 1).

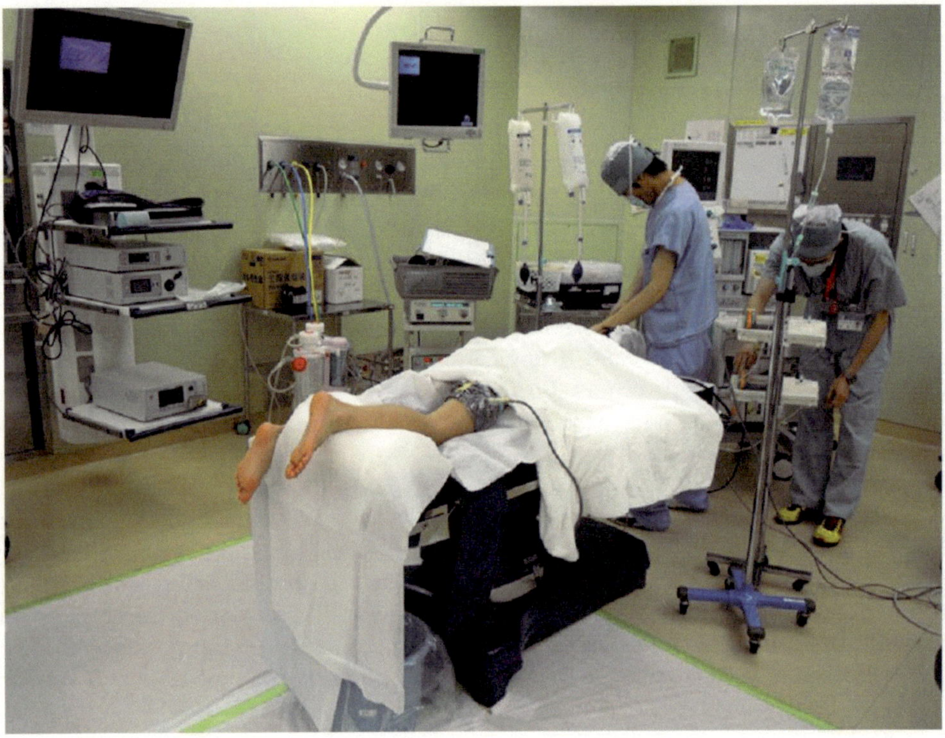

Fig. 1. Position of the patient.

A small support was placed under the lower leg. A pneumotourniquet is inflated to a pressure of 300 mm Hg. An arthroscope 4.0 mm in diameter with a 30 degree angle and the irrigation of saline with a pressure of 50 to 80 mmHg is used. Although any distraction device may not be needed in most cases, the bandage distraction technique[4] with a force of 78.4 Newtons (Figure 2) is beneficial in cases where it is needed to be widen the posterior talocrural joint (Figure 3).

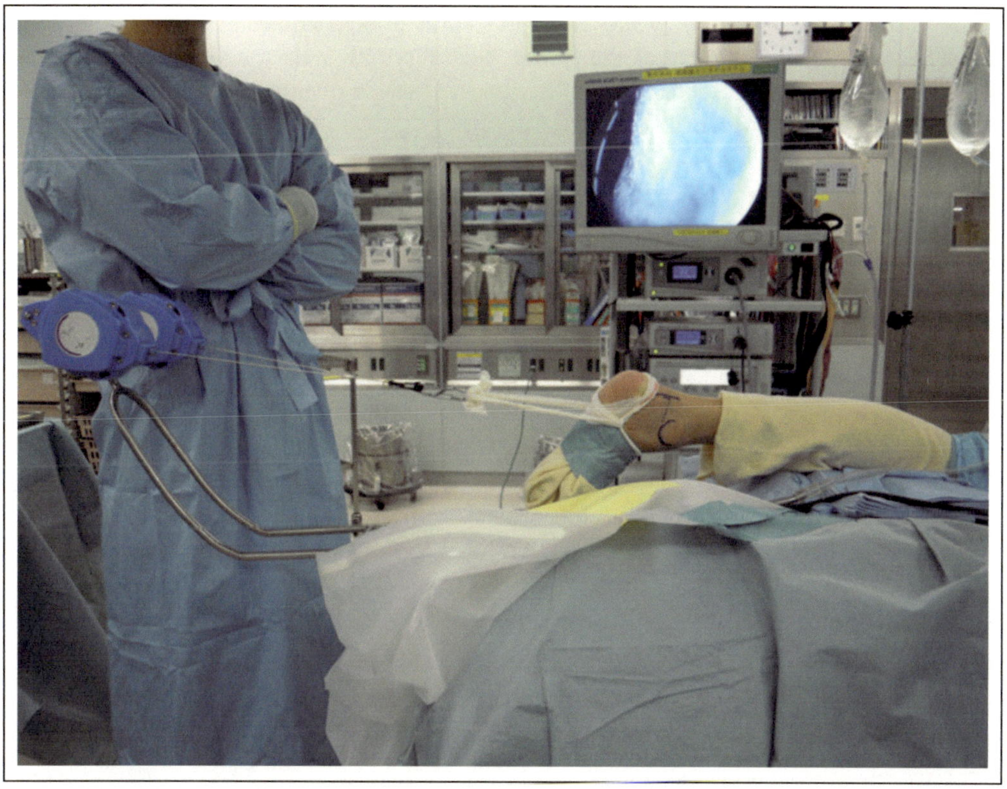

Fig. 2. Bandage distraction technique.

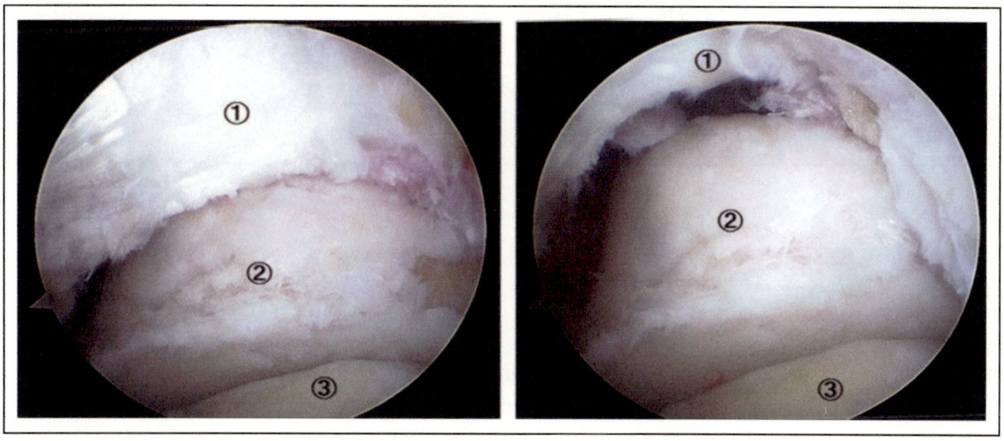

Fig. 3. Arthroscopic view of the posterior talocrural joint before distraction (left) and after distraction (right).
1. Tibia; 2. Talus; 3. Calcaneus

2.2.2 Making the portal and the working space

A line was drawn from the tip of the lateral malleolus to the Achilles tendon, parallel to the sole of the foot. The posterolateral and posteromedial portals were made just above this line and 3 mm medial and lateral of the Achilles tendon using a pneumotourniquet inflated to a pressure of 300 mm Hg (Figure 4).

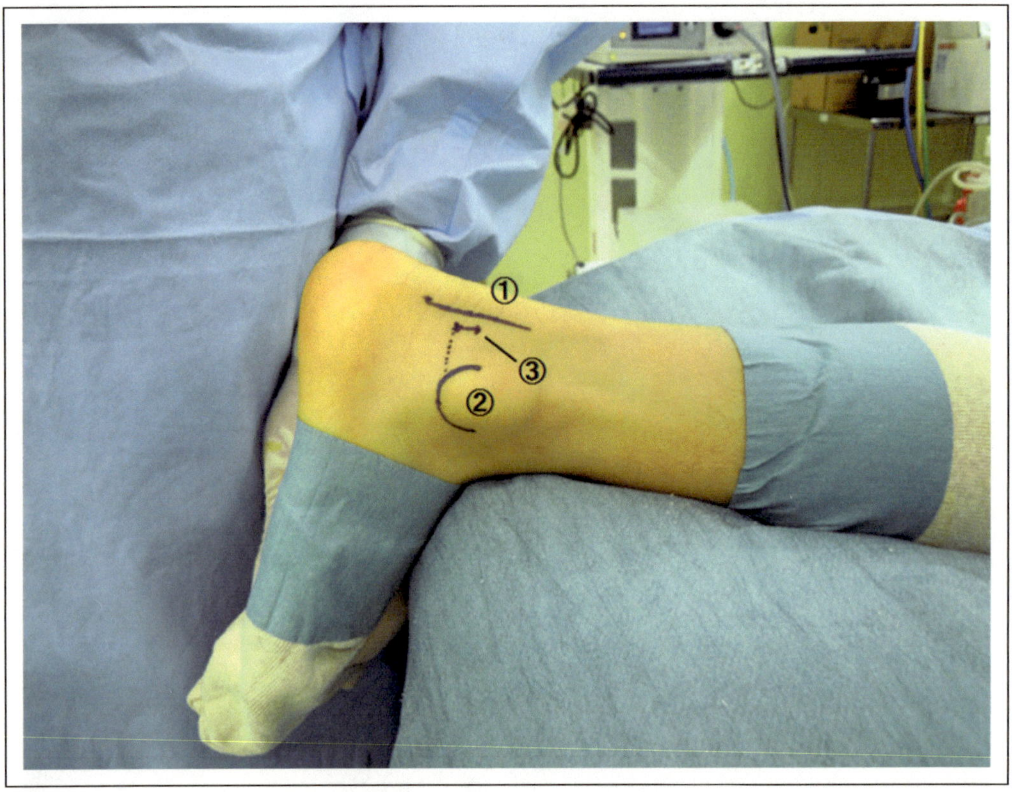

Fig. 4. Posterolateral portal.
1. Achilles tendon; 2. Lateral malleolus; 3. Posterolateral portal

If the portals are close to the Achilles tendon it may lead to tenosynovitis of the Achilles tendon. On the other hand, if the portals are too far from the Achilles tendon, it is difficult to watch the field fully. The deep layer is split by mosquito clamp via a posterolateral portal that is directed to the first web or second toe through the 1 cm vertical skin incision (Figure 5). When the tip of the clamp touches the bone, it is exchanged for a 4.5 mm arthroscope shaft with the blunt trocar to direct to the first web or second toe (Figure 6).

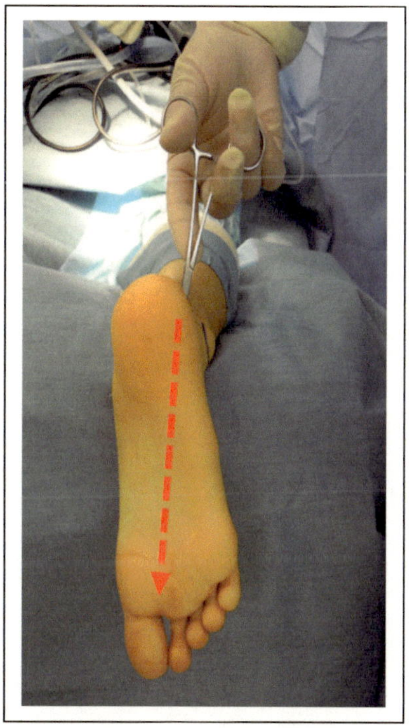

Fig. 5. Split of the deep layer by mosquito clamp directing to the first web.

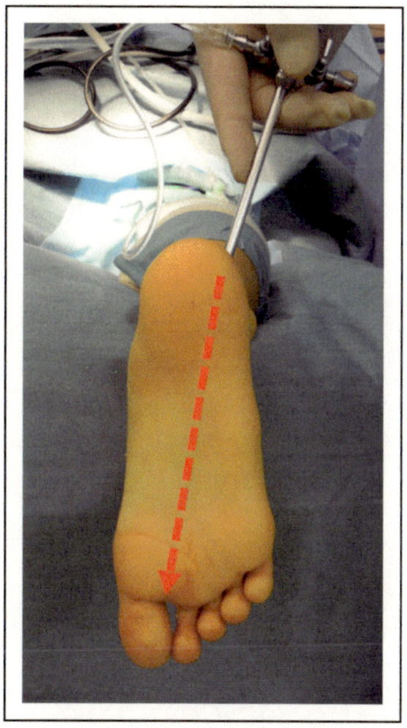

Fig. 6. Insert an arthroscope shaft with the blunt trocar directing to the first web.

The trocar is exchanged to an arthroscope 4.0 mm in diameter with a 30 degree angle. Next, a mosquito clamp is introduced via a posteromedial portal. A mosquito clamp touches the shaft of the arthroscope and the deep layer around the arthroscope is split. A 4.0 to 5.0 mm motorized shaver (full radius shaver) is inserted through the posteromedial portal in order to make the working space (Figure 7).

For bringing the shaver into the field of vision of the arthroscopy, it is helpful that the tip of the shaver touches the shaft of the arthroscope and slide distally (Figure 8).

Adipose tissue and the posterior joint capsule are removed by motorized shaver. First of all, the surgeon must show the FHL tendon (Figure 9). The neurovascular bundle lies medial to the FHL tendon, so the surgeon should perform the arthroscopic surgery laterally to the FHL tendon (Figure 10).

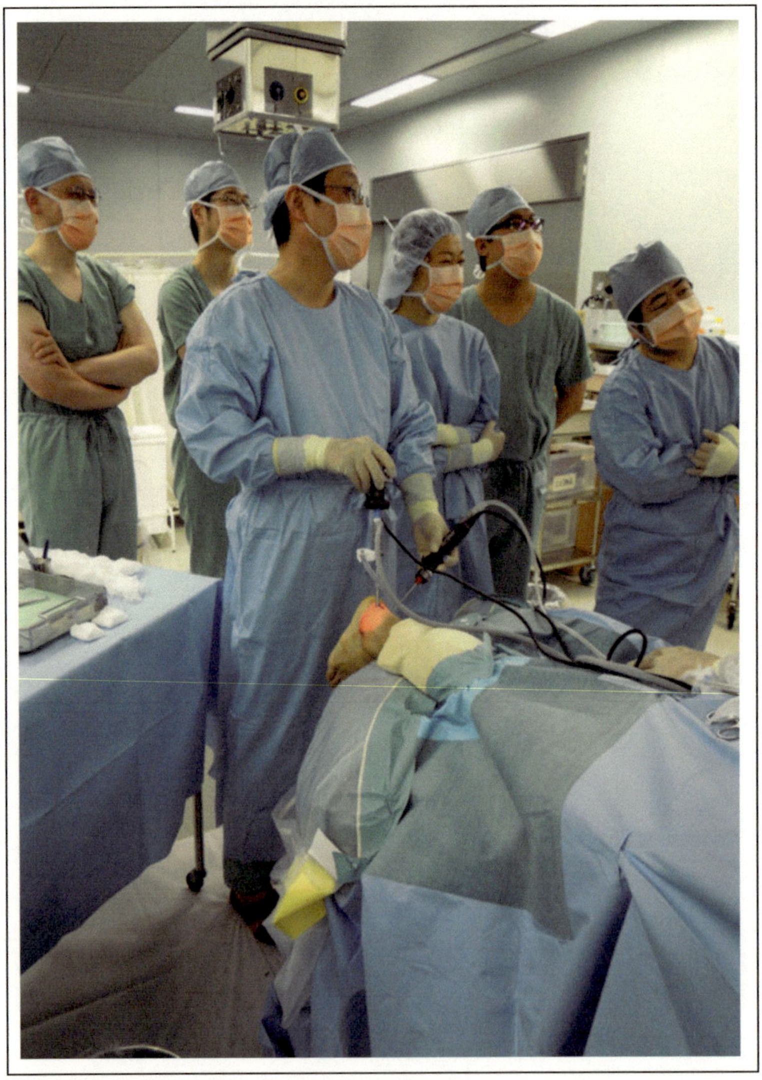

Fig. 7. Hindfoot endoscopy.

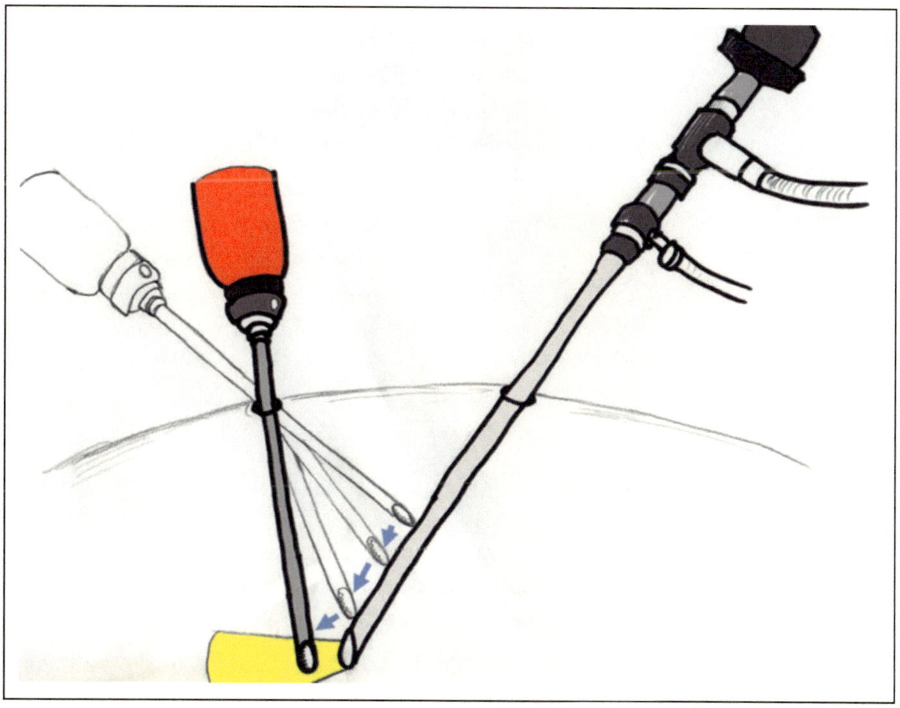

Fig. 8. Introducing the shaver into the field of vision of the arthroscopy.

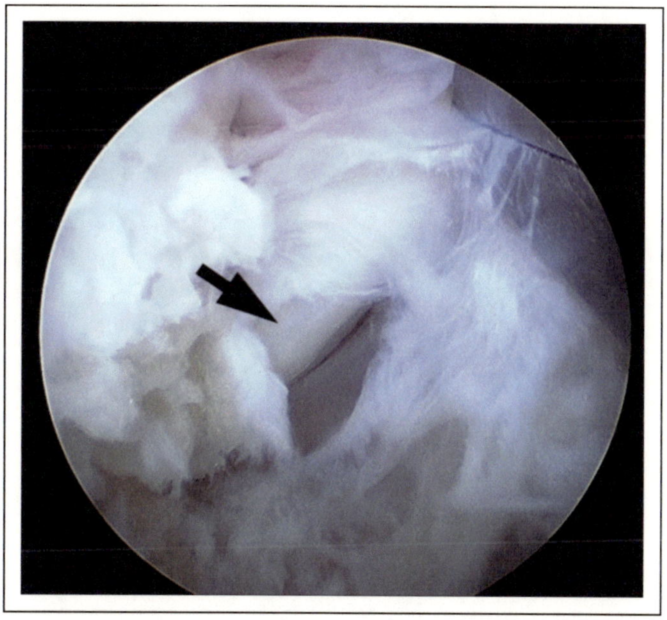

Fig. 9. Flexor hallucis longus tendon (arrow).

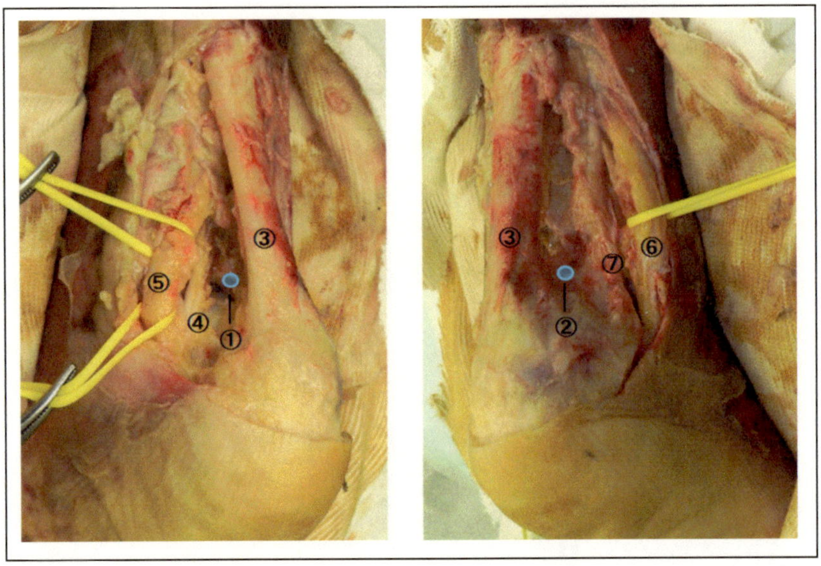

Fig. 10. Anatomic dissection of the posterior ankle around the posteromedial portal (left) and the posterolateral portal (right).

1. Posteromedial portal; 2. Posterolateral portal; 3. Achilles tendon; 4. Flexor hallucis longus tendon; 5. Tibian nerve and posterior tibial artery; 6. Sural nerve; 7. Peroneal tendon

2.2.3 Normal anatomy

Normal structures which can be observed via posterior two portals are shown in Figure 11[5].

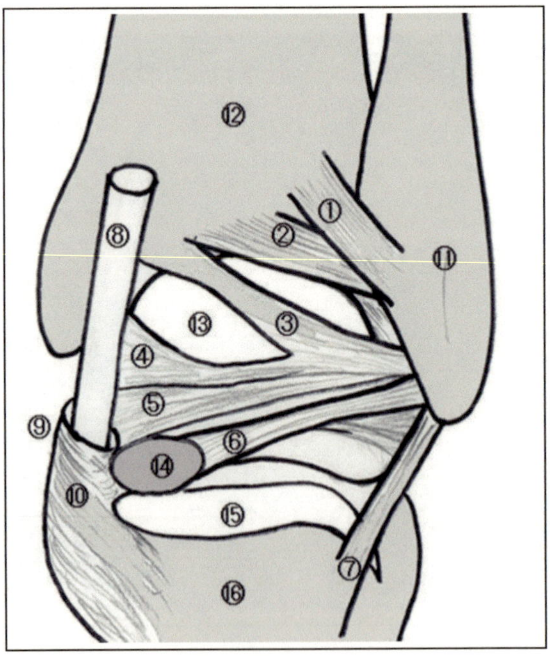

Fig. 11. Normal anatomy of the posterior ankle.

1. Superficial component of the posterior tibiofibular ligament; 2. Deep component of the posterior tibiofibular ligament or transvers ligament; 3. Tibial insertion of the posterior intermalleolar ligament; 4. Tibial malleolar insertion of the posterior intermalleolar ligament; 5. Talar insertion of the posterior intermalleolar ligament; 6. Posterior talofibular ligament; 7. Calcaneofibular ligament; 8. Flexor hallucis longus (FHL) tendon; 9. Entrance of the tarsal tunnel; 10. FHL retinaculum; 11. Lateral malleolus; 12. Tibia; 13. Posterior talar dome; 14. Posterolateral talar process; 15. Subtalar joint; 16. Calcaneus

2.3 Clinical applications

2.3.1 Posterior ankle impingement syndrome

Posterior ankle impingement syndrome (PAIS) is generally considered to be the clinical disorder characterized by posterior ankle pain in forced plantar flexion[6]. The etiology of this syndrome is varied and may involve any part of the posterior ankle anatomy, including bony and soft tissue structures. Among them, os trigonum and large posterior talar process are frequent (Figure 12).

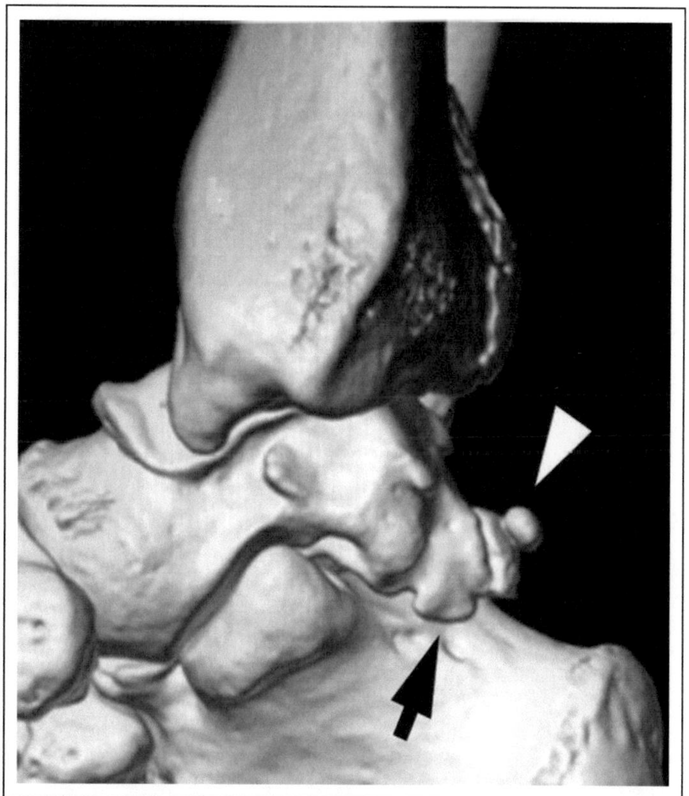

Fig. 12. Three dimensional computed tomogram of the hindfoot.

An arrow shows a large posterolateral process of the talus and an arrow head shows an os trigonum.

According to the author's experiences gained in approximately 200 cases, it should be noted that hindfoot endoscopies have shown that large posterolateral talar processes compress a

FHL tendon in most cases (Figure 13) and in some cases constrict the FHL tendon at the posteromedial part of the fibro-osseous tunnel leading to tenosynovitis of the FHL (Figure 14).

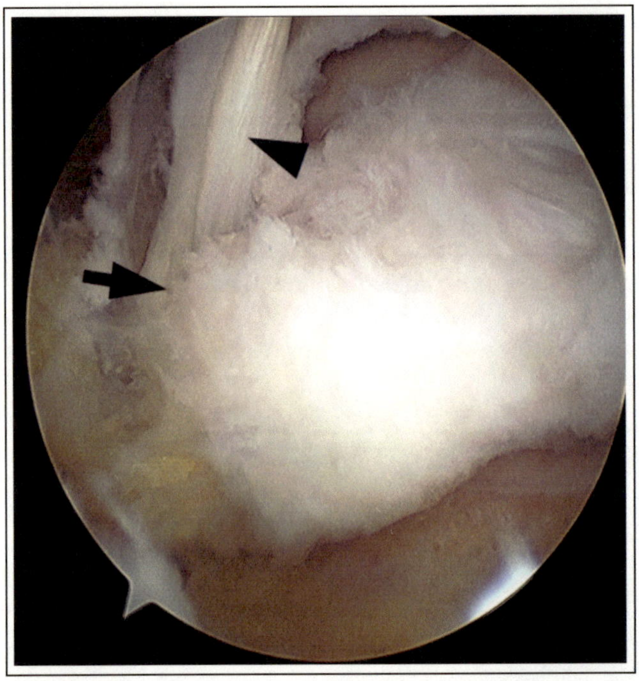

Fig. 13. Flexor hallucis longus tendon (arrow head) compressed by large posterolateral talar process (arrow).

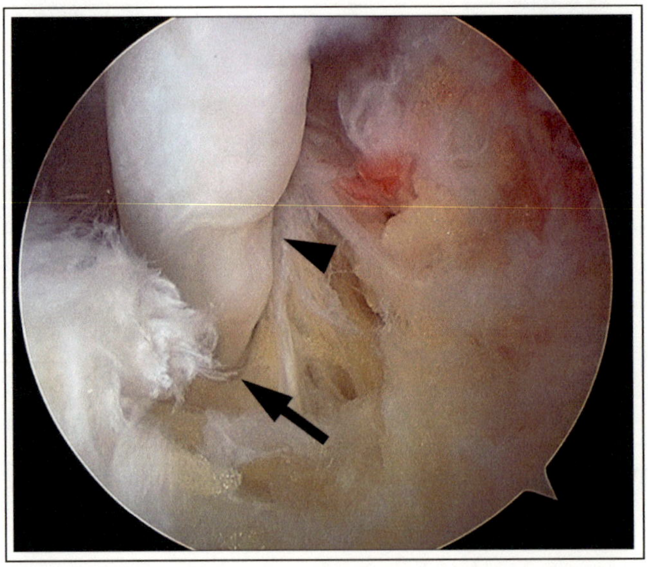

Fig. 14. Constriction of the flexor hallucis longus tendon (arrow head) at the posteromedial part of the fibro-osseous tunnel (cut, arrow).

Care should be taken as it is difficult for diagnosis of tenosynovitis of the FHL with preoperative imaging[7], especially in the early stage cases. For treating this disorder, operative release of the FHL is recommended when disabling symptoms persist despite non-operative treatment[8-12], and hindfoot endoscopic surgery is beneficial, especially for athletes who expect to return to their initial athletic activities with a shorter recovery time. After removing the hypertrophic synovium over the FHL tendon with forceps, the hypertrophic flexor retinaculum, which lays at the insertion of the tarsal tunnel and/or abnormal bony structures, were removed with curved forceps and motorized shaver for decompression of the constricted FHL tendon (Figure 15).

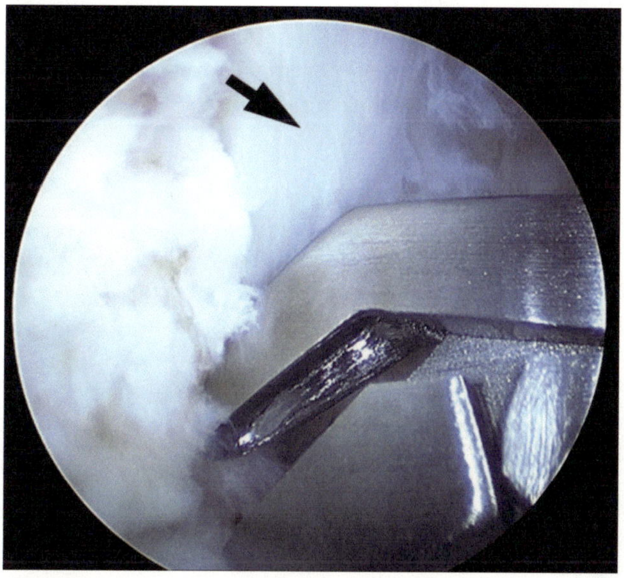

Fig. 15. Decompression of the flexor hallucis longus tendon (arrow) with curved forceps.

After surgery, the ankle was immobilized with an elastic bandage for two days. One day after the surgery, an active range of motion was allowed, and a passive range of motion was allowed two weeks after the surgery. Full weight bearing was allowed at 2 days after the surgery. Athletic activity was allowed if the patients feel no pain and no limitation of range of motion of their affected foot. They will return to the full athletic activity at four to seven weeks after surgery.

2.3.2 Osteoarthritis of the subtalar joint

Recently, arthroscopic subtalar arthrodesis has been reported as an alternative to traditional open methods for intractable hindfoot disorders, such as subtalar arthritis after fracture of the calcaneus or talus, primary arthritis, talocalcaneal coalition or inflammatory arthritis[13-17], because of its advantages, including minimizing invasion to the soft tissue around the hindfoot and preserving blood supply to the talus. Although the lateral approach using anterolateral and posterolateral portals in the supine or lateral decubitus position was initially introduced for arthroscopic subtalar arthrodesis[18, 19], the recent trend is the use of

the posterior two portals with patients in the prone position, permitting surgeons to access the posterior subtalar joint easily, as compared to the lateral approach[13, 17]. Accompanying techniques, such as the use of a third accessory portal[14, 15, 17] or bone substitute for grafting[13, 15], have been reported to result in successful prognosis without complications. The author recommends arthroscopic subtalar arthrodesis via a posterior approach using two portals accompanied by grafting of autologous cancellous bone, which is harvested by means of a tube harvester and grafted thorough these arthroscopic portals.
First, the shaver is inserted through the posteromedial portal and the soft tissue is removed until the FHL tendon is identified by arthroscopic visualization. If tenosynovitis is present around the FHL tendon, release of the flexor retinaculum and synovectomy are performed. After identification of the FHL tendon, the soft tissue overlying the posterior facet of the subtalar joint is removed from the lateral field of the FHL tendon. Next, the articular cartilage of the posterior facet of the subtalar joint is removed using a small chisel and a shaver until subchondral bone is exposed (Figure 16).

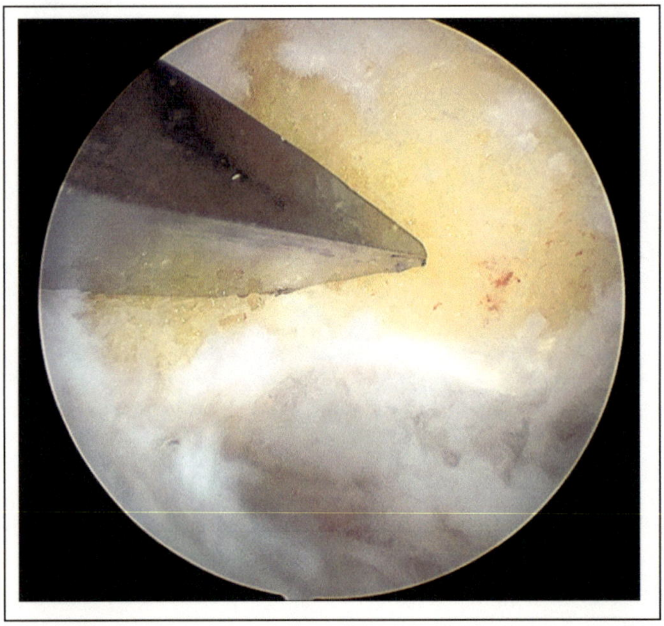

Fig. 16. Debridement of the subtalar joint with a small chisel.

After curettage of the anterior region of the posterior facet is confirmed arthroscopically, temporary fixation is performed using guide wires with the hindfoot in a neutral position. Subsequently, cancellous autograft bone is harvested from the ipsilateral iliac crest by using a tube harvester (OATS system, Arthrex, Naples, Florida) (Figure 17).
Two or three rigid cancellous bone plugs harvested through an approximately 1.5-cm skin incision are cut by a blade into small bone columns (Figure 18) so that autologous bone grafting is easily performed via arthroscopic portals.

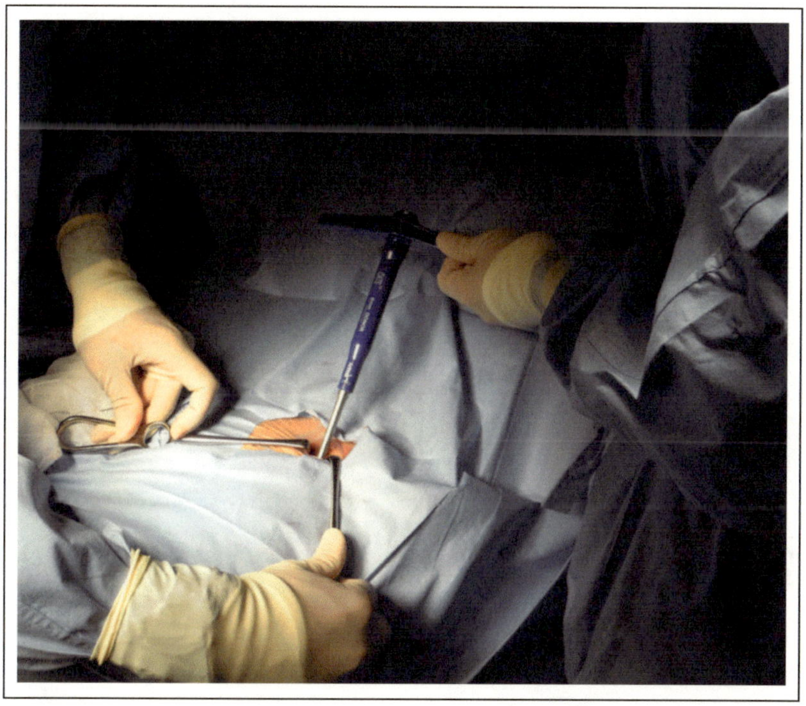

Fig. 17. Harvesting cancellous bone from the ipsilateral iliac crest using a tube harvester.

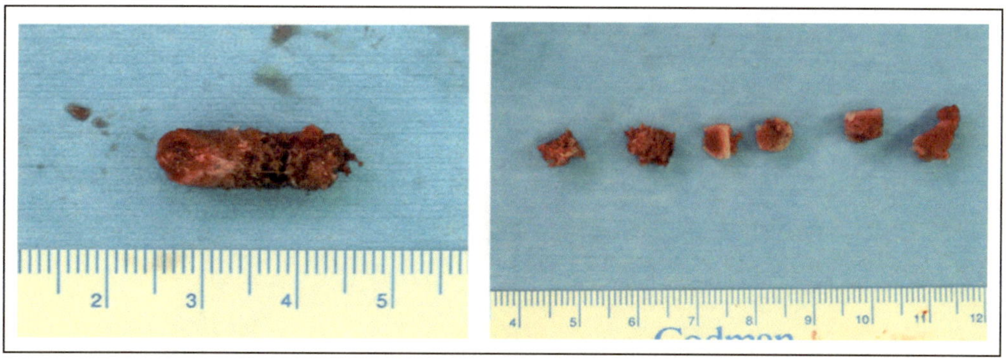

Fig. 18. Harvested cancellous bone plug (left) is cut into small bone columns (right).

Under arthroscopic visualization, two guide wires of the headless cannulated screws (Acutrak plus, Acumed, Hillsboro, Oregon) are inserted from the plantar of the heel to the talus body through the posterior facet of the subtalar joint and was followed by the over-drilling (Figure 19).

After autologous bone is grafted to the void after curettage of the posterior facet of the subtalar joint via portals (Fugure 20), the headless cannulated screws with a diameter of 6.5 mm are inserted (Figure 21).

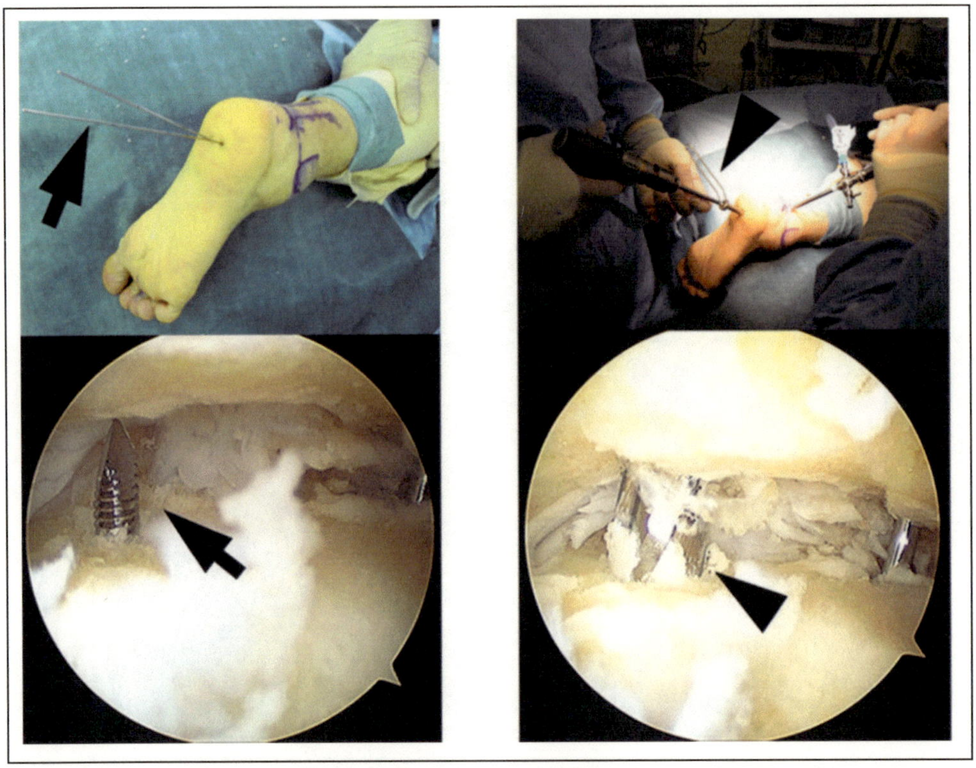

Fig. 19. Inserted guide wire through the subtalar joint (left, arrow) followed by the over drilling (right, arrowhead).

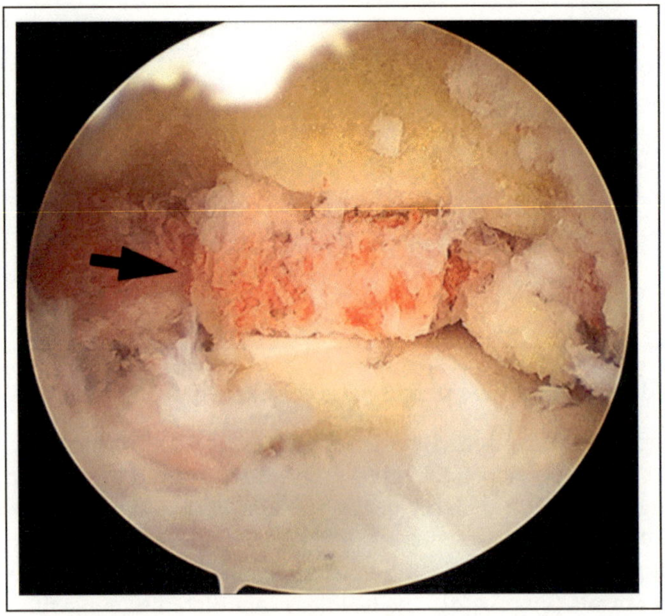

Fig. 20. Grafted cancellous bone on the subtalar joint (arrow).

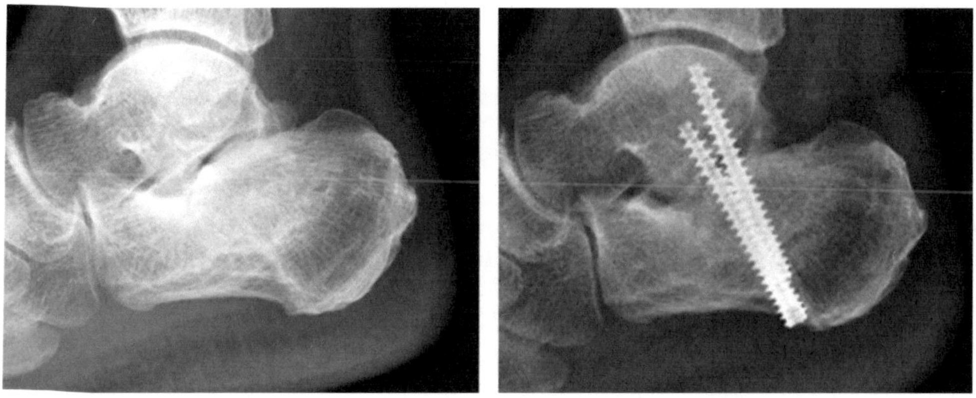

Fig. 21. Lateral view of the standard X-ray of the ankle before surgery (left) and after surgery (right).

After surgery, operated feet are not placed in casts, and active range-of-motion exercise of the talocrural joint is allowed the next day. Partial weight-bearing is allowed six weeks after surgery and full weight- bearing is permitted after a bridging callus is confirmed between posterior facets by radiological investigation.

3. Conclusion

Since 1997, the author has performed about 300 hindfoot endoscopic procedures utilizing posterior two portals without any complications. The patients complained of less pain after surgery and recovered earlier than those who underwent open surgery. The author believes that hindfoot endoscopic surgery, performed by an experienced arthroscopist who has enough knowledge for local anatomy and become skillful in this art, is safe and reliable method for posterior ankle disorders.

4. References

[1] Van Dijk, CN.; Scholten, PE. & Krips, R. (2000). A 2-portal endoscopic approach for diagnosis and treatment of posterior ankle pathology. *Arthroscopy,* Vol.16, pp. 871-876.

[2] Parisien, JS. & Vangsness, T. (1985). Arthroscopy of the subtalar joint: An experimental approach. *Arthroscopy,* Vol.1, pp. 53-57.

[3] Van Dijk, CN. (2006). Hindfoot endoscopy for posterior ankle pain. *Instr Course Lect,* Vol.55, pp. 545-554.

[4] Takao, M; Ochi, M; Shu, N; Naito, K; Matsusaki, M; Tobita, M & Kawasaki, K. (1999). Bandage distraction technique for ankle arthroscopy. *Foot Ankle Int,* Vol. 20, pp. 389-91.

[5] Golano, P; Vega, J; de Leeuw, PA; Malagelada, F; Manzanares, MC; Gotzens V & van Fijk, CN. (2010). Anatomy of the ankle ligaments: a pictorical essay. *Knee Surg Sports Traumatol Arthrosc,* Vol. 18, pp. 557-569.

[6] Maquirriain, J. (2005). Posterior ankle impingement syndrome. *J Am Acad Orthop Surg,* Vol. 13, pp. 365-371.
[7] Link, SC; Erickson, SJ & Timins ME. (1993). MR imaging of the ankle and foot: normal structures and anatomic variants that may simulate disease. *Am J Roentgenol,* Vol. 161, pp. 607-612.
[8] Cowell, HR; Elener, V & Lawhon SM. (1982). Bilateral tendinitis of the flexor hallucis longus in a ballet dancer. *J Pediat,* Vol. 2, pp. 582-586.
[9] Hamilton, HG. (1982). Stenosing tenosynovitis of the flexor hallucis longus tendon and posterior impingement upon the os trigonum in ballet dancers. *Foot Ankle,* Vol. 3, pp. 74-80.
[10] Lereim, P. (1985). Trigger toe in classical-ballet dancers. *Arch Orthop Trauma Surg,* Vol. 104, pp. 325-326.
[11] Lynch, T & Pupp GR. (1990). Stenosing tenosynovitis of the flexor hallucis longus at the ankle joint. *J Foot Surg,* Vol. 29, pp. 345-348.
[12] McCarroll, JR; Ritter, MA & Becker, TE. (1983). Triggering of the great toe. A case report. *Clin Orthop,* Vol. 175, pp. 184-185.
[13] Amendola, A; Leun-Bae, L; Charles, LS & Jin-Soo, S. (2007). Technique and early experience with posterior arthroscopic subtalar arthrodesis. *Foot Ankle Int,* Vol. 28, pp. 298-302.
[14] Beimers, L; Leeuw, PAJ & Van Dijk, CN. (2009). A 3-portal approach for arthroscopic subtalar arthrodesis. *Knee Surg Sports Traumatol Arthrosc,* Vol. 17, pp. 830-834.
[15] Lee, KB; Saltzman CL; Suh, JS; Wasserman, L & Amendola, A. (2008). A posterior 3-portal arthroscopic approach for isolated subtalar arthrodesis. *Arthroscopy,* Vol. 24, pp. 1306-1310.
[16] Lee, KB; Park, CH; Seon, JK & Kim, MS. (2010). Arthroscopic subtalar arthrodesis using a posterior 2-portal approach in the prone position. *Arthroscopy,* Vol. 26, pp. 230-238.
[17] Perez Carro, L; Golano, P & Vega, J. (2007). Arthroscopic subtalar arthrodesis: the posterior approach in the prone position. *Arthroscopy,* Vol. 23, pp. e l-4.
[18] Glanzmann, MC & Sanhueza-Hernandez, R. (2007). Arthroscopic subtalar arthrodesis for symptomatic osteoarthritis of the hindfoot: a prospective study of 41 cases. *Foot Ankle Int,* Vol. 28, pp. 2-7.
[19] Tasto, JP. (2003). Arthroscopic subtalar arthritis. *Tech Foot Ankle Surg,* Vol. 2, pp. 122-128.